T0227264

Pain Management

Editors

MILIND DEOGAONKAR
ANDRE G. MACHADO
ASHWINI SHARAN

NEUROSURGERY CLINICS OF NORTH AMERICA

www.neurosurgery.theclinics.com

Consulting Editors
RUSSELL LONSER
ISAAC YANG

October 2014 • Volume 25 • Number 4

ELSEVIER

1600 John F. Kennedy Boulevard • Suite 1800 • Philadelphia, Pennsylvania, 19103-2899

http://www.theclinics.com

NEUROSURGERY CLINICS OF NORTH AMERICA Volume 25, Number 4
October 2014 ISSN 1042-3680, ISBN-13: 978-0-323-32618-6

Editor: Jennifer Flynn-Briggs
Developmental Editor: Yonah Korngold

Neurosurgery Clinics of North America (ISSN 1042-3680) is published quarterly by Elsevier Inc., 360 Park Avenue South, New York, NY 10010-1710. Months of issue are January, April, July, and October. Business and Editorial Offices: 1600 John F. Kennedy Blvd., Suite 1800, Philadelphia, PA 19103-2899. Customer Service Office: 11830 Westline Industrial Drive, St. Louis, MO 63146. Periodicals postage paid at New York, NY, and additional mailing offices. Subscription prices are $380.00 per year (US individuals), $572.00 per year (US institutions), $415.00 per year (Canadian individuals), $711.00 per year (Canadian institutions), $525.00 per year (international individuals), $711.00 per year (international institutions), $185.00 per year (US students), and $255.00 per year (international and Canadian students). International air speed delivery is included in all *Clinics* subscription prices. All prices are subject to change without notice. **POSTMASTER:** Send address changes to *Neurosurgery Clinics of North America*, Elsevier Periodicals Customer Service, 11830 Westline Industrial Drive, St. Louis, MO 63146. **Customer Service: 1-800-654-2452 (US and Canada). From outside the US and Canada, call: 1-314-453-7041. Fax: 1-314-453-5170. E-mail: JournalsCustomerService-usa@elsevier.com (for print support) and journalsonlinesupport-usa@elsevier.com (for online support).**

Reprints. For copies of 100 or more, of articles in this publication, please contact the Commercial Reprints Department, Elsevier Inc., 360 Park Avenue South, New York, NY 10010-1710. Tel. 212-633-3874; Fax: 212-633-3820; E-mail: reprints@elsevier.com.

Neurosurgery Clinics of North America is covered in *MEDLINE/PubMed (Index Medicus)*, *EMBASE/Excerpta Medica*, and *Current Contents/Clinical Medicine (CC/CM)*.

Contributors

CONSULTING EDITORS

RUSSELL LONSER, MD
Chair, Department of Neurological Surgery, The Ohio State University, Columbus, Ohio

ISAAC YANG, MD
Assistant Professor, Department of Neurosurgery, David Geffen School of Medicine, Jonsson Comprehensive Cancer Center, University of California Los Angeles, Los Angeles, California

EDITORS

MILIND DEOGAONKAR, MD
Associate Professor, Department of Neurological Surgery, Wexner Medical Center, Center for Neuromodulation, The Ohio State University, Columbus, Ohio

ANDRE G. MACHADO, MD, PhD
Staff Neurosurgeon, Department of Neurosurgery, Center for Neurological Restoration; Associate Professor, Cleveland Clinic Lerner College of Medicine, Cleveland Clinic, Cleveland, Ohio

ASHWINI SHARAN, MD
Professor, Department of Neurosurgery and Neurology, Jefferson Medical College, Thomas Jefferson University, Philadelphia, Pennsylvania

AUTHORS

GENE H. BARNETT, MD, MBA
Associate Dean for Faculty Affairs, Cleveland Clinic Lerner College of Medicine of Case Western Reserve University; The Rose Ella Burkhardt Chair in Neurosurgical Oncology; Professor and Director, Department of Neurosurgery, Neurological Institute, The Rose Ella Burkhardt Brain Tumor and Neuro-Oncology Center, Cleveland Clinic, Cleveland, Ohio

ROBERT BOLASH, MD
Staff Physician, Department of Pain Management, Cleveland Clinic, Cleveland, Ohio

NICHOLAS M. BOULIS, MD
Associate Professor, Department of Neurosurgery, School of Medicine, Emory University, Atlanta, Georgia

SARAH BOURNE, MD
Resident, Department of Neurosurgery, Cleveland Clinic, Cleveland, Ohio

SARA DAVIN, PhD
Pain Medicine and Rehabilitation, Cleveland Clinic, Cleveland, Ohio

MILIND DEOGAONKAR, MD
Associate Professor, Department of Neurological Surgery, Wexner Medical Center, Center for Neuromodulation, The Ohio State University, Columbus, Ohio

JUANMARCO GUTIERREZ, MD, MSc
Postgraduate Research Fellow, Department of Neurosurgery, School of Medicine, Emory University, Atlanta, Georgia

SALIM M. HAYEK, MD, PhD
Chief, Division of Pain Medicine; Professor,
Department of Anesthesiology, University
Hospitals of Cleveland, Case Western Reserve
University, Cleveland, Ohio

ORION PAUL KEIFER Jr, PhD
MD/PhD Candidate, MD/PhD Program,
School of Medicine, Emory University,
Atlanta, Georgia

PETER KONRAD, MD, PhD
Professor and Director, Functional
Neurosurgery, Neurological Surgery and
Biomedical Engineering, Vanderbilt University,
Nashville, Tennessee

JOUNG H. LEE, MD
The Hycy and Howard Neuroscience Institute,
Providence St. Joseph Medical Center,
Burbank, California

SCOTT F. LEMPKA, PhD
Department of Neurosurgery, Center for
Neurological Restoration, Neurological
Institute, Cleveland Clinic; Research Service,
Louis Stokes Cleveland Veterans Affairs
Medical Center, Cleveland, Ohio

LINDSAY J. LIPINSKI, MD
Department of Neurologic Surgery, Mayo
Clinic, Rochester, Minnesota

ANDRE G. MACHADO, MD, PhD
Staff Neurosurgeon, Department of
Neurosurgery, Center for Neurological
Restoration; Associate Professor, Cleveland
Clinic Lerner College of Medicine, Cleveland
Clinic, Cleveland, Ohio

MANU MATHEWS, MD
Pain Medicine and Rehabilitation, Cleveland
Clinic, Euclid Avenue, Cleveland, Ohio

NAGY MEKHAIL, MD, PhD
Carl E. Wasmuth Endowed Chair; Director of
Evidence Based Pain Medicine Research,
Department of Pain Management, Cleveland
Clinic, Cleveland, Ohio

JAYANT P. MENON, MD, MEng
Medical Specialist and Bioengineer, IDEO;
Clinical Instructor, Stanford Neurosurgery,
Stanford, California

JONATHAN P. MILLER, MD
Director, Center for Functional and
Restorative Neurosurgery; Associate
Professor of Neurological Surgery; George R.
and Constance P. Lincoln Endowed Chair,
Department of Neurological Surgery,
University Hospitals Case Medical Center,
Cleveland, Ohio

SYMEON MISSIOS, MD
Neurosurgical Oncology Fellow, Department
of Neurosurgery, Neurological Institute,
The Rose Ella Burkhardt Brain Tumor and
Neuro-Oncology Center, Cleveland Clinic,
Cleveland, Ohio

ALIREZA M. MOHAMMADI, MD
Clinical Associate, Department of
Neurosurgery, Neurological Institute,
The Rose Ella Burkhardt Brain Tumor and
Neuro-Oncology Center, Cleveland Clinic,
Cleveland, Ohio

CHARLES MUNYON, MD
Fellow, Functional and Stereotactic
Neurosurgery, Department of Neurological
Surgery, University Hospitals Case Medical
Center, Cleveland, Ohio

SEAN J. NAGEL, MD
Staff Neurosurgeon, Department of
Neurosurgery, Center for Neurological
Restoration, Assistant Professor, Cleveland
Clinic Lerner College of Medicine, Cleveland
Clinic, Cleveland, Ohio

THOMAS OSTERGARD, MD, MS
Resident, Department of Neurological Surgery,
University Hospitals Case Medical Center,
Cleveland, Ohio

ERIKA A. PETERSEN, MD
Assistant Professor, Department
of Neurosurgery, University of Arkansas
for Medical Sciences, Little Rock,
Arkansas

SUKREET RAJU, MD
Roy Bakay Visiting Research Scholar,
Department of Neurosurgery, School
of Medicine, Emory University, Atlanta,
Georgia

ALI REZAI, MD
Professor of Neurosurgery; Stanley and
Ross Chair of Neuromodulation; Director of
Neuromodulation; Director of Neuroscience
Program; Associate Dean of Neuroscience,
Department of Neurological Surgery, Wexner
Medical Center, Center for Neuromodulation,
Ohio State University, Columbus, Ohio

JONATHAN P. RILEY, MD, MS
Senior Resident Physician, Department of
Neurosurgery, School of Medicine, Emory
University, Atlanta, Georgia

BURAK SADE, MD, FACS
Professor, Department of Neurosurgery, Beyin
ve Sinir Cerrahisi ABD, Dokuz Eylul Universitesi
Hastanesi, Balcova, Izmir, Turkey

ATIT SHAH, MD
Pain Management Fellow, Department of
Anesthesiology, Case Western University,
Chicago, Illinois

MAYUR SHARMA, MD, MCh
Clinical Fellow, Department of Neurosurgery,
Center for Neuromodulation, Wexner
Medical Center, The Ohio State University,
Columbus, Ohio

ANDREW SHAW, MD
Resident, Department of Neurosurgery, Center
for Neuromodulation, Wexner Medical Center,
The Ohio State University, Columbus, Ohio

KONSTANTIN V. SLAVIN, MD, FAANS
Professor, Department of Neurosurgery,
University of Illinois at Chicago, Chicago, Illinois

ROBERT J. SPINNER, MD
Department of Neurologic Surgery, Mayo
Clinic, Rochester, Minnesota

NICOLE A. YOUNG, PhD
Research Assistant Professor, Department
of Neuroscience, Center for Neuromodulation,
Wexner Medical Center, The Ohio State
University, Columbus, Ohio

Contents

This article provides an integrated review of the basic anatomy and physiology of the pain processing pathways. The transmission and parcellation of noxious stimuli from the peripheral nervous system to the central nervous system is discussed. In addition, the inhibitory and excitatory systems that regulate pain along with the consequences of dysfunction are considered.

Chronic pain impairs the quality of life for millions of individuals and therefore presents a serious ongoing challenge to clinicians and researchers. Debilitating chronic pain syndromes cost the US economy more than $600 billion per year. This article provides an overview of the epidemiology, clinical presentation, and treatment outcomes for craniofacial, spinal, and peripheral neurologic pain syndromes. Although the authors recognize that the diagnosis and treatment of the chronic forms of neuropathic pain syndromes represent a clinical challenge, there is an urgent need for standardized classification systems, improved epidemiologic data, and reliable treatment outcomes data.

Three main techniques delineate a possible role for intracranial ablative procedures in patients with chronic pain. Recent studies demonstrate a continued need for clinical investigation into central mechanisms of neuroablation to best define its role in the care of patients with otherwise intractable and severe pain syndromes. Cingulotomy can result in long-term pain relief. Although it can be associated with subtle impairments of attention, there is little risk to other cognitive domains.

For over half a century, neurosurgeons have attempted to treat pain from a diversity of causes using acute and chronic intracranial stimulation. Targets of stimulation have included the sensory thalamus, periventricular and periaqueductal gray, the septum, the internal capsule, the motor cortex, posterior hypothalamus, and more recently, the anterior cingulate cortex. The current work focuses on presenting and evaluating the evidence for the efficacy of these targets in a historical context while also highlighting the major challenges to having a double-blind placebo-controlled clinical trial. Considerations for pain research in general and use of intracranial targets specifically are included.

Trigeminal neuralgia (TN) is a neurologic disorder, defined by paroxysmal electric shocklike painful attacks in 1 or more trigeminal nerve branches. Treatment of TN is diverse and includes minimally invasive percutaneous techniques, which consist of balloon compression, glycerol rhizotomy, and radiofrequency thermocoagulation. Although all 3 techniques are generally safe, efficient, and effective, a clear consensus has not been reached regarding their specific indications and degree of efficacy. The aim of this article is to describe the percutaneous treatments available for TN and outline their characteristics, technique, indications and efficacy.

Complex craniofacial pain can be a challenging condition to manage both medically and surgically, but there is a resurgence of interest in the role of neurostimulation therapy. Surgical options for complex craniofacial pain syndromes include peripheral nerve/field stimulation, ganglion stimulation, spinal cord stimulation, dorsal nerve root entry zone lesioning, motor cortex stimulation, and deep brain stimulation. Peripheral nerve/field stimulation is rapidly being explored and is preferred by both patients and surgeons. Technological advances and improved understanding of the interactions of pain pathways with its affective component will widen the scope of neurostimulation therapy for craniofacial pain syndromes.

Neuropathic pain may be a result of focal injury to a peripheral nerve. The treatment algorithm begins with nonoperative, then operative, options. In our practice, first-line surgical treatment should directly treat the injured nerve. Nerve decompression or neurolysis is useful in patients with entrapment syndromes and in cases where the course and/or the function of the nerve is altered by local scar or pathoanatomy. Neurectomy is an option in primary cases where numbness is an acceptable alternative to dysesthetic pain, or as an alternative following failed neurolysis. Nerve repair or reconstruction may improve pain by guiding axons past the neuroma.

Peripheral nerve stimulation and peripheral nerve field stimulation involve the delivery of electrical stimulation using implanted electrodes either over a target nerve or over the painful area with the goal of modulating neuropathic pain. The selection of appropriate candidates for this therapy hinges on skillful application of inclusion and exclusion criteria, psychological screening, and an invasive screening trial. Patients with significant improvement in pain severity and pain-related disability during the trial are considered candidates for implantation of a permanent system. As with other implanted devices for neuromodulation, risks of mechanical failures, infection, and neurologic complications exist.

The article discusses chronic pain rehabilitation and describes its components and some of the core operating principles. Outcomes in chronic pain are best when multiple treatment strategies with a focus on functional restoration are employed, and this is often best done in an interdisciplinary pain rehabilitation program.

Chronic pain is a complex disorder with extensive overlap in sensory and limbic pathways. It needs systemic therapy in addition to focused local treatment. This article discusses treatment modalities other than surgical and interventional approaches and also discusses the literature regarding these treatment modalities, including pharmacotherapy, physical and occupational therapy, psychological approaches including cognitive behavior therapy, and other adjunctive treatments like yoga and tai chi.

Nerve blocks are often performed as therapeutic or palliative interventions for pain relief. However, they are often performed for diagnostic or prognostic purposes. When considering nerve blocks for chronic pain, clinicians must always consider the indications, risks, benefits, and proper technique. Nerve blocks encompass a wide variety of interventional procedures. The most common nerve blocks for chronic pain and that may be applicable to the neurosurgical patient population are reviewed in this article. This article is an introduction and brief synopsis of the different available blocks that can be offered to a patient.

Current data suggest that transcranial magnetic stimulation (TMS) has the potential to be an effective and complimentary treatment modality for patients with chronic neuropathic pain syndromes. The success of TMS for pain relief depends on the parameters of the stimulation delivered, the location of neural target, and duration of treatment. TMS can be used to excite or inhibit underlying neural tissue that depends on long-term potentiation and long-term depression, respectively. Long-term randomized controlled studies are warranted to establish the efficacy of repetitive TMS in patients with various chronic pain syndromes.

The field of pain management has experienced tremendous growth in implantable therapies secondary to the innovations of bioengineers, implanters, and industry. Every aspect of neuromodulation is amenable to innovation from implanting devices to anchors, electrodes, programming, and even patient programmers. Patients with previously refractory neuropathic pain syndromes have new and effective pain management strategies that are a direct result of innovations in implantable devices.

NEUROSURGERY CLINICS OF NORTH AMERICA

RELATED INTEREST

Anesthesiology Clinics, June 2014 (Vol. 32, Issue 2)
Ambulatory Anesthesiology
Jeffrey L. Apfelbaum, MD, Thomas W. Cutter, MD, MAEd, *Editors*
http://www.anesthesiology.theclinics.com

**DOWNLOAD
Free App!**

Review Articles
THE CLINICS

NOW AVAILABLE FOR YOUR iPhone and iPad

NEUROSURGERY CLINICS OF NORTH AMERICA

Preface
Pain Management

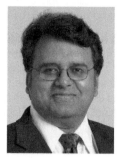
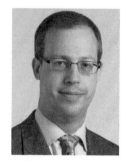
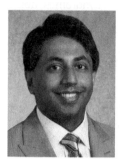

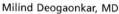

Milind Deogaonkar, MD   Andre G. Machado, MD   Ashwini Sharan, MD

Editors

Chronic pain is a complex problem to treat. Pain is at the crossroads of affective, cognitive, and somatic disorders not only symptomatically but also in terms of neural networks. That adds a complex and amorphous dimension of "sorrow" to pain disorders, making it more difficult to treat. In the last two decades, treatment of chronic pain has evolved. This evolution can be noted primarily in two main categories: conceptual evolution and technological evolution. This issue of *Neurosurgery Clinics of North America* is an attempt to provide a glimpse into how pain can be assessed and managed by several medical disciplines and approaches. We have covered classical or conventional techniques as well as innovative techniques in this issue.

Conceptually, the theories of pain have evolved from single pain pathway to duality of pain to a complex neural network of "pain matrix." Pain is no more thought to be a sensory phenomenon but a multidimensional expression that emerges from collaborative actions of sensory, cognitive, and emotional cortical and subcortical circuits. Accordingly, the medical and surgical pain management approaches have also changed from focused treatment to multimodality management. Lesioning procedures have given way to neuromodulation. The nodal points of neuromodulation have also expanded, leading to targeting of various nodes outside the conventional pain pathways. A second conceptual shift in treatment of chronic pain is a "move to periphery." Peripheral neuromodulation is being used more often. Treatments have evolved, in some cases, to minimize the invasiveness of interventions. Noninvasive neuromodulating techniques like transcranial magnetic stimulation are also being used more often.

Technologically, the ability to access, deliver, and power neuromodulation implants has evolved significantly. The implants have become smaller, more adaptive, and more diverse. Newer leads are able to cover larger areas and are able to steer the stimulation. Newer access devices have made placing leads easier. Newer pulse generators are longer lasting and have an ability to deliver stimulation using complex programs. In this era of nanotechnology, it will not be surprising if microcoils and microimplants are used in recent future.

neurosurgery.theclinics.com

In this issue, we have included the classical, contemporary classical, and innovative topics to discuss the origin, network, interventions, and outcomes of chronic pain. This issue has articles describing theories of pain, pain syndromes, ablative procedures, neuromodulation procedures, noninvasive therapies, multimodal therapies, and technological innovations to give a 360-degree look at the evolution of the treatment of chronic pain.

Milind Deogaonkar, MD
Department of Neurological Surgery
Wexner Medical Center
Center for Neuromodulation
Ohio State University
410 West 10th Avenue
Columbus, OH 43210, USA

Andre G. Machado, MD
Department of Neurosurgery
Center for Neurological Restoration
Cleveland Clinic
9500 Euclid Avenue, S31
Cleveland, OH 44195, USA

Ashwini Sharan, MD
Department of Neurosurgery
and Neurology
Jefferson Medical College
Thomas Jefferson University
909 Walnut Street, 2nd Floor
Philadelphia, PA 19107, USA

E-mail addresses:
Milind.deogaonkar@osumc.edu (M. Deogaonkar)
machada@ccf.org (A.G. Machado)
ashwini.sharan@jefferson.edu (A. Sharan)

Basic Anatomy and Physiology of Pain Pathways

Sarah Bourne, MD[a], Andre G. Machado, MD, PhD[b],
Sean J. Nagel, MD[b],*

KEYWORDS

- Hyperalgesia • Allodynia • Peripheral sensitization • Spino-thalamic tract • Gait control theory
- Descending systems

KEY POINTS

- Pain signals are transmitted along Aδ and C nociceptive nerve fibers to the central nervous system.
- Most peripheral nerve fibers will synapse in the Rexed lamina and then ascend in the contralateral spinothalamic tract before terminating in the ventral posterior nuclei and central nuclei of the thalamus.
- The receptive fields of the thalamus may reorganize following injury.
- The primary and secondary somatosensory cortex receive the bulk of direct projections from the thalamus; the insula, orbitofrontal cortex, dorsolateral prefrontal cortex, amygdala and cingulate are additional early relay sites important in pain processing.
- The rostral ventromedial medulla, the dorsolateral pontomesencephalic tegmentum, and the periaquaductal gray region are important structures in the descending regulation of noxious stimuli at the dorsal horn.
- The neuromatrix theory of pain incorporates the gate control theory of pain that focused on pain regulation at the spinal cord with more recent evidence that expands the role of the cortex.

INTRODUCTION

The pain pathways form a complex, dynamic, sensory, cognitive, and behavioral system that evolved to detect, integrate, and coordinate a protective response to incoming noxious stimuli that threatens tissue injury or organism survival.[1] This defense system includes both the primitive spinal reflexes that are the only protection for simple organisms all the way up to the complex emotional responses humans consciously and subconsciously experience as pain. The mental representation of pain is stored as both short-term and long-term memory and serves as an early warning avoidance system for future threats.[1] When severe, mental anguish may be projected with a physical complaint or symptom. Although many of the basic structures of the pain pathways have been defined, a more complete understanding of the interactions that would enable the development of targeted therapies remains elusive.

PERIPHERAL SENSORY SYSTEM AND MECHANISMS OF SENSITIZATION

The location, intensity, and temporal pattern of noxious stimuli are transduced into a recognizable signal through unmyelinated nociceptors at the

[a] Department of Neurosurgery, Cleveland Clinic, 9500 Euclid Avenue, S4, Cleveland, OH 44195, USA;
[b] Department of Neurosurgery, Center for Neurological Restoration, Cleveland Clinic Lerner College of Medicine, Cleveland Clinic, 9500 Euclid Avenue, S31, Cleveland, OH 44195, USA
* Corresponding author.
E-mail address: nagels@ccf.org

Neurosurg Clin N Am 25 (2014) 629–638
http://dx.doi.org/10.1016/j.nec.2014.06.001
1042-3680/14/$ – see front matter © 2014 Elsevier Inc. All rights reserved.

terminal end of sensory neurons. Through physical deformation or molecular binding, membrane permeability and, consequently, the membrane potential fluctuate.[2] If depolarization reaches a critical threshold, an action potential is propagated along the length of a sensory nerve toward the spinal cord.

Most sensory receptors respond to a single stimulus modality. Nociceptors, designed to detect tissue injury, are excited by three noxious stimuli: mechanical, thermal, and chemical. Mechanical stimuli deform the receptor to augment receptor ion permeability,[3] whereas chemicals such as bradykinin, serotonin, histamine, potassium ions, acids, acetylcholine, and proteolytic enzymes[2] bind directly to receptors to influence membrane permeability. Prostaglandins and substance P (SP) do not directly activate pain receptors but indirectly influence membrane permeability.

Nociceptive receptors sit at the ends of pseudounipolar sensory neurons with cell bodies in the dorsal root, trigeminal, or nodose ganglia (Fig. 1).[4] Pain receptors are unencapsulated free nerve endings. Sensory nerve fibers range from 0.5 to 20 μm in diameter and can conduct impulses at speeds ranging from 0.5 to 120 m/sec. Larger diameter neurons conduct information at a faster speed.[2] Nerve fibers are divided up into two main categories: type A, which are medium to large diameter myelinated neurons, and type C, small diameter unmyelinated neurons.[2] Pain transmission is divided into two categories, fast and slow. A-delta fibers detect and transmit pain quickly. These fibers are relatively small (1–6 m), thinly myelinated neurons that can conduct at speeds of 6 to 30 m/sec.[3] C fibers are small (<1.5 m) and unmyelinated, conducting pain at 0.5 to 2 m/sec.[2] A-beta are large (6–12 m) myelinated fibers that are high speed (30–70 m/sec).[2] They have encapsulated receptors and transmit information about touch, pressure, and vibration.[3] Most A-delta fibers are associated with thermo or mechanoreceptors. C fibers can be associated with polymodal receptors, suggesting a role in monitoring the overall tissue condition.[3]

Innocuous stimuli may elicit excitation of neurons in the peripheral nociceptive system following repeated injury or inflammation. These pathologic changes contribute to phenomena such as sensitization, allodynia, or hyperalgesia. In peripheral sensitization, neurons fire at a lower threshold and have greater response magnitude to a given stimuli,[5] may fire spontaneously, or may even have altered receptive field areas.[6,7] This occurs via inflammatory mediators, including bradykinin, prostaglandins, serotonin,

tumor necrosis factor alpha, and histamine.[8] After integration in the brainstem, descending pronociceptive and antinociceptive pathways contribute to peripheral sensitization. When the function of these pathways becomes abnormal, chronic pain may occur.

The expression of molecules, including GABA, histamine, serotonin, and opiate receptors in nociceptive neurons, may be modulated by inflammation or injury.[8] Near the receptor there is a high concentration of sodium channels. Increased channel expression can alter sensitivity of nerve endings to noxious stimuli by modulating integration of stimuli and threshold potential for action potential generation.[3] Increased sodium channel expression has been reported after nerve injury and may contribute to hyperexcitability and associated abnormal sensation.[9] C fibers have long response times and are slow to adapt. Because of this, they show summation of response to noxious stimuli in the presence of tissue injury,[10] perhaps contributing to sensitization and hyperalgesia.

Inflammation results in an upregulation of SP, including in A-beta fibers.[11] In this setting, A fibers may play a role in central sensitivity, perhaps contributing to hypersensitivity.[11,12] A-beta fibers terminate in lamina III of the spinal cord where SP receptors are present. They may contribute to ongoing activation of SP expressing nociceptive neurons in chronic pain states.[12]

DORSAL ROOT GANGLIA

Sensory neuron cell bodies are located in the dorsal root ganglia (DRG). DRG neurons are classically pseudounipolar; one process extends into the peripheral nerve and the other process extends centrally, transmitting information through the dorsal root into the spinal cord. Each DRG contains thousands of unique sensory neuron cell bodies that are capable of encoding and then transmitting specific information gathered from external stimuli.[13] Cells in the DRG are subclassified into peptidergic neurons and non-peptidergic neurons. Peptidergic neurons contain peptides such as SP, calcitonin gene–related peptide (CGRP), and somatostatin.[14] Each DRG neuron is surrounded by glial cell cytoplasm. The surface of the DRG neuron cell bodies are covered with perikaryal projections that are invested in the surrounding glial cytoplasm, increasing the surface area.[15]

The soma of DRG neurons synthesizes and transports the substances needed for neuron functioning to the far reaches of the axon terminals, including receptors, ion channels, as well as

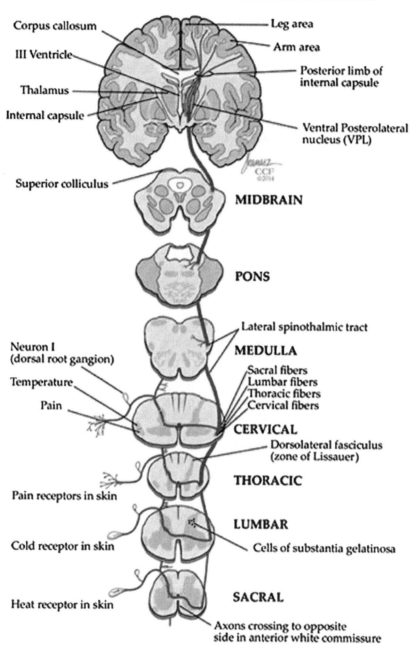

Fig. 1. Pain and temperature transmission from receptors in the skin ascend in the spinal cord to the postcentral gyrus via the lateral spinothalamic tract. First-order neurons transmit this sensory information via pseudounipolar neurons that enter the spinal cord in the Lissauer tract where they synapse in the Rexed lamina. Second-order neurons from the dorsal horn then decussate at the ventral commissure and ascend in the lateral spinothalamic tract before ending in the ventral posterolateral nuclei of the thalamus. Third-order neurons then project to the postcentral gyrus. (*Courtesy of* the Cleveland Clinic Foundation, Cleveland, Ohio.)

molecules essential for synaptic transmission.[13] The most common neurotransmitter that is synthesized by DRG cells is glutamate; however, many DRG cells also express SP, which facilitates pain transmission.[3] There are no direct synaptic connections between DRG neurons but their activity is indirectly modulated.[16] After injury, DRG neurons may become innervated by postganglionic axons in a neurotrophin-mediated process.[8] C fibers may also modulate DRG sensitivity by altering intracellular calcium concentration affecting N-methyl-d-aspartate receptor configuration and sensitivity.[11] Therefore, plastic reorganization of the DRG is one of the many mechanisms involved in pain sensitization and chronification.

SPINAL CORD

Most sensory fibers project from the DRG through the dorsal root and into the dorsal root entry zone (DREZ). There is evidence that the ventral roots also receive projections from unmyelinated fibers originating from DRG cells that are involved in sensation, including nociception, violating the Bell-Magendie law.[17–20] At the DREZ, most unmyelinated and small myelinated axons project laterally to enter. Lissauer tract (see **Fig. 1**)[21] fibers then extend vertically in this tract for several spinal segments before synapsing. Second-order neurons then cross to the opposite side, in the ventral decussation of the central canal of the spinal cord.[22] The Lissauer tract contains both unmyelinated C fibers and myelinated A-delta fibers. A-delta fibers may ascend 3 to 4 segments in the Lissauer tract before finally terminating in lamina of Rexed I, II_o, or V. C fibers typically ascend one segment before terminating, most often in Rexed lamina II.[21]

Rexed lamina I, or the marginal layer, is composed of two main types of cells, nociceptive-specific neurons, and wide dynamic range neurons (WDRs). Nociceptive-specific neurons respond to noxious stimuli and express neuropeptides such as SP, CGRP, enkephalin, and serotonin.[3] WDRs dynamic range neurons transmit both noxious and nonnoxious information.[10] WDR display graded responses, proportional to the input stimulus by firing at a higher frequency.[3] WDR neurons have a large receptive field, including a center that responds to both noxious and nonnoxious stimuli and surrounding area responds to noxious stimuli only.[4] The large receptive fields of WDR neurons reflect its proposed integrative function that may contribute to allodynia through increased and disproportionate responsiveness to nonnoxious stimuli.[8]

Lamina II (substantia gelatinous) may play a role modulating spinothalamic and spinobulbar projection neurons via its numerous inhibitory interneurons that primarily release GABA. C fibers and A-delta fibers are the primary afferent inputs of lamina II. Lamina II inhibitory neurons then arborize locally to other lamina, including I, II, III, and IV.[3,23] There are very few projection neurons in lamina II. It has been hypothesized that disinhibition related to the functional loss of lamina II inhibitory neurons facilitates chronic neuropathic pain.

A-beta fibers project to lamina III and IV. Layer III also receives A-delta fiber mechanoreceptive input and may have sprouting of A-category neurons to lamina I and II after injury, possibly contributing to chronic pain and allodynia.[10,24] Some layer IV neurons project to layer I, which contributes to integration of sensation.[3] Lamina V receives input from A-delta and C fibers and neurons project to the spinothalamic tract (STT). Lamina V also contains a large number of WDR neurons with projections to reticular formation, periaqueductal gray, and medial thalamic nuclei, forming part of the mesial pathways that mediate the emotional characteristics of pain.[3,8] Lamina X surrounds the spinal cord central canal. The function of this region is less well defined but likely is involved in visceral pain. It receives some direct input from A-delta fibers and may play a role in integration of nociception.[3]

Dorsal horn (DH) nociceptive neurons form glutamatergic synapses that may also release neuropeptides, including SP, CGRP, vasoactive intestinal peptide (VIP), and somatostatin. Expression of these substances may be altered in the setting of injury,[8] leading to sensitization, allodynia, and secondary hyperalgesia. WDR neurons have also been implicated in the development of these phenomena. Secondary hyperalgesia may occur due to central sensitization which is, in turn, mediated by abnormal connections between nonnociceptive neurons and centrally transmitting nociceptive pathways, as well as receptive field plasticity of DH neurons.[25]

SPINOTHALAMIC PATHWAYS

The STT is oriented vertically along the ventrolateral portion of the spinal cord (see **Fig. 1**). It serves as the main conduit from the peripheral nerves to the brain by transmitting pain, temperature and deep touch signals to the thalamus. It receives projections from contralateral lamina I and IV-VI[26] and is composed of two tracts: one dorsolateral, carrying axons from the superficial lamina, and the other ventrolateral, carrying axons from deeper lamina.[27] Most projections are contralateral, although there is also an ipsilateral contribution.[8] There is somatotopic organization of the STT with the lower limbs dorsolaterally and upper body and limbs positioned ventromedially. Cells projecting to ventral posterolateral nuclei originate from laminae I and V. Lateral STT neurons have small contralateral receptive fields and are most likely involved in sensory-discriminative aspects of pain signaling.[8] Cells projecting to the medial thalamic nuclei originate from the deep dorsal laminae (ie, layer V; see above discussion) and ventral horn. The medial STT relays the motivational and affective components of noxious stimuli.[28] These neurons have large receptive fields to support this purpose.

The paleospinothalamic tract projects to brainstem reticular formation, hypothalamus, and thalamic nuclei.[3] Neurons in lamina VI, VII, and VIII have direct projections to reticular formation nuclei, some of which are bilateral.[29] Neurons in lamina I, VII, and VIII project to pons.[29] Neurons in the marginal zone, nucleus proprius, and lateral reticulated area project both to thalamus and hypothalamus. These neurons include both WDR neurons and nociceptive-specific neurons.[30] They project to reticular formation, periaquaductal gray (PAG), and medial thalamic nuclei, and may also be involved in motivational-affective component of pain.

Most of the projections to the reticular formation arise from A fibers, although A and C fiber innervation has been described.[29] Reticular formation response is proportional to noxious characteristics of the stimulus.[29] The spinoreticular tract travels with STT in ventrolateral spinal cord. Fibers largely terminate in ventral medial portion of the medulla

reticular formation, medullae oblongatae centralis, pars ventralis, and nucleus gigantocellularis.[29,31] These cells have large receptive fields and exhibit heterotopic convergence. This tract functions to activate homeostatic mechanisms in brainstem autonomic centers as well as to provide input to antinociceptive systems and motivational-affective systems.

The spinomesencephalic tract originates in laminae I and IV-VI, with some contribution from lamina X and ventral horn. It projects to areas including periaqueductal gray, pretectal nuclei, red nucleus, Edinger-Westphal nucleus, and interstitial nucleus of Cajal. Neurons in this tract are nociceptive, and generally have large, complex receptive fields.[8] They are involved in aversive behavior and orientation responses, and may activate descending antinociceptive systems.

The 1965 gate control theory of pain by Melzack and Wall[32] proposed that there were three spinal cord systems involved in pain transmission: the substantia gelatinosa, dorsal column fibers, and central transmission cells in the DH (**Fig. 2**). The substantia gelatinosa functions as a gate that modulates signals before they reach the brain.

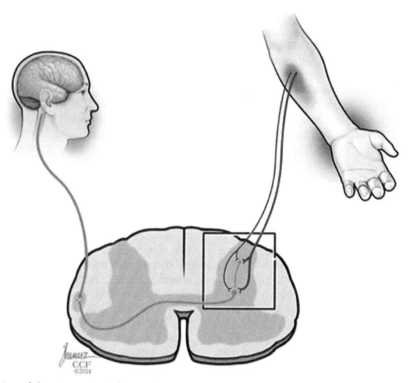

Fig. 2. Illustration of the gate control theory of pain. The substantia gelatinosa (SG) serves as a gate in the spinal cord that closes in response to large fiber (L) inputs, suppressing pain transmission. Alternatively, small fiber inputs open the gate or facilitate pain transmission. The summated pain signal then ascends in a projection neuron (P) via the spinothalamic (S) tract. This theory has since been revised to include the role of higher cortical processing to explain pain perception. (*Courtesy of* the Cleveland Clinic Foundation, Cleveland, Ohio.)

Large diameter fibers have inhibitory effects to "shut the gate" whereas small diameter fibers carrying noxious stimuli open the gate to pain transmission. In a simplistic view of this model, rubbing of the injured area promotes proprioceptive (ie, large diameter) fiber input and reduces pain perception.[32] The gate-control theory has been criticized and revisited because it is inherently incomplete in its view of the nervous system. Nevertheless, it needs to be recognized for its key role in advancing the understanding of pain perception five decades ago and promoting the development of modern neurostimulation for pain management.

THALAMUS

The sensory thalamus is divided into nuclei that roughly maintain the segmentation of the noxious and innocuous divisions from the periphery. The ventral caudal (Hassler's nomenclature) or ventroposterior (VP) nucleus thalamic nuclei are the most direct subcortical relay site for the STT and the trigeminal thalami ctract (TTT)[27,33] before relaying pain signals to the primary sensory cortex and other cortical regions.[34] Glutaminergic projections from the dorsal column nuclei and from the DH via the STT synapse on neurons in the VP.[33] The VP is somatotopically organized with neurons excited by face stimulation medially (VPM) and arm and leg laterally (VPL). Cutaneous sensation from the distal extremities is located ventrally and truncal representation dorsally in the VP.[8] The VP can be further subdivided into a core that responds to mechanical, nonnoxious stimuli and a posterior inferior region that transmits nociceptive signals.[35] Deep brain stimulation (DBS) of VP (Vc [Ventralis caudalis]) has been studied as a target to treat intractable, chronic pain.[35]

VP also receives WDR nociceptive neurons with large receptive fields and responses proportional to stimulus intensity.[26] Some of these neurons project to areas 3b and 1.

The ventralis posterior inferior (VPI) nucleus, which lies inferior to VPL and lateral to VPM, has larger receptive fields than VPL but retains somatotopic organization. It projects to SII.[26] The ventromedial posterior (VMpo) nucleus plays an important role in pain processing.[33] It receives projections from lamina I STT neurons and is composed of nociceptive-specific neurons with small, contralateral, receptive fields.[26] VMpo neurons project to the insula and area 3a.

The central nuclei of the thalamus are also involved in pain transmission. Neurons from the STT terminate in the intralaminar nuclei, including the central medial nuclei, parafasicularis, medial dorsal nucleus, and in the centralis lateralis.[27] These midline intralaminar thalamic nuclei also receive indirect projections important in pain processing from the parabrachial nucleus and brainstem reticular nuclei. Neurons in these thalamic nuclei have large and nonspecific receptive fields that integrate pain signals and initiate protective responses such as arousal in response to noxious stimuli.[36]

The receptive fields of the specific nuclei of the thalamus have been shown to reorganize following injury. This thalamic reorganization subsequently influences downstream cortical reorganization.[35] Thalamic neurons with receptive fields adjacent to the receptive fields of an injured area gain a larger representation in the homunculus.[35,37] Decreased excitatory input or increased inhibitory input leads to neuronal hyperpolarization and aberrant bursting.[26] For example, membrane hyperpolarization secondary to loss of excitatory STT input following spinal cord injury contributes to cell bursting interspersed with periods of low firing between bursts.[35] This irregular firing is associated with development of central pain following spinal cord injury. Patients with neuropathic pain also demonstrate detrimental thalamic reorganization that may lead to innocuous thermal stimuli encoded as nociceptive signals.[37]

In some patients with chronic pain, the surface encephalographic recordings demonstrate a recognizable shift from normal alpha rhythms to low-frequency theta rhythms.[38] This cortical dysrhythmia is best observed between the medial thalamic nuclei and the insular, parietal opercular, and cingulate cortices.[38] Simultaneous thalamic recordings in patients with chronic pain show an increase in low frequency, coherent thalamocortical activity.[38]

CORTICAL AREAS

Painful stimuli activate distant cortical regions, including the primary somatosensory cortex (SI; Brodmann areas 3a/b, 2, 1, postcentral gyrus), secondary somatosensory cortex (SII), insula, orbitofrontal cortex, dorsal-lateral prefrontal cortex, extended amygdala, and cingulate cortex.[27] The SI is arranged with somatotopic organization of nociceptive signals that follows Penfield's homuncular pattern.[39] Projections from the VPM and VPL nuclei synapse directly in the SI. These neurons in SI demonstrate a graded response according to intensity of noxious stimulus.[27] This suggests that SI is involved in the discriminative quality of pain. The SII (parietal operculum) receives projections from ventrobasal thalamus, the VPM-VPL, and from the SI, as well as contralateral input.[27]

Neurons in both the SII and Broadmann's area 7 also show responses proportional to magnitude of noxious stimuli.[27]

C fibers stimulation is associated with activation of the contralateral SI, in particular area 3a, the SII, and ipsilateral SII.[34] Similarly, activation of A-group fibers causes activation of the contralateral SI followed by SII.[34] This nociceptive input mainly projects to cortical layers III and IV.[3] The insula receives input from SI, SII, VPI, pulvinar, central median and parafascicular nuclei, medial dorsal nucleus, and Vmpo.[27] It demonstrates a graded response proportional to intensity of noxious stimulus and is likely involved in the sensory-discriminative processing of pain.[27] The insula projects to limbic structures such as amygdala and perirhinal cortex.[27] These widespread connections of the insula are involved in higher order pain processing and require consciousness for activation with painful stimuli.[3] Insula lesions have been associated with altered motivational-affective responses to pain.

The anterior cingulate cortex (ACC) and middle cingulate cortex receive projections from the medial and intralaminar thalamic nuclei and the VPI. These areas are activated with noxious stimuli that elicit an affective or motivational response to pain. Lesioning of the cingulate cortex attenuates these motivational-affective characteristics of pain, particularly in patients with chronic cancer pain.[27] Increased ACC activity may be seen in those with chronic pain.[39]

In the late 1990s, Melzack[1] revisited the original gate control theory and proposed the neuromatrix theory, adding higher cortical functions as key elements of pain transmission and interpretation. It postulates that individuals possess a genetically determined neural matrix that is shaped and modulated by sensory input. The neuromatrix contains parallel and interacting thalamocortical and limbic loops. Nodes in the sensory signaling circuitry are predetermined pattern generators and contribute to abnormal nociception. The structure and output of the neuromatrix is also controlled by cognitive and affective spheres. Thus, the final pain experience is determined not only by sensory input but also by behavioral and cognitive interpretation of pain, which includes prior experiences, injuries, and cultural background.

DESCENDING SYSTEMS

Descending pathways originating in the brain regulate incoming signals from noxious stimuli primarily through synapses on DH neurons (**Fig. 3**). Facilitative regulation amplifies the response as observed in sensitization. Alternatively, inhibitory regulation suppresses ascending pain signals during life-threatening events and other periods of extraordinary stress. These descending pathways include several relevant supraspinal structures: the rostral ventromedial medulla (RVM), the dorso-lateral pontomesencephalic tegmentum, and the PAG region. The descending systems exert their effect predominantly in lamina I and II in the DH through the release of the monamine-serotonin, norepinephrine, and dopamine.[40] The monoamine released and receptor subtype will dictate an antinociceptive or pronociceptive effect. Dysregulation of these descending systems are believed to play a major role in chronic pain states.

The PAG-RVM-DH pathway is a descending pain modulatory system that has been well characterized. Stimulation of the PAG, first reported in the 1960s, induces analgesia and blocks the response of lamina V interneurons to noxious stimuli.[41,42] This net analgesic effect of PAG stimulation depends, in part, on the release of serotonin from neurons activated in the RVM.[43] Functional depletion of 5-hydroxytryptamine (5-HT) from RVM neurons has been shown to inhibit persistent pain in a rat model.[44] In addition to these serotonergic neurons, three additional neuron subtypes found in the RVM regulate pain transmission. Unlike the 5-HT neurons, the bulk of these neurons are GABA-ergic. ON-cells are inhibited by opioids and excite DH neurons to facilitate nociceptive pain. OFF-cells are excited by opioids and inhibit DH neurons to attenuate nociceptive pain. The function of the third population of neurons, NEUTRAL-cells, is not known. These three neuron types project to the spine and branch locally within the RVM.

The PAG also has direct projections to the spinal cord and additional indirect projections via the reticular formation and the parabrachial nuclei. Furthermore, the PAG has widespread connections with structures in rostral midbrain, diencephalon, and telencephalon.[28] The PAG projects to central nuclei of the thalamus, including centrolateral, paraventricular, parafascicular, and central medial areas, along with several dopaminergic areas, including ventral tegmental area and substantia nigra pars compacta. The PAG is likely also involved in the ascending modulation of nociception and integration of behavioral responses.[28]

Descending noradrenergic systems originating from the pontine A7 cell group (subcoerulus) and A5, A6 (locus coerulus) also show bidirectional pain control.[45] This pontine noradrenergic system is at least partly influenced by direct projections from neurons that release SP located in the RVM.[46] The regulation of pain signals transiting through the DH of the spinal cord is also under

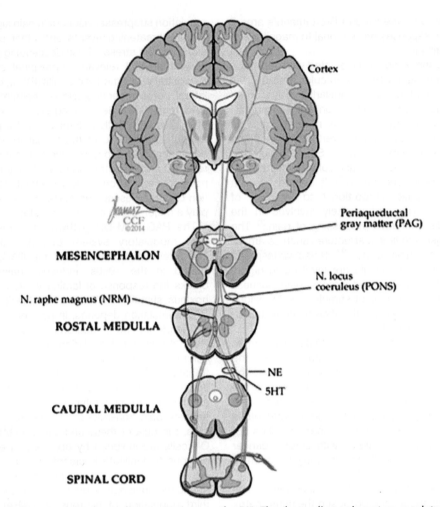

Cortex

Periaqueductal gray matter (PAG)

MESENCEPHALON

N. locus coeruleus (PONS)

N. raphe magnus (NRM)

ROSTAL MEDULLA

NE

5HT

CAUDAL MEDULLA

SPINAL CORD

Fig. 3. The influence of the descending projections on the DH. The descending pain system regulates incoming pain signals at the DH. Input into the descending pain system is encoded at several sites in the brainstem including the PAG, dorsolateral pontine tegmentum (DLPT) and the RVM. The PAG exerts both direct and indirect descending control at the DH. The indirect pathway induces the release of 5-HT from neurons in the nucleus raphe magnus (NRM) located in the RVM. The descending noradrenergic system includes the nucleus locus coeruleus in the DLPT. (*Courtesy of* the Cleveland Clinic Foundation, Cleveland, Ohio.)

the control of dopaminergic descending neurons from the periventricular region of the hypothalamus (A11).[47] The dopamine receptor subtype expressed by primary afferents or DH neurons in lamina I dictate an antinociceptive or pronociceptive effect.[47] Dysfunction of this descending pain system may lead to chronic pain conditions; however, this descending dopaminergic system is another potential target for treatment.[47]

The descending endogenous opioid pain modulation system also augments pain processing. Activation of opioid receptors in the brain, specifically the mu receptor, blocks pain transmission centrally in the brain but also will activate descending systems. Opioid receptor binding alters membrane conductance and protein phosphorylation states.[3] Dynorphin is found in laminae I and V

as well as PAG and midbrain reticular formation. It hypothesized that dynorphin contributes to pain centralization.

The interactions of the descending systems are still being defined although several hypothesis have been proposed to explain certain abnormal pain states. For example, central sensitization is believed to involve an increase in the activity of the ascending pain pathway coupled with a decrease in activity in the descending inhibitory pathway. Similarly, the release of tonic inhibition at the DH is associated with chronic pain.

SUMMARY

Although the details underpinning the pain systems are debatable, the evolutionary advantage to having an integrative pain system culminating in the conscious recognition of pain is not. When studied using modern neuroimaging or electrophysiological studies, the nature of the perceptual experience of pain still remains fragmented. This has unfortunately delayed the development of novel neurosurgical approaches to treat chronic non-cancer pain. Nevertheless, the surgical treatments represented in this issue have taken advantage of what is known currently and represent an important step forward for those patients with chronic pain.

REFERENCES

1. Melzack R. From the gate to the neuromatrix. Pain 1999;(Suppl 6):S121–6.
2. Hall JE, Guyton AC. Guyton and Hall textbook of medical physiology. 12th edition. Philadelphia: Saunders/Elsevier; 2011.
3. Rosenow JM, Henderson JM. Anatomy and physiology of chronic pain. Neurosurg Clin N Am 2003; 14(3):445–62, vii.
4. Fishman S, Ballantyne J, Rathmell JP, et al. Bonica's management of pain. 4th edition. Baltimore (MD): Lippincott, Williams & Wilkins; 2010.
5. Cooper B, Ahlquist M, Friedman RM, et al. Properties of high-threshold mechanoreceptors in the goat oral mucosa. II. Dynamic and static reactivity in carrageenan-inflamed mucosa. J Neurophysiol 1991;66(4):1280–90.
6. Handwerker HO, Anton F, Reeh PW. Discharge patterns of afferent cutaneous nerve fibers from the rat's tail during prolonged noxious mechanical stimulation. Exp Brain Res 1987;65(3):493–504.
7. Thalhammer JG, LaMotte RH. Spatial properties of nociceptor sensitization following heat injury of the skin. Brain Res 1982;231(2):257–65.
8. Willis WD, Westlund KN. Neuroanatomy of the pain system and of the pathways that modulate pain. J Clin Neurophysiol 1997;14(1):2–31.
9. England JD, Happel LT, Kline DG, et al. Sodium channel accumulation in humans with painful neuromas. Neurology 1996;47(1):272–6.
10. Benzel EC, Francis TB. Spine surgery: techniques, complication avoidance, and management. 3rd edition. Philadelphia: Elsevier/Saunders; 2012.
11. Neumann S, Doubell TP, Leslie T, et al. Inflammatory pain hypersensitivity mediated by phenotypic switch in myelinated primary sensory neurons. Nature 1996;384(6607):360–4.
12. Pitcher GM, Henry JL. Nociceptive response to innocuous mechanical stimulation is mediated via myelinated afferents and NK-1 receptor activation in a rat model of neuropathic pain. Exp Neurol 2004;186(2):173–97.
13. Devor M. Unexplained peculiarities of the dorsal root ganglion. Pain 1999;(Suppl 6):S27–35.
14. McMahon SB. Wall and Melzack's textbook of pain. 6th edition. Philadelphia: Elsevier/Saunders; 2013.
15. Pannese E, Ledda M, Conte V, et al. The perikaryal projections of rabbit spinal ganglion neurons. A comparison of thin section reconstructions and scanning microscopy views. Anat Embryol (Berl) 1990;181(5):427–32.
16. Amir R, Devor M. Chemically mediated cross-excitation in rat dorsal root ganglia. J Neurosci 1996;16(15):4733–41.
17. Applebaum ML, Clifton GL, Coggeshall RE, et al. Unmyelinated fibres in the sacral 3 and caudal 1 ventral roots of the cat. J Physiol 1976;256(3):557–72.
18. Coggeshall RE, Applebaum ML, Fazen M, et al. Unmyelinated axons in human ventral roots, a possible explanation for the failure of dorsal rhizotomy to relieve pain. Brain 1975;98(1):157–66.
19. Coggeshall RE, Maynard CW, Langford LA. Unmyelinated sensory and preganglionic fibers in rat L6 and S1 ventral spinal roots. J Comp Neurol 1980; 193(1):41–7.
20. Sykes MT, Coggeshall RE. Unmyelinated fibers in the human L4 and L5 ventral roots. Brain Res 1973;63:490–5.
21. Traub RJ, Mendell LM. The spinal projection of individual identified A-delta- and C-fibers. J Neurophysiol 1988;59(1):41–55.
22. Earle KM. The tract of Lissauer and its possible relation to the pain pathway. J Comp Neurol 1952;96(1):93–111.
23. Gobel S. Golgi studies of the neurons in layer II of the dorsal horn of the medulla (trigeminal nucleus caudalis). J Comp Neurol 1978;180(2):395–413.
24. Mannion RJ, Doubell TP, Gill H, et al. Deafferentation is insufficient to induce sprouting of A-fibre central terminals in the rat dorsal horn. J Comp Neurol 1998;393(2):135–44.
25. Treede RD, Meyer RA, Raja SN, et al. Peripheral and central mechanisms of cutaneous hyperalgesia. Prog Neurobiol 1992;38(4):397–421.
26. Dostrovsky JO. Role of thalamus in pain. Prog Brain Res 2000;129:245–57.
27. Lenz FA, Weiss N, Ohara S, et al. The role of the thalamus in pain. Suppl Clin Neurophysiol 2004;57:50–61.
28. Cameron AA, Khan IA, Westlund KN, et al. The efferent projections of the periaqueductal gray in the rat: a Phaseolus vulgaris-leucoagglutinin study. I. Ascending projections. J Comp Neurol 1995;351(4):568–84.
29. Bowsher D. Role of the reticular formation in responses to noxious stimulation. Pain 1976;2(4):361–78.
30. Dado RJ, Katter JT, Giesler GJ Jr. Spinothalamic and spinohypothalamic tract neurons in the cervical enlargement of rats. II. Responses to innocuous and noxious mechanical and thermal stimuli. J Neurophysiol 1994;71(3):981–1002.

31. Bowsher D, Mallart A, Petit D, et al. A bulbar relay to the centre median. J Neurophysiol 1968;31(2):288–300.

32. Melzack R, Wall PD. Pain mechanisms: a new theory. Science 1965;150(3699):971–9.

33. Ralston HJ 3rd. Pain and the primate thalamus. Prog Brain Res 2005;149:1–10.

34. Tran TD, Inui K, Hoshiyama M, et al. Cerebral activation by the signals ascending through unmyelinated C-fibers in humans: a magnetoencephalographic study. Neuroscience 2002;113(2):375–86.

35. Anderson WS, O'Hara S, Lawson HC, et al. Plasticity of pain-related neuronal activity in the human thalamus. Prog Brain Res 2006;157:353–64.

36. Krout KE, Belzer RE, Loewy AD. Brainstem projections to midline and intralaminar thalamic nuclei of the rat. J Comp Neurol 2002;448(1):53–101.

37. Lenz FA, Lee JI, Garonzik IM, et al. Plasticity of pain-related neuronal activity in the human thalamus. Prog Brain Res 2000;129:259–73.

38. Llinas RR, Ribary U, Jeanmonod D, et al. Thalamocortical dysrhythmia: a neurological and neuropsychiatric syndrome characterized by magnetoencephalography. Proc Natl Acad Sci U S A 1999;96(26):15222–7.

39. Jones AK, Kulkarni B, Derbyshire SW. Pain mechanisms and their disorders. Br Med Bull 2003;65:83–93.

40. Møller AR. Textbook of tinnitus. New York: Springer; 2011.

41. Oliveras JL, Woda A, Guilbaud G, et al. Inhibition of the jaw opening reflex by electrical stimulation of the periaqueductal gray matter in the awake, unrestrained cat. Brain Res 1974;72(2):328–31.

42. Reynolds DV. Surgery in the rat during electrical analgesia induced by focal brain stimulation. Science 1969;164(3878):444–5.

43. Mayer DJ, Liebeskind JC. Pain reduction by focal electrical stimulation of the brain: an anatomical and behavioral analysis. Brain Res 1974;68(1):73–93.

44. Wei F, Dubner R, Zou S, et al. Molecular depletion of descending serotonin unmasks its novel facilitatory role in the development of persistent pain. J Neurosci 2010;30(25):8624–36.

45. Yeomans DC, Proudfit HK. Antinociception induced by microinjection of substance P into the A7 catecholamine cell group in the rat. Neuroscience 1992;49(3):681–91.

46. Yeomans DC, Clark FM, Paice JA, et al. Antinociception induced by electrical stimulation of spinally projecting noradrenergic neurons in the A7 catecholamine cell group of the rat. Pain 1992;48(3):449–61.

47. Kwon M, Altin M, Duenas H, et al. The role of descending inhibitory pathways on chronic pain modulation and clinical implications. Pain Pract 2013. [Epub ahead of print].

Introduction to Neuropathic Pain Syndromes

Juanmarco Gutierrez, MD, MSc*, Sukreet Raju, MD*,
Jonathan P. Riley, MD, MS, Nicholas M. Boulis, MD

KEYWORDS

• Pain • Neuropathic • Nociceptive • Chronic • Epidemiology • Treatment outcomes

KEY POINTS

- Chronic pain impairs the quality of life for millions of individuals and therefore presents a serious ongoing challenge to clinicians and researchers.
- Debilitating chronic pain syndromes cost the US economy more than $600 billion per year. This article provides an overview of the epidemiology, clinical presentation, and treatment outcomes for craniofacial, spinal, and peripheral neurologic pain syndromes.
- Although the authors recognize that the diagnosis and treatment of the chronic forms of neuropathic pain syndromes represent a clinical challenge, there is an urgent need for standardized classification systems, improved epidemiologic data, and reliable treatment outcomes data.

Chronic pain impairs the quality of life for millions of people, and therefore presents a serious ongoing challenge to clinicians and researchers.[1] Debilitating chronic pain syndromes cost the US economy more than $600 billion per year.[2] The annual cost of pain treatment is greater than the combined annual costs of heart disease, cancer, and diabetes. A recent epidemiology review reports that prevalence rates of neuropathic pain as a global clinical entity range from 0.9% to 17.9%.[3]

For many years, clinicians have understood that nociceptive pain sensation serves as a crucial, adaptive physiologic response to noxious stimuli through primary nociceptive afferent activation. In contrast, neuropathic pain arises by activity generated within the somatosensory system without adequate stimulation of peripheral afferents.[4] This maladaptive plasticity in the neuropathic pain state is often a consequence of lesions to the peripheral or central nervous system. Alterations such as ectopic generation of action potentials, facilitation and disinhibition of synaptic transmission, loss of synaptic connectivity and formation of new synaptic circuits, and neuroimmune interactions contribute to the multifaceted pathogenesis of complex neuropathic pain syndromes.[5,6]

Historically, neuropathic pain syndromes have been classified based on their cause or on the anatomic distribution of pain. Although this classification has some use for diagnostic purposes, it offers no good framework for the clinical management of pain or for the evaluation of the available therapies.[7] A range of positive and negative neurosensory symptoms usually characterize

Disclosure of relationships with drug or equipment trademarks: No disclosures to declare for any of the authors or coauthors.

Department of Neurosurgery, School of Medicine, Emory University, 101 Woodruff Circle, Lab 6339, Atlanta, GA 30322, USA

* Corresponding authors.

E-mail addresses: juanmarco.gutierrez@emory.edu; sraju8@emory.edu

these syndromes.[8] This clinical heterogeneity makes the development of standardized diagnostic and evaluation tools for pain increasingly challenging. Consequently, patients are frequently misclassified and treatment outcomes are not recorded in a reliable and efficient manner.[3,9–11] Modern pain research has explored genetic and molecular modulation of nociceptive systems to develop new analgesic strategies. Such examples of backward translation from the clinic to basic science are starting to become increasingly important. For this approach to be successful, it is of utmost importance to first develop an effective way of assessing treatment outcomes in the clinic. Successful exploration of genetic and molecular tools to better define neuropathic pain syndromes requires the tandem improvement of clinical outcome measurements.[12,13] This article categorizes the existing literature for neuropathic pain, focusing on craniofacial, spinal, and peripheral pain syndromes.

CRANIOFACIAL PAIN SYNDROMES

Epidemiologists estimate that approximately 39 million adult Americans are suffering from chronic craniofacial pain.[14] Despite the high prevalence, in the last few years, the classification of craniofacial pain disorders has been a matter of active debate, and there are no established criteria to evaluate the efficacy or effectiveness of available pharmacologic and nonpharmacologic therapies.[15] This section details recently reported epidemiology and neurosurgical treatment outcomes for craniofacial pain syndromes.

Primary Headaches

Primary headaches, such as tension-type, migraine, and cluster headaches, are prevalent conditions that affect the US population. **Table 1** provides a comprehensive overview of the available neurosurgical interventions for cluster and migraine headaches.

Patients suffering from cluster or migraine headache often do not find pain relief from conventional management. Considerable progress has been made in neurostimulative and neuroablative approaches to treat chronic headache syndromes. However, the effectiveness of each treatment approach varies widely in terms of pain relief. Some of the studies that were reviewed report moderate to significant pain reduction, whereas others report decrease in frequency of pain attacks. The level of evidence for the treatment outcomes ranges from case reports to quasi-randomized studies, thus unmasking a clear need for prospective randomized controlled studies to rigorously

evaluate current surgical treatment interventions effective for craniofacial neuropathic pain.

Cranial Neuralgias

Cranial neuralgias comprise various painful paroxysmal disorders of the head. Although trigeminal neuralgia has an incidence that ranges from 3 to 5 new cases for 100,000 persons per year and a prevalence that ranges from 12.6 to 28.9 per 100,000 persons, it is still a rare disease that is easily misdiagnosed among the duplicative and inconsistent nomenclature of craniofacial neuralgias (**Table 2**).[3,16]

Despite the low incidence and prevalence of cranial neuralgias, a wide range of surgical and nonsurgical interventions are available, most of which have good success rates. Classification criteria (eg, International Headache Society, International Classification of Headache Disorders 2nd edition) have long been purely based on the clinical presentation of pain, which can sometimes be subjective. Thus, it makes it easy to misdiagnose or misclassify patients with chronic conditions. To have more reliable outcomes data, one must first have a more effective classification system for these conditions. Classification systems, such as the one proposed by Burchiel in 2003, attempt to reduce misclassification by standardizing the nomenclature.[17] However, this system is based on empirical observations rather than on prospective data.

Other Types of Craniofacial Pain

Other types of craniofacial pain, such as temporomandibular joint (TMJ) disorders, are not uncommon; however, most of the available treatment options do not fall in the scope of the neurosurgery practice. Persistent idiopathic facial pain (PIFP), also known as atypical facial pain, is a rare condition that includes facial pain that does not have the characteristics or distribution of any of the cranial neuralgias. Likewise, anesthesia dolorosa (AD) is a pain syndrome that arises as a complication of the surgical treatments of neuralgias and trauma, among other causes. PIFP and AD are rare chronic pain conditions that are commonly treatment refractory; consequently, there is a limited literature on success rates of the available treatments (**Table 3**).

Neuroablative and neurostimlative approaches used to treat these conditions have had questionable success rates that can be attributed to the rarity of these conditions, as well as the limited body of published literature on successful intervention. The level of evidence that supports the effectiveness of the available treatments for PIFP, AD, and TMJ disorders ranges from case

Table 1
Clinical presentation, epidemiology and treatment outcomes for primary headaches

Pain Syndrome	Epidemiology	Clinical Presentation	Treatments	Outcomes	References
Cluster headaches	Prevalence of 53 per 100,000 Male to female ratio is 1.7:1 for chronic cluster headache	• Pain attacks of severe or very severe unilateral orbital, supraorbital, and/or temporal pain lasting 15–180 min if untreated. May be accompanied by ipsilateral conjunctival injection and/or lacrimation, nasal congestion, and/or rhinorrhea, eyelid edema, forehead and facial sweating, miosis and/or ptosis and a sense of restlessness or agitation • Attacks have a frequency from 1 every other day to 8 per day • Chronic cluster headache has attacks occurring for >1 y without remission or with remissions lasting <1 mo • Episodic form is 6 times more common than the chronic form	Occipital nerve stimulation Sphenopalatine ganglion stimulation Radiofrequency ablation of sphenopalatine ganglion Gamma Knife stereotactic radiosurgery to trigeminal nerve root Hypothalamic deep brain stimulation Transection of the nervus intermedius	Significant, long-term benefit in 67% of patients with refractory chronic cluster headache Pain relief seen in 67.1% of attacks treated with full stimulation. Mean attack frequency decreased from 17.4 per week at baseline to 12.5 per week during treatment Reported to reduce attack intensity and frequency in patients with refractory chronic cluster headache A case series with 15 patients showed decrease in mean attack intensity (8.6 vs 4.2) and mean attack frequency (17 vs 8.3 attacks/wk) at 18 mo follow-up vs baseline On comparing complete pain relief vs partial pain relief (medication <50% preoperative requirement) vs no pain relief, in a study of 10 patients with medication-resistant chronic cluster headache, outcome was 30% vs 30% vs 40% A review of 43 patients followed for 12–40 mo reported pain relief rated as excellent in 28%, good in 21%, fair in 12%, and poor in 39% Total positive response rate of around 60% High early success rate for pain relief, with potential for long-lasting pain relief. Rowed reported a 75% success rate	23–33
Migraine headaches	Prevalence in the US population: Acute: 18% (women) and 6% (men) Chronic: 4%	Moderate to severe headache attacks, with or without accompanying vegetative symptoms	Botulinum toxin A prophylactic injections Trigger site deactivation surgery Occipital nerve stimulation	Small to modest pain reduction Pain elimination or significant reduction in 29%–57% Overall improvement in 50 to >90%	34–43

Table 2
Clinical presentation, epidemiology and treatment outcomes for cranial neuralgias

Pain Syndrome	Epidemiology	Clinical Presentation	Treatments	Outcomes	References
Occipital neuralgia	• Prevalence and incidence estimates not available • The major occipital nerve is more frequently involved (90%) as compared with the minor occipital nerve (10%)	Paroxysmal stabbing pain, with or without persistent aching between paroxysms, in the distribution of the greater, lesser, and/or third occipital nerves	Peripheral neurectomy	Outcome of 95 neurectomies: excellent 15%, good 71%, poor 9% Initial pain relief reported to be durable in only approximately 50% of cases in a series	25,44–59
			C2 dorsal root ganglionectomy	One series reports that >80% of patients with trauma as a precipitant achieved good or excellent results. Results were poorer with nontraumatic occipital pain. >50% of these patients did not experience worthwhile improvement (>50% reduction in pain) with their surgery. In patients with a history of migraine headaches, surgery produced a satisfactory result in only 30% Extended follow-up of another series noted pain recurrence in 65% of patients by 12 mo and no recurrences after 24 mo	
			Microvascular decompression	Pain relief: complete in 89.5% and significant in 6.6%. Recurrence in 3.9% (89 procedures performed in 76 Chinese patients)	
			Percutaneous neurolysis of C-2 nerve root	Case report of a patient being free of pain for more than 12 mo, after alcohol-induced rhizotomy	
			Occipital nerve stimulation	Success rates of 70%–100% (mean 88%)	
			Radiofrequency lesioning of greater and lesser occipital nerves	Traumatic cause: 72%; excellent pain relief. Nontraumatic cause: 76%; excellent	
			Botulinum toxin type A	Reports of effectiveness exist, but botulinum toxin cannot be firmly recommended as an evidence-based treatment in secondary headaches or cranial neuralgias	

	Prevalence/Characteristics	Treatment	Outcome	Ref
		Nerve decompression and fixation of the atlantoaxial joint	In patients with subluxation of the atlantoaxial joint causing compression of the C2 nerve, reliable benefit was achieved	
		Partial posterior rhizotomy at C1–3 or selective posterior rhizidiotomy or microsurgical DREZ-otomy	Likelihood of long-term pain relief ~71%. Complete pain relief in 44% (4 of 9) of patients who underwent intradural C1-C3 and C1-C4 selective dorsal rhizotomies. Chambers reported 22 patients, 6 of whom had 75% improvement and 10 complete relief	
		Pulsed radiofrequency treatment of occipital nerve	19 patients included in the prospective trial, 68.4%, 57.9%, and 52.6% reported an improvement of 50% or more 1, 2, and 6 mo after pulsed radiofrequency treatment, respectively.	
		Pulsed radiofrequency treatment of C-2 dorsal root ganglion	2 of 4 patients had a long-term effect (18 and >24 mo), no improvement observed in the other 2 patients	
Trigeminal neuralgia	Prevalence: 12.6–28.9 per 100,000 • Brief strong, sharp, unilateral shooting pain in 1 or more branches of cranial nerve. Quality of pain is sharp, shooting, electric-like • Distribution: V1, 4%; V2, 17%; V3, 15%; V2 + V3, 32%; V1 + V2, 14%; V1 + V2 + V3, 17%	Gasserian ganglion radiofrequency thermocoagulation, glycerol, balloon compression Gamma Knife Microvascular decompression	Pain relief: significant in 50% of cases for 5 y Pain relief: significant in 52% of cases for 3 y Pain relief: significant in 73% of cases for 5 y	3,60,61

(continued on next page)

Table 2
(continued)

Pain Syndrome	Epidemiology	Clinical Presentation	Treatments	Outcomes	References
Glossopharyngeal neuralgia	• Incidence: 0.2 and 0.7 per 100,000 people per year • Average annual recurrence rate for a second episode is low (3.6%)	• Paroxysmal attacks of facial pain lasting from a fraction of a second to 2 min Characterized by unilateral, sharp, stabbing, and severe pain in the distribution within the posterior part of the tongue, tonsillar fossa, pharynx, or beneath the angle of the lower jaw and/or in the ear • Triggers: swallowing, chewing, talking, coughing, and yawning	Microvascular decompression Rhizotomy of cranial nerve IX and with or without upper rootlets of X Gamma Knife Motor cortex stimulation Computed tomography–guided percutaneous trigeminal tractotomy-nucleotomy Selective trigeminal tractotomy Percutaneous radiofrequency neurolysis (pulsed-mode, low-temperature, and conventional radiofrequency)	Highest initial and long-term success rates. Complete pain relief in the range of 76%–97% Long-term relief is 96.4% 13 of 15 (87%) reported patients treated have achieved significant pain relief >50% pain relief noted to last for 18–72 mo 14 patients, half of them experienced recurrent pain during the long-term follow-up period (5–12 y); 4 underwent a second procedure, 3 of them with rhizotomy; 3 of the 4 in this recurrent group had no pain after the second surgical intervention All 6 patients were cured of neuralgia. Tractotomy was repeated in 1 within 12 d because the analgesia was not complete. 1 patient has been followed up for 6 y, 2 for 3 y, 1 for 1 y, and 2 for a few months 5 patients pain free 4 mo to 3 y. About 10 other patients have been reported to be pain free after the procedure[a]	25,62–71
Geniculate neuralgia	Data not available because it is an uncommon condition	Brief paroxysms of pain felt deep in the auditory canal. A trigger area is present in the posterior wall of the auditory canal	Transection of nervus intermedius (with or without geniculate ganglion removal) Microvascular decompression	An author reports that in 64 patients who underwent nervus intermedius transaction and geniculate ganglion removal, excellent results were obtained, except in 1 patient Based on case reports and small series, long-term pain control can be seen after nerve sectioning or microvascular decompression, but no prospective studies exist	25,72,73

Abbreviation: DREZ, dorsal root entry zone.

[a] Because of the high incidence of complications, it was recommended that this procedure be reserved for patients whose condition is secondary to malignancy or who are unable to withstand intracranial procedures.

Table 3
Clinical presentation, epidemiology, and treatment outcomes of other types of craniofacial pain

Pain Syndrome	Epidemiology	Clinical Presentation	Treatments	Outcomes	References
Persistent idiopathic facial pain	Prevalence: 3.2–5.9 per 100,000 people	• Persistent facial pain that does not have the characteristics of cranial neuralgias or cannot be attributed to another disorder • Described as throbbing pain situated deep in the eye and malar region, often radiating to the ear, neck, and shoulders	CT-guided percutaneous trigeminal tractotomy-nucleotomy Nucleus caudalis DREZ lesioning Experimental procedures: pulsed radiofrequency to the sphenopalatine ganglion	Largest case series shows pain relief in 16 of 17 patients Not available Pain relief: complete in 21% of cases and significant in 65% of cases	74–78
Anesthesia dolorosa	Incidence rate: 0.8%	• Uncommon complication of surgical treatments for neuralgias • Described as excruciating pain perceived in an insensate region of the face	Neuromodulation by motor cortex stimulation Deep brain stimulation Nucleus caudalis DREZ lesioning	Pain relief: minimal, high recurrence Mixed reports of efficacy Pain relief: significant in >60% of cases. Postprocedure ataxia of 90%	68,79–82
TMJ disorders	Estimated 15%–16% prevalence of treatment need for temporomandibular disorder in general adult population	• Recurrent pain in one or more regions of the head and/or face • Pain is precipitated by jaw movements and/or chewing of hard or tough food • Reduced range of or irregular jaw opening • Noise from one or both TMJs during jaw movements • Tenderness of the joint capsule of one or both TMJs • Headache resolves within 3 mo, and does not recur, after successful treatment of the TMJ disorder	Botulinum toxin Arthrocentesis and arthroscopy Open surgery: disk repositioning, disk repair, discectomy, discectomy with graft replacement Joint replacement Denervation of TMJ	90% patients treated with botulinum toxin had mean 3.2-point reduction in pain on visual analog scale. Pain significantly reduced in patients with botulinum toxin compared with placebo (P<.01) Both affect mandibular movement, reduce pain intensity and mandibular functioning to the same degree. Success rates were often high, independent of treatment mode. The effect of maxillofacial surgery is still unclear Improvement in pain is generally seen Intended primarily at restoration of form and function, and any pain relief gained is only a secondary benefit Pain free for 12 mo after surgery (patient with recurrent dislocations of TMJ articular disc. History of 2 arthroscopic surgeries and 1 open attempt to treat TMJ pain)	25,83–87

Abbreviations: CT, computed tomography; DREZ, dorsal root entry zone.

Table 4
Clinical presentation, epidemiology, and treatment outcomes of pain syndromes involving the spine and/or spinal cord

Pain Syndrome	Epidemiology	Clinical Presentation	Treatments	Outcomes	References
Low back pain	Prevalence: 8.1%–10.2% of the US population	Chronic, recurrent, or long-lasting pain localized below the costal margin and above the inferior gluteal folds lasting for at least 6 mo	Lumbar fusion	15% pain free out of 152 patients in a randomized trial	88–94
			Total disc replacement	30% pain free out of 152 patients in a randomized trial	
				Pain relief >50% for 7 mo	
			Spinal endoscopic adhesiolysis	Pain relief 33% for 1 mo	
			Caudal epidural steroid injection	45% out of 33 patients in an RCT reported a pain relief of >50% for 12 mo	
			Spinal cord stimulation	A review of 72 case series reported a pain relief of >50% in 62% of the patients	
FBSS	• Incidence of FBSS has increased with increasing rates of spine surgery • 10%–40% patients may develop FBSS after lumbar spinal surgery • Success rate of lumbar spinal surgery falls with each successive surgery on the same patient	• Persistent or recurring low back pain, with or without sciatica, after one or more spine surgeries • FBSS can be a result of the outcome of lumbar spinal surgery not meeting the presurgical expectations of the patient and surgeon	Lumbar epidural steroid injection	>50% reduction in pain reported, with analgesia ranging from 15 d up to 180 d. Adjuvant hyaluronidase may prolong analgesia	95–103
				Transforaminal injection has the strongest evidence for short- and long-term improvement when compared with interlaminar and caudal injections	
			Percutaneous epidural adhesiolysis	Strong evidence for short- and long-term pain relief, with 1 study reporting effectiveness in 73% of patients during a 12-mo period	
			Ozone therapy	43.7% reduction in lumbar pain and a 60.9% reduction in leg pain, with a 44.0% of improvement in ODI scores after 6 mo has been reported. Nonneuropathic pain responded better than neuropathic pain	
			Facet medial branch RF rhizotomy	At 12 mo follow-up, >90% pain relief in 60% and >60% pain relief in 87% of patients. (Facet joints may be responsible for persistent pain in up to 16% of patients)	
			Intrathecal drug delivery	67.4% pain reduction at 6 mo; mean pain reduction of 64%	
			Peripheral nerve field stimulation	>50% pain relief sustained for at least 12 mo, in a significant number of patients	

Syndrome	Epidemiology	Clinical features	Treatment	Evidence	References
			Spinal cord stimulation	More effective at controlling radicular or radiating pain vs axial pain, with RCTs demonstrating clinical effectiveness. 47%–62% response rate reported	
			Spinal cord stimulation in conjunction with peripheral nerve field stimulation	Pain control is better with the combination than either modality alone	
			Deep brain stimulation	54 of 59 patients in a study had success on initial stimulation. 46 had success on chronic stimulation. 85.2% success rate reported in the cases internalized	
			Revision surgery	22%–50% successful outcomes reported after a revision surgery. An initial success rate of >50% can reduce to 5% after the fourth revision surgery. A small prospective study, with 1-y follow-up, suggests that a 90% success rate is possible with proper patient selection, correct diagnosis, and indicated surgical procedure targeted at the pain generator. Other studies have shown trend to poor outcome at 2-y follow-up	
Postherpetic neuralgia	Acute: Incidence: 3.9–41.8 per 100,000 people. Prevalence in the general population: 7%–27% Chronic: not available	Pain after acute rash has healed accompanied by pain, allodynia, paresthesia, or dysesthesia. The pain usually affects a single dermatome	Botulinum toxin A	Significant pain relief in 87% of 30 patients in a small RCT	3,94,104–111
			Sympathetic nerve block	No RCTs have been conducted. May be effective in refractory cases	
			Spinal cord stimulation	Good to excellent pain relief in case series and case reports	
			Gamma Knife stereotactic radiosurgery	Excellent and good pain relief in 44% of the patients in a case series with 15 patients Multicenter study including 500 patients reported pain relief in 50%–90% of patients	
			Peripheral nerve stimulation	Excellent and good pain relief reported in case series and case reports	
			DREZ lesioning	Effective pain relief in most patients in case series	

(continued on next page)

Table 4
(continued)

Pain Syndrome	Epidemiology	Clinical Presentation	Treatments	Outcomes	References
Postthoracotomy pain syndrome	• Incidence: 15% and 80% • Incidence of severe pain: 3%–5% • Prevalence: highly variable, but high (about 50%) • Prevalence may be higher for thoracotomy (45%) than it is for video-assisted thoracotomy (41%)	• "Pain that recurs or persists along a thoracotomy incision at least 2 mo after the surgical procedure" (International Association for the Study of Pain definition) • Nature: burning and stabbing, with dysesthesia • Pain is mild to moderate in most, 5% of patients experience severe and disabling pain. The gentlest of stimulation can trigger intense pain	Peripheral nerve field stimulation Peripheral nerve stimulation Intercostal nerve block Intercostal nerve (ICN) cryoablation Microsurgical DREZ lesion Pulsed RF of the ICN Pulsed RF of the DRG Spinal cord stimulation	80%–100% pain relief reported. One case was followed up to 26 mo Relative reduction in pain intensity (>80%) reported in 2 cases after neurostimulation of the thoracic paravertebral plexus Provides significant pain relief. Complete pain relief lasting for >9 mo reported in 1 case. Average pain score decreased to 4.1 ± 1.7 from a preprocedural pain score of 7.5 ± 2.0, after a mean follow-up period of 51 d, in a study of 18 patients undergoing CT-guided percutaneous cryoneurolysis In another study, 50% of patients continued to report significant pain relief at 3-mo follow-up. Complete pain relief in 2 patients In a study of 31 patients, after 3 mo of follow-up: 2 of 13 (15%) managed medically continued to have a positive outcome compared with 10% (1 of 10) in the ICN group and half the patients in the DRG group (4 of 8) Improved treatment outcomes with Pulsed RF of the DRG at 3 mo postprocedure, when compared with medical management alone or pulsed RF of the ICN (see earlier above) 5 of 9 patients experienced long term amelioration of pain in one study 75%–100% pain relief reported up to 24 mo follow up in other case reports	112–127

Pain after spinal cord injury	Approximately 65%–85% of people have pain (nociceptive and neuropathic) after spinal cord injury. One-third of them report the pain as severe	Neuropathic pain and dysesthesia in areas with sensory deficit and can be spontaneous or stimulus evoked. Quality can be burning, smarting, shooting, aching, pricking, and tingling. Might be accompanied by paresthesia	DREZ lesioning	In most studies 50%–88% of patients obtain good pain relief	3,94,108, 109,128–133
			Spinal cord stimulation	In most studies <25% of patients who received stimulators had pain relief	
			Cordotomy or cordomyelotomy	Case reports and case series showed modest effectiveness.	
			Intrathecal drug delivery devices	Baclofen has proved to have modest effectiveness on central pain but no pain relief for neuropathic pain	
				An RCT (15 patients) using morphine and clonidine showed good short-term pain relief	
			Invasive and noninvasive motor cortex stimulation	Promising alternative for the treatment of central pain	

Abbreviations: CT, computed tomography; DREZ, dorsal root entry zone; DRG, dorsal root ganglia; ICN, intercostals nerve; ODI, oswestry disability index; RCT, randomized controlled trial; RF, radiofrequency.

Table 5
Clinical presentation, epidemiology and treatment outcomes of pain syndromes involving peripheral nerves

Pain Syndrome	Epidemiology	Clinical Presentation	Treatments	Outcomes	References
CRPS	• 5–25 cases per 100,000 person-years • High rates after events such as fracture or surgery (up to 36%) • 4:1 female to male ratio reported	• CRPS type I: formerly called Reflex Sympathetic Dystrophy; has no definable nerve lesion. CRPS type II: formerly called Causalgia; a peripheral nerve lesion can be demonstrated • Presents with severe pain that is disproportionate to the inciting event, most commonly affecting the hand or foot but that can spread to other body regions • The affected body parts may display sensory disturbances, temperature changes, abnormal patterns of sweating, edema, reduced joint range of motion, movement abnormalities such as weakness, tremor, or dystonia, trophic changes such as skin atrophy or altered hair and nail growth, and localized osteoporotic changes • Alterations in body perception or schema may be present	Epidural clonidine	300 or 600 µg clonidine reported to reduce pain greater than placebo for 6 h posttreatment	103,134–155
			Intravenous regional anesthetic blocks	2 RCTs (17 patients totally) using ketanserin and bretylium demonstrated significant relief when compared with control	
			Local anesthetic sympathetic blockade (lidocaine or bupivacaine)	Not effective (low quality evidence)	
			Local anesthetic sympathetic blockade along with botulinum toxin A	Longer duration of pain relief with the combination (71 d) than with local anesthetic sympathetic blockade alone (<10 d)	
			Intrathecal baclofen	4 of 6 women with an implanted subcutaneous pump for continuous intrathecal baclofen showed marked improvement in dystonia after being followed up for a mean of 1.7 y	
			Sympathectomy Surgical	No evidence from controlled trials from which to draw conclusions on efficacy. Reported to be helpful for pain in 12%–97% of patients; persistent mild hyperpathia, tenderness, joint stiffness, and trophic changes have been noted in 30%–40%	
			Radiofrequency lumbar sympathectomy or Phenol lumbar sympathectomy	No significant difference between groups for significant reduction in pain from baseline	
			Repair of injured nerve in CRPS type II	Repair of nerve lesion and of adjacent axial artery reported to eliminate pain in 32 patients	
			Amputation	Pain improved in 2 of 5 patients. Residual function improved in 9 of 15 patients CRPS type I recurred in the stump in 28 amputations of 34 amputations in 31 limbs	

Spinal cord stimulation	Pain: 50%–91% effectiveness for pain relief. Diminished pain relief over 5 y reported by one RCT Function: May not improve function in CRPS type I, but a prospective study of 29 patients found that significant reduction of deep pain and allodynia ultimately resulted in functional improvements
Transcutaneous electrical nerve stimulation	Insufficient evidence for treatment effectiveness in CRPS type I
Repetitive TMS	An RCT of 23 patients with CRPS type I of upper limb demonstrated a mean reduction in visual analog scale scores 1 wk after last stimulation of 50.9% with TMS vs 24.7% with placebo
Peripheral nerve stimulation	Good relief for CRPS I that is limited to the distribution of 1 major nerve. Good or fair pain relief, during a period of 1–4 y reported CRPS II: Good pain relief with improved function reported for CRPS II
Stimulation of Dorsal Root Ganglia	Short-term reduction in average self-reported pain to 62% relative to baseline values, with relief persisting through 12 mo in most. Improvement in function, edema, and trophic skin changes in some
Combined spinal cord and peripheral nerve field stimulation	Coutilization of both cervical spinal cord and peripheral nerve field stimulation provided 95% pain relief in 1 case study
Deep brain stimulation	Significant reduction in dystonia and pain in CRPS I reported in a case series with 2 patients A meta-analysis reports long-term success in 80%
Motor cortex stimulation	Mean VAS decrease of 75% with associated decreases in hyperalgesia, allo dynia, and sympathetic dysfunction reported in 2 patients each with CRPS I and II

(continued on next page)

Table 5
(continued)

Pain Syndrome	Epidemiology	Clinical Presentation	Treatments	Outcomes	References
DPNP	Prevalence among adults with diabetes in the US population: 27%–50%. Among these, 11% are affected with neuropathic pain	DPNP presents with burning-type pain, paresthesia, and numbness of mild to moderate severity. These symptoms may be accompanied by loss of proprioception, temperature sensitivity, and eventually pain sensation	Surgical decompression Electrical Spinal Cord Stimulation	Modest improvement in 67%–79% of patients in one small prospective study and nonblinded case series Case series and prospective studies have shown sustained pain relief and a good safety profile	156–162
Posttraumatic pain	• Posttraumatic neuropathic pain (from accidental or surgical injury) is one of the most common causes of chronic pain • 5%–50% estimated incidence of chronic postoperative pain • 79%–83% of patients with post-traumatic/postsurgical pain classify the pain as moderate to severe pain • Cervical root avulsion: 27%–40% of patients experience long term significant or intolerable pain levels	• Symptoms such as hypesthesia, paresthesia, allodynia, hyperpathia, and hyperalgesia may be seen within days of nerve damage or months later • Two main subgroups of patients have been identified: one with a minor sensory deficit plus hyperalgesia/mechanical allodynia and the other with hypoesthesia and a pronounced deficit in thermal and pain sensitivity	Nerve resection Relocation of end neuromas Neurovascular island flaps Neurolysis (external epineurectomy and interfascicular dissection) Neurotenolysis followed by wrapping in autogenous tissue DREZ lesioning DREZ combined with selective rhizotomy	Resection of part of an injured peripheral nerve yielded fair to excellent results Degree of pain relief varies from excellent to ineffective. After resection, nerves may be relocated into muscle, bone, or vein Good pain control and recovery of hand function after surgery for painful neuromas at the digit tip Pain declined by 78% in 28 patients with brachial plexus traction injuries. Repair of the brachial plexus lesions included neurolysis, repair with autologous grafts, extraplexual and/or intraplexual nerve transfers, and partial section of the traumatized root Unpredictable effectiveness with low success rates i. Fascial flap wrapping: failure rate of 10% or more ii. Vein wrapping: only short-term pain relief. Failure to achieve long-term pain relief Degree of pain reduction varies from 75% to 62%, depending on the length of the follow-up period and the rating scale used 87% improvement in patients monitored for an average of 47.5 mo	21,22,103, 145,163–187

Peripheral nerve stimulation	Complete to poor pain relief with PNS reported. One series reports considerable relief of pain in 79% and complete pain relief in 57% of patients followed up to 29 mo. PNS can decrease analgesic use, facilitate return to work, and improve quality of life
Percutaneous Implantation of PNS	>50% pain relief, decreased dependence on analgesics and improved functionality observed in most of the cases reported. One study reports >80% relief in 43% of permanent systems
Subcutaneous peripheral nerve stimulation	>50% reduction in VAS reportedly sustained at 12 mo. 50%–100% pain relief reported to last for 2.5–6 mo
Deep brain stimulation	55%–70% long-term success for peripheral nerve injury 50%–66.7% long-term success for cervical root/brachial plexus damage/avulsion
Motor cortex stimulation	50–80% pain relief reported up to 31 mo Reported to restore tactile and thermal sensory loss
Spinal cord stimulation	85% good and excellent results reported at 2 y or more. Reports of 50% analgesia up to 20 mo in other studies
Epidural steroid injections	A study reports reduction in VAS 1 mo after treatments, from pretreatment values of 78.7 to 15.2, which were further reduced to 11.6 after 1 y when 59% of patients were completely pain free
Brachial plexus grafting	A study reports pain reduction of i. 56% on the first day after surgery ii. 80% 3 wk after surgery iii. 90% 12 mo after surgery iv. 95% 24 mo after surgery 80% of patients reported either no or minimal pain, at the final evaluation
Botulinum toxin	Probably effective

(continued on next page)

Table 5
(continued)

Pain Syndrome	Epidemiology	Clinical Presentation	Treatments	Outcomes	References
Phantom Limb Pain	Prevalence of phantom pain among amputated patients: 50%–90%	The pain presents as short-lasting and rarely occurring painful shocks or as constant, excruciatingly painful experience in the missing body part	Surgical treatments: sympathectomy, DREZ lesions, cordotomy, and rhizotomy, neurostimulation methods	Short-term uncontrolled studies using these surgical approaches report a maximum benefit of about 32%	188–195
Brachial Plexus Avulsion Pain	Most occur as a consequence in approximately 5% motorcycle accidents. Prevalence of neuropathic pain ranges from 34%–95% of cases. 20%–30% of patients experience intractable long-term pain of the upper limb	The typical root avulsion pain is a constant dull, crushing, or burning pain with superimposed lightening jolts of severe sharp pain shooting down the arm	DREZ lesion Rhizotomy, cordotomy, segmental cordectomy, mescencephalotomy, medullary tractotomy, cingulotomy and sympathectomy	Long-term significant pain relief has been reported in 50%–70% of patients in case series Have shown no benefit for chronic neuropathic pain after avulsion	164,165,196–200

Abbreviations: CRPS, complex regional pain syndrome; DPNP, diabetic peripheral neuropathic pain; DREZ, dorsal root entry zone; PNS, peripheral nerve stimulator; VAS, visual analogue scale.

reports to prospective studies lacking randomization or control cohorts.

PAIN SYNDROMES OF THE SPINE AND SPINAL CORD

Mechanical low back pain was found to be the fourth most expensive condition for employers in the United States.[18,19] A high rate of spinal surgery also sets the stage for an increased incidence of failed back surgery syndrome (FBSS).[20] Neurosurgical interventions have been developed for various pain syndromes of the spine and spinal cord as listed in **Table 4**.

Good epidemiologic data and reliable diagnostic criteria have been generated for pain syndromes involving the spine and/or spinal cord. Many randomized controlled trials (RCTs) have been conducted for low back pain, with pain relief reported in many. Correct diagnosis is essential for the management of FBSS. Most treatment modalities for FBSS demonstrate decreasing pain relief over time, except neuromodulatory techniques, which demonstrate better long-term pain control. More studies are needed on invasive and noninvasive motor cortex stimulation for pain after spinal cord injury. A low number of RCTs with a predominance of case reports and series, inconsistent style of reporting results, and variable periods of follow-up are the main drawbacks identified.

PAIN SYNDROMES INVOLVING PERIPHERAL NERVES

Peripheral pain syndromes continue to present a significant challenge to physicians. These syndromes are known to adversely affect quality of life and lead to an increased use of health resources.[21] A study of patients in the United States with postpostsur/postsurgical neuropathic pain calculated the total mean annualized adjusted direct and indirect costs per subject as $11,846 and $29,617, respectively.[22] This section provides epidemiologic and outcomes data for neurosurgical interventions available for the management of peripheral pain syndromes (**Table 5**).

There are not any reports of a particular treatment modality consistently achieving a complete decrease in pain, improvement in function, and other outcome measures. The vast number of treatment modalities, few RCTs comparing them, and an inconsistent style of reporting data make it difficult to compare the effectiveness of the different modalities. However, the results of the various studies provide reasonable confidence for their consideration in the treatment of pain syndromes involving the peripheral nerves.

DISCUSSION AND SUMMARY

This review provides an overview of the epidemiology, clinical presentation, and treatment outcomes for craniofacial, spinal, and peripheral neurologic pain syndromes. Although the diagnosis and treatment of the chronic forms of these neurologic pain syndromes represent a clinical challenge, there is an urgent need for standardized classification systems, better epidemiologic data, and reliable treatment outcomes data.

Historically, classification systems have relied on the characteristics or localization of pain and other clinical criteria, making them somewhat subjective. Thus, development of new assessment tools is a critical step toward making the evaluation of these patients more objective and consistent. The availability of better epidemiologic data will result from improved classification systems worldwide. Creating databases specifically designed to hold the information on treatment outcomes would enable clinicians to better assess the application of specific therapies for each condition. All these will allow clinicians and researchers to have a better understanding of the real efficacy and effectiveness of the currently available pain surgery treatments, thus providing a basis for the development of the next generation of therapies.

REFERENCES

1. Weiss K, Boulis N. Herpes simplex virus-based gene therapies for chronic pain. J Pain Palliat Care Pharmacother 2012;26:291–3.
2. Gaskin DJ, Richard P. The economic costs of pain in the United States. J Pain 2012;13(8):715–24.
3. van Hecke O, Austin SK, Khan RA, et al. Neuropathic pain in the general population: a systematic review of epidemiological studies. Pain 2014; 155(4):654–62.
4. Mao J. Translational pain research: achievements and challenges. J Pain 2009;10(10):1001–11.
5. Costigan M, Scholz J, Woolf CJ. Neuropathic pain: a maladaptive response of the nervous system to damage. Annu Rev Neurosci 2009;32:1–32.
6. Scholz J, Woolf CJ. Can we conquer pain? Nat Neurosci 2002;5:1062–7.
7. Woolf CJ, Mannion RJ. Neuropathic pain: aetiology, symptoms, mechanisms, and management. Lancet 1999;353(9168):1959–64.
8. Backonja MM, Galer BS. Pain assessment and evaluation of patients who have neuropathic pain. Neurol Clin 1998;16(4):775–90.
9. Finnerup NB, Otto M, McQuay HJ, et al. Algorithm for neuropathic pain treatment: an evidence based proposal. Pain 2005;118(3):289–305.

10. Akram H, Mirza B, Kitchen N, et al. Proposal for evaluating the quality of reports of surgical interventions in the treatment of trigeminal neuralgia: the Surgical Trigeminal Neuralgia Score. Neurosurg Focus 2013;35(3):E3.

11. Bennett M. The LANSS Pain Scale: the Leeds assessment of neuropathic symptoms and signs. Pain 2001;92(1–2):147–57.

12. Baron R, Wasner G, Binder A. Chronic pain: genes, plasticity, and phenotypes. Lancet Neurol 2012; 11(1):19–21.

13. Nickel FT, Seifert F, Lanz S, et al. Mechanisms of neuropathic pain. Eur Neuropsychopharmacol 2012;22(2):81–91.

14. Renton T, Durham J, Aggarwal VR. The classification and differential diagnosis of orofacial pain. Expert Rev Neurother 2012;12(5):569–76.

15. Basser DS. Chronic pain: a neuroscientific understanding. Med Hypotheses 2012;78(1):79–85.

16. Katusic S, Williams DB, Beard CM, et al. Epidemiology and clinical features of idiopathic trigeminal neuralgia and glossopharyngeal neuralgia: similarities and differences, Rochester, Minnesota, 1945-1984. Neuroepidemiology 1991; 10(5–6):276–81.

17. Burchiel KJ. A new classification for facial pain. Neurosurgery 2003;53(5):1164–6 [discussion: 1166–7].

18. Slipman CW, Shin CH, Patel RK, et al. Etiologies of failed back surgery syndrome. Pain Med 2002;3(3): 200–14.

19. Taylor VM, Deyo RA, Cherkin DC, et al. Low back pain hospitalization. Recent United States trends and regional variations. Spine 1994;19(11):1207–12 [discussion: 1213].

20. Goetzel RZ, Hawkins K, Ozminkowski RJ, et al. The health and productivity cost burden of the "top 10" physical and mental health conditions affecting six large U.S. employers in 1999. J Occup Environ Med 2003;45(1):5–14.

21. Freynhagen R, Bennett MI. Diagnosis and management of neuropathic pain. BMJ 2009;339:b3002.

22. Parsons B, Schaefer C, Mann R, et al. Economic and humanistic burden of post-trauma and post-surgical neuropathic pain among adults in the United States. J Pain Res 2013;6:459–69.

23. Fischera M, Marziniak M, Gralow I, et al. The incidence and prevalence of cluster headache: a meta-analysis of population-based studies. Cephalalgia 2008;28(6):614–8.

24. Manzoni GC, Maffezzoni M, Lambru G, et al. Late-onset cluster headache: some considerations about 73 cases. Neurol Sci 2012;33(Suppl 1):S157–9.

25. Headache Classification Subcommittee of the International Headache Society. The International Classification of Headache Disorders: 2nd edition. Cephalalgia 2004;24(Suppl 1):9–160.

26. Magis D, Schoenen J. Advances and challenges in neurostimulation for headaches. Lancet Neurol 2012;11(8):708–19.

27. Schoenen J, Jensen RH, Lantéri-Minet M, et al. Stimulation of the sphenopalatine ganglion (SPG) for cluster headache treatment. Pathway CH-1: a randomized, sham-controlled study. Cephalalgia 2013;33(10):816–30.

28. Narouze S, Kapural L, Casanova J, et al. Sphenopalatine ganglion radiofrequency ablation for the management of chronic cluster headache. Headache 2009;49(4):571–7.

29. Sanders M, Zuurmond WW. Efficacy of sphenopalatine ganglion blockade in 66 patients suffering from cluster headache: a 12- to 70-month follow-up evaluation. J Neurosurg 1997;87(6): 876–80.

30. Kano H, Kondziolka D, Niranjan A, et al. γ knife stereotactic radiosurgery in the management of cluster headache. Curr Pain Headache Rep 2011; 15(2):118–23.

31. Pedersen JL, Barloese M, Jensen RH. Neurostimulation in cluster headache: a review of current progress. Cephalalgia 2013;33(14):1179–93.

32. Rowed DW. Chronic cluster headache managed by nervus intermedius section. Headache 1990; 30(7):401–6.

33. Morgenlander JC, Wilkins RH. Surgical treatment of cluster headache. J Neurosurg 1990;72(6):866–71.

34. Bigal ME, Lipton RB. The epidemiology, burden, and comorbidities of migraine. Neurol Clin 2009; 27(2):321–34.

35. Guyuron B, Kriegler JS, Davis J, et al. Five-year outcome of surgical treatment of migraine headaches. Plast Reconstr Surg 2011;127(2):603–8.

36. Jackson JL, Kuriyama A, Hayashino Y. Botulinum toxin A for prophylactic treatment of migraine and tension headaches in adults: a meta-analysis. JAMA 2012;307(16):1736–45.

37. Lambru G, Matharu MS. Occipital nerve stimulation in primary headache syndromes. Ther Adv Neurol Disord 2012;5(1):57–67.

38. Manack AN, Buse DC, Lipton RB. Chronic migraine: epidemiology and disease burden. Curr Pain Headache Rep 2011;15(1):70–8.

39. Mathew PG. A critical evaluation of migraine trigger site deactivation surgery. Headache 2014;54(1): 142–52.

40. Palmisani S, Al-Kaisy A, Arcioni R, et al. A six year retrospective review of occipital nerve stimulation practice–controversies and challenges of an emerging technique for treating refractory headache syndromes. J Headache Pain 2013;14(1):67.

41. Schurks M, Rist PM, Bigal ME, et al. Migraine and cardiovascular disease: systematic review and meta-analysis. BMJ 2009;339:b3914.

42. Skaer TL. Clinical presentation and treatment of migraine. Clin Ther 1996;18(2):229–45 [discussion: 228].

43. Vargas BB, Dodick DW. The face of chronic migraine: epidemiology, demographics, and treatment strategies. Neurol Clin 2009;27(2):467–79.

44. Hammond SR, Danta G. Occipital neuralgia. Clin Exp Neurol 1978;15:258–70.

45. Linde M, Hagen K, Stovner LJ. Botulinum toxin treatment of secondary headaches and cranial neuralgias: a review of evidence. Acta Neurol Scand Suppl 2011;(191):50–5.

46. Oh S, Tok S, Allemann J, et al. Exeresis in occipital neuralgia. Neurochirurgia (Stuttg) 1983;26(2):47–50 [in German].

47. Cox CL Jr, Cocks GR. Occipital neuralgia. J Med Assoc State Ala 1979;48(7):23–7, 32.

48. Lozano AM, Vanderlinden G, Bachoo R, et al. Microsurgical C-2 ganglionectomy for chronic intractable occipital pain. J Neurosurg 1998;89(3):359–65.

49. Acar F, Miller J, Golshani KJ, et al. Pain relief after cervical ganglionectomy (C2 and C3) for the treatment of medically intractable occipital neuralgia. Stereotact Funct Neurosurg 2008;86(2):106–12.

50. Li F, Ma Y, Zou J, et al. Micro-surgical decompression for greater occipital neuralgia. Turk Neurosurg 2012;22(4):427–9.

51. Reed KL. Peripheral neuromodulation and headaches: history, clinical approach, and considerations on underlying mechanisms. Curr Pain Headache Rep 2013;17(1):305.

52. Koch D, Wakhloo AK. CT-guided chemical rhizotomy of the C1 root for occipital neuralgia. Neuroradiology 1992;34(5):451–2.

53. Ehni G, Benner B. Occipital neuralgia and C1-C2 arthrosis. N Engl J Med 1984;310(2):127.

54. Dubuisson D. Treatment of occipital neuralgia by partial posterior rhizotomy at C1-3. J Neurosurg 1995;82(4):581–6.

55. Horowitz MB, Yonas H. Occipital neuralgia treated by intradural dorsal nerve root sectioning. Cephalalgia 1993;13(5):354–60 [discussion: 307].

56. Chambers WR. Posterior rhizotomy of the second and third cervical nerves for occipital pain. J Am Med Assoc 1954;155(5):431–2.

57. Blume HG. Radiofrequency denaturation in occipital pain: a new approach in 114 cases. In: Bonica JJ, Alse-Fessard D, editors. Advances in pain research and therapy, vol. 1. New York: Raven Press; 1976. p. 691–8.

58. Vanelderen P, Rouwette T, De Vooght P, et al. Pulsed radiofrequency for the treatment of occipital neuralgia: a prospective study with 6 months of follow-up. Reg Anesth Pain Med 2010;35(2):148–51.

59. Van Zundert J, Lamé IE, de Louw A, et al. Percutaneous pulsed radiofrequency treatment of the cervical dorsal root ganglion in the treatment of chronic cervical pain syndromes: a clinical audit. Neuromodulation 2003;6(1):6–14.

60. van Kleef M, van Genderen WE, Narouze S, et al. 1. Trigeminal neuralgia. Pain Pract 2009;9(4):252–9.

61. Zakrzewska JM, McMillan R. Trigeminal neuralgia: the diagnosis and management of this excruciating and poorly understood facial pain. Postgrad Med J 2011;87(1028):410–6.

62. Katusic S, Williams DB, Beard CM, et al. Incidence and clinical features of glossopharyngeal neuralgia, Rochester, Minnesota, 1945-1984. Neuroepidemiology 1991;10(5–6):266–75.

63. Rey-Dios R, Cohen-Gadol AA. Current neurosurgical management of glossopharyngeal neuralgia and technical nuances for microvascular decompression surgery. Neurosurg Focus 2013;34(3):E8.

64. Blumenfeld A, Nikolskaya G. Glossopharyngeal neuralgia. Curr Pain Headache Rep 2013;17(7):343.

65. O'Connor JK, Bidiwala S. Effectiveness and safety of Gamma Knife radiosurgery for glossopharyngeal neuralgia. Proc (Bayl Univ Med Cent) 2013;26(3):262–4.

66. Rainov NG, Fels C, Heidecke V, et al. Epidural electrical stimulation of the motor cortex in patients with facial neuralgia. Clin Neurol Neurosurg 1997;99(3):205–9.

67. Rainov NG, Heidecke V. Motor cortex stimulation for neuropathic facial pain. Neurol Res 2003;25(2):157–61.

68. Kanpolat Y, Kahilogullari G, Ugur HC, et al. Computed tomography-guided percutaneous trigeminal tractotomy-nucleotomy. Neurosurgery 2008;63(1 Suppl 1):ONS147–53 [discussion: ONS153–5].

69. Kunc Z. Treatment of essential neuralgia of the 9th nerve by selective tractotomy. J Neurosurg 1965;23(5):494–500.

70. Tew JM Jr. Percutaneous rhizotomy in the treatment of intractable facial pain (trigeminal, glossopharyngeal, and vagal nerves). In: Schmidek HH, Sweet WH, editors. Operative neurosurgical techniques: indications, methods, and results. New York: Grune & Stratton; 1988. p. 1083–106.

71. Giorgi C, Broggi G. Surgical treatment of glossopharyngeal neuralgia and pain from cancer of the nasopharynx. A 20-year experience. J Neurosurg 1984;61(5):952–5.

72. Tubbs RS, Steck DT, Mortazavi MM, et al. The nervus intermedius: a review of its anatomy, function, pathology, and role in neurosurgery. World Neurosurg 2013;79(5–6):763–7.

73. Pulec JL. Geniculate neuralgia: long-term results of surgical treatment. Ear Nose Throat J 2002;81(1): 30–3.

74. Agostoni E, Frigerio R, Santoro P. Atypical facial pain: clinical considerations and differential diagnosis. Neurol Sci 2005;26(Suppl 2):s71–4.

75. Bayer E, Racz GB, Miles D, et al. Sphenopalatine ganglion pulsed radiofrequency treatment in 30 patients suffering from chronic face and head pain. Pain Pract 2005;5(3):223–7.

76. Kanpolat Y, Savas A, Ugur HC, et al. The trigeminal tract and nucleus procedures in treatment of atypical facial pain. Surg Neurol 2005;64(Suppl 2):S96–100 [discussion: S100–1].

77. Koopman JS, Dieleman JP, Huygen FJ, et al. Incidence of facial pain in the general population. Pain 2009;147(1–3):122–7.

78. Nguyen CT, Wang MB. Complementary and integrative treatments: atypical facial pain. Otolaryngol Clin North Am 2013;46(3):367–82.

79. Bullard DE, Nashold BS Jr. The caudalis DREZ for facial pain. Stereotact Funct Neurosurg 1997; 68(1–4 Pt 1):168–74.

80. Eller JL, Raslan AM, Burchiel KJ. Trigeminal neuralgia: definition and classification. Neurosurg Focus 2005;18(5):E3.

81. Sandwell SE, El-Naggar AO. Nucleus caudalis dorsal root entry zone lesioning for the treatment of anesthesia dolorosa. J Neurosurg 2013;118(3): 534–8.

82. Tatli M, Keklikci U, Aluclu U, et al. Anesthesia dolorosa caused by penetrating cranial injury. Eur Neurol 2006;56(3):162–5.

83. Al-Jundi MA, John MT, Setz JM, et al. Meta-analysis of treatment need for temporomandibular disorders in adult nonpatients. J Orofac Pain 2008; 22(2):97–107.

84. von Lindern JJ, Niederhagen B, Bergé S, et al. Type A botulinum toxin in the treatment of chronic facial pain associated with masticatory hyperactivity. J Oral Maxillofac Surg 2003;61(7):774–8.

85. List T, Axelsson S. Management of TMD: evidence from systematic reviews and meta-analyses. J Oral Rehabil 2010;37(6):430–51.

86. Liu F, Steinkeler A. Epidemiology, diagnosis, and treatment of temporomandibular disorders. Dent Clin North Am 2013;57(3):465–79.

87. William PM. Paper presented at: vision 2010-the North American Neuromodulation Society. Las Vegas (NV), December 2–5, 2010.

88. Berg S, Tullberg T, Branth B, et al. Total disc replacement compared to lumbar fusion: a randomised controlled trial with 2-year follow-up. Eur Spine J 2009;18(10):1512–9.

89. Freburger JK, Holmes GM, Agans RP, et al. The rising prevalence of chronic low back pain. Arch Intern Med 2009;169(3):251–8.

90. Johannes CB, Le TK, Zhou X, et al. The prevalence of chronic pain in United States adults: results of an Internet-based survey. J Pain 2010;11(11):1230–9.

91. Koes BW, van Tulder MW, Thomas S. Diagnosis and treatment of low back pain. BMJ 2006; 332(7555):1430–4.

92. Manchikanti L, Boswell MV, Rivera JJ, et al. [ISRCTN 16558617] A randomized, controlled trial of spinal endoscopic adhesiolysis in chronic refractory low back and lower extremity pain. BMC Anesthesiol 2005;5:10.

93. North RB, Kidd DH, Farrokhi F, et al. Spinal cord stimulation versus repeated lumbosacral spine surgery for chronic pain: a randomized, controlled trial. Neurosurgery 2005;56(1):98–106 [discussion: 106–7].

94. Taylor RS, Van Buyten JP, Buchser E. Spinal cord stimulation for chronic back and leg pain and failed back surgery syndrome: a systematic review and analysis of prognostic factors. Spine 2005;30(1): 152–60.

95. Chan CW, Peng P. Failed back surgery syndrome. Pain Med 2011;12(4):577–606.

96. Nachemson AL. Evaluation of results in lumbar spine surgery. Acta Orthop Scand Suppl 1993;251:130–3.

97. Rahimzadeh P, Sharma V, Imani F, et al. Adjuvant hyaluronidase to epidural steroid improves the quality of analgesia in failed back surgery syndrome: a prospective randomized clinical trial. Pain Physician 2014;17(1):E75–82.

98. de Nêuton F, Magalhães O, Soares SC, et al. Effects of ozone applied by spinal endoscopy in patients with chronic pain related to failed back surgery syndrome: a pilot study. Neuropsychiatr Dis Treat 2013;9:1759–66.

99. Yakovlev AE, Resch BE, Yakovleva VE. Peripheral nerve field stimulation in the treatment of postlaminectomy syndrome after multilevel spinal surgeries. Neuromodulation 2011;14(6):534–8 [discussion: 538].

100. Chen Y, Bramley G, Unwin G, et al. Stimulation of peripheral nerves for the treatment of refractory pain (including peripheral nerve field). Systematic Reviews referred by the NICE Interventional Procedures Programme on behalf of the NICE Interventional Procedures Advisory Committee (IPAC). 2012.

101. Taylor RS, Desai MJ, Rigoard P, et al. Predictors of pain relief following spinal cord stimulation in chronic back and leg pain and failed back surgery syndrome: a systematic review and meta-regression analysis. Pain Pract 2013;13:2–17.

102. Bernstein CA, Paicius RM, Barkow SH, et al. Spinal cord stimulation in conjunction with peripheral nerve field stimulation for the treatment of low back and leg pain: a case series. Neuromodulation 2008;11(2):116–23.

103. Bittar RG, Kar-Purkayastha I, Owen SL, et al. Deep brain stimulation for pain relief: a meta-analysis. J Clin Neurosci 2005;12(5):515–9.

104. Friedman AH, Nashold BS Jr, Ovelmen-Levitt J. Dorsal root entry zone lesions for the treatment of post-herpetic neuralgia. J Neurosurg 1984;60(6): 1258–62.

105. Harke H, Gretenkort P, Ladleif HU, et al. Spinal cord stimulation in postherpetic neuralgia and in acute herpes zoster pain. Anesth Analg 2002; 94(3):694–700. Table of contents.

106. Kanpolat Y, Tuna H, Bozkurt M, et al. Spinal and nucleus caudalis dorsal root entry zone operations for chronic pain. Neurosurgery 2008;62(3 Suppl 1): 235–42 [discussion: 242–4].

107. Sadosky A, McDermott AM, Brandenburg NA, et al. A review of the epidemiology of painful diabetic peripheral neuropathy, postherpetic neuralgia, and less commonly studied neuropathic pain conditions. Pain Pract 2008;8(1):45–56.

108. Wu CL, Raja SN. An update on the treatment of postherpetic neuralgia. J Pain 2008;9(1 Suppl 1): S19–30.

109. Yakovlev AE, Peterson AT. Peripheral nerve stimulation in treatment of intractable postherpetic neuralgia. Neuromodulation 2007;10(4):373–5.

110. Kondziolka D, Lunsford LD, Flickinger JC, et al. Stereotactic radiosurgery for trigeminal neuralgia: a multiinstitutional study using the gamma unit. J Neurosurg 1996;84(6):940–5.

111. Urgosik D, Vymazal J, Vladyka V, et al. Treatment of postherpetic trigeminal neuralgia with the Leksell gamma knife. J Neurosurg 2011;115:113–6.

112. Perttunen K, Tasmuth T, Kalso E. Chronic pain after thoracic surgery: a follow-up study. Acta Anaesthesiol Scand 1999;43(5):563–7.

113. Gerner P. Postthoracotomy pain management problems. Anesthesiol Clin 2008;26(2):355–67, vii.

114. Koehler RP, Keenan RJ. Management of postthoracotomy pain: acute and chronic. Thorac Surg Clin 2006;16(3):287–97.

115. Wildgaard K, Ravn J, Kehlet H. Chronic postthoracotomy pain: a critical review of pathogenic mechanisms and strategies for prevention. Eur J Cardiothorac Surg 2009;36(1):170–80.

116. Maguire MF, Ravenscroft A, Beggs D, et al. A questionnaire study investigating the prevalence of the neuropathic component of chronic pain after thoracic surgery. Eur J Cardiothorac Surg 2006; 29(5):800–5.

117. Rogers ML, Duffy JP. Surgical aspects of chronic post-thoracotomy pain. Eur J Cardiothorac Surg 2000;18(6):711–6.

118. Goyal GN, Gupta D, Jain R, et al. Peripheral nerve field stimulation for intractable post-thoracotomy scar pain not relieved by conventional treatment. Pain Pract 2010;10(4):366–9.

119. Goroszeniuk T, Kothari S, Hamann W. Subcutaneous neuromodulating implant targeted at the site of pain. Reg Anesth Pain Med 2006;31(2):168–71.

120. Hegarty D, Goroszeniuk T. Peripheral nerve stimulation of the thoracic paravertebral plexus for chronic neuropathic pain. Pain Physician 2011; 14(3):295–300.

121. Doi K, Nikai T, Sakura S, et al. Intercostal nerve block with 5% tetracaine for chronic pain syndromes. J Clin Anesth 2002;14(1):39–41.

122. Green CR, de Rosayro AM, Tait AR. The role of cryoanalgesia for chronic thoracic pain: results of a long-term follow up. J Natl Med Assoc 2002; 94(8):716–20.

123. Moore W, Kolnick D, Tan J, et al. CT guided percutaneous cryoneurolysis for post thoracotomy pain syndrome: early experience and effectiveness. Acad Radiol 2010;17(5):603–6.

124. Esposito S, Delitala A, Nardi PV. Microsurgical DREZ-lesion in the treatment of deafferentation pain. J Neurosurg Sci 1988;32(3):113–5.

125. Cohen SP, Sireci A, Wu CL, et al. Pulsed radiofrequency of the dorsal root ganglia is superior to pharmacotherapy or pulsed radiofrequency of the intercostal nerves in the treatment of chronic postsurgical thoracic pain. Pain Physician 2006;9(3): 227–35.

126. Wininger KL, Bester ML, Deshpande KK. Spinal cord stimulation to treat postthoracotomy neuralgia: non-small-cell lung cancer: a case report. Pain Manag Nurs 2012;13(1):52–9.

127. Graybill J, Conermann T, Kabazie AJ, et al. Spinal cord stimulation for treatment of pain in a patient with post thoracotomy pain syndrome. Pain Physician 2011;14(5):441–5.

128. Falci S, Best L, Bayles R, et al. Dorsal root entry zone microcoagulation for spinal cord injury-related central pain: operative intramedullary electrophysiological guidance and clinical outcome. J Neurosurg 2002;97(Suppl 2):193–200.

129. Fregni F, Boggio PS, Lima MC, et al. A sham-controlled, phase II trial of transcranial direct current stimulation for the treatment of central pain in postsur spinal cord injury. Pain 2006;122(1–2): 197–209.

130. Siddall PJ. Management of neuropathic pain following spinal cord injury: now and in the future. Spinal Cord 2009;47(5):352–9.

131. Siddall PJ, Loeser JD. Pain following spinal cord injury. Spinal Cord 2001;39(2):63–73.

132. ten Vaarwerk IA, Staal MJ. Spinal cord stimulation in chronic pain syndromes. Spinal Cord 1998; 36(10):671–82.

133. Warms CA, Turner JA, Marshall HM, et al. Treatments for chronic pain associated with spinal cord injuries: many are tried, few are helpful. Clin J Pain 2002;18(3):154–63.

134. Sandroni P, Benrud-Larson LM, McClelland RL, et al. Complex regional pain syndrome type I: incidence and prevalence in Olmsted county, a population-based study. Pain 2003;103(1–2): 199–207.

135. Van Buyten JP, Smet I, Liem L, et al. Stimulation of dorsal root ganglia for the management of complex regional pain syndrome: a prospective case series. Pain Pract 2014;14:1–9.

136. Bean DJ, Johnson MH, Kydd RR. The outcome of complex regional pain syndrome type 1: a systematic review. J Pain 2014;15(7):677–90.

137. Perez RS, Zollinger PE, Dijkstra PU, et al. Evidence based guidelines for complex regional pain syndrome type 1. BMC Neurol 2010;10:20.

138. Stanton-Hicks MD, Burton AW, Bruehl SP, et al. An updated interdisciplinary clinical pathway for CRPS: report of an expert panel. Pain Pract 2002;2(1):1–16.

139. O'Connell NE, Wand BM, McAuley J, et al. Interventions for treating pain and disability in adults with complex regional pain syndrome. Cochrane Database Syst Rev 2013;(4):CD009416.

140. Tran DQ, Duong S, Bertini P, et al. Treatment of complex regional pain syndrome: a review of the evidence. Can J Anaesth 2010;57(2):149–66.

141. Jadad AR, Carroll D, Glynn CJ, et al. Intravenous regional sympathetic blockade for pain relief in reflex sympathetic dystrophy: a systematic review and a randomized, double-blind crossover study. J Pain Symptom Manage 1995;10(1):13–20.

142. Carroll I, Clark JD, Mackey S. Sympathetic block with botulinum toxin to treat complex regional pain syndrome. Ann Neurol 2009;65(3):348–51.

143. Birch R. Causalgia: a restatement. Neurosurgery 2009;65(Suppl 4):A222–8.

144. van Hilten BJ, van de Beek WJ, Hoff JI, et al. Intrathecal baclofen for the treatment of dystonia in patients with reflex sympathetic dystrophy. N Engl J Med 2000;343(9):625–30.

145. Cruccu G, Aziz TZ, Garcia-Larrea L, et al. EFNS guidelines on neurostimulation therapy for neuropathic pain. Eur J Neurol 2007;14(9):952–70.

146. de Leon-Casasola OA. Spinal cord and peripheral nerve stimulation techniques for neuropathic pain. J Pain Symptom Manage 2009;38(Suppl 2): S28–38.

147. Stojanovic MP. Stimulation methods for neuropathic pain control. Curr Pain Headache Rep 2001;5(2): 130–7.

148. Dielissen PW, Claassen AT, Veldman PH, et al. Amputation for reflex sympathetic dystrophy. J Bone Joint Surg Br 1995;77(2):270–3.

149. Picarelli H, Teixeira MJ, de Andrade DC, et al. Repetitive transcranial magnetic stimulation is efficacious as an add-on to pharmacological therapy in complex regional pain syndrome (CRPS) type I. J Pain 2010;11(11):1203–10.

150. Hassenbusch SJ, Stanton-Hicks M, Schoppa D, et al. Long-term results of peripheral nerve stimulation for reflex sympathetic dystrophy. J Neurosurg 1996;84(3):415–23.

151. Eric GC, Lynsday B, Alanna R, et al. Ultrasound-guided infraclavicular peripheral nerve stimulation for the treatment of complex regional pain syndrome (CRPS) type II of the upper extremity. Paper presented at: Neuromodulation: Vision 2010. Las Vegas (NV), December 2-5, 2010.

152. Rezai AR, Rozano AM. Deep brain stimulation (DBS) for pain. In: Burchiel KJ, editor. Surgical management of pain. New York: Thieme Medical Publishers; 2002. p. 565–76.

153. Javed S, Sharples PM, Khan S, et al. Recovery from fixed dystonia in complex regional pain syndrome type 1 (CRPS-1) following deep brain stimulation (DBS) surgery. Arch Dis Child 2011; 96(Suppl 1):A81.

154. Levy RM. Evidence-based review of neuromodulation for complex regional pain syndrome: a conflict between faith and science? Neuromodulation 2012;15(6):501–6.

155. McRoberts WP, Cairns KD. Combined Spinal Cord and Peripheral Nerve Field Stimulation for the Control of Chronic Regional Pain Syndrome (CRPS) [Poster]. Presented at Neuromodulation Annual Meeting: Vision 2010. Las Vegas (NV), December 2-5, 2010.

156. Argoff CE, Cole BE, Fishbain DA, et al. Diabetic peripheral neuropathic pain: clinical and quality-of-life issues. Mayo Clin Proc 2006;81(Suppl 4): S3–11.

157. Barrett AM, Lucero MA, Le T, et al. Epidemiology, public health burden, and treatment of diabetic peripheral neuropathic pain: a review. Pain Med 2007;8(Suppl 2):S50–62.

158. Chiles NS, Phillips CL, Volpato S, et al. Diabetes, peripheral neuropathy, and lower-extremity function. J Diabetes Complications 2014;28(1):91–5.

159. Daousi C, Benbow SJ, MacFarlane IA. Electrical spinal cord stimulation in the long-term treatment of chronic painful diabetic neuropathy. Diabet Med 2005;22(4):393–8.

160. de Vos CC, Rajan V, Steenbergen W, et al. Effect and safety of spinal cord stimulation for treatment of chronic pain caused by diabetic neuropathy. J Diabetes Complications 2009;23(1):40–5.

161. Tesfaye S, Selvarajah D. Advances in the epidemiology, pathogenesis and management of diabetic peripheral neuropathy. Diabetes Metab Res Rev 2012;28(Suppl 1):8–14.

162. Therapeutics and Technology Assessment Subcommittee of the American Academy of Neurology, Chaudhry V, Stevens JC, et al. Practice Advisory: utility of surgical decompression for treatment of diabetic neuropathy: report of the Therapeutics

and Technology Assessment Subcommittee of the American Academy of Neurology. Neurology 2006;66(12):1805–8.

163. Akkaya T, Ozkan D. Chronic post-surgical pain. Agri 2009;21(1):1–9.

164. Ciaramitaro P, Mondelli M, Logullo F, et al. Traumatic peripheral nerve injuries: epidemiological findings, neuropathic pain and quality of life in 158 patients. J Peripher Nerv Syst 2010;15(2):120–7.

165. Samii M, Bear-Henney S, Ludemann W, et al. Treatment of refractory pain after brachial plexus avulsion with dorsal root entry zone lesions. Neurosurgery 2001;48(6):1269–75 [discussion: 1275–7].

166. Finnerup NB, Sindrup SH, Jensen TS. Chronic neuropathic pain: mechanisms, drug targets and measurement. Fundam Clin Pharmacol 2007; 21(2):129–36.

167. Schüning J, Scherens A, Haussleiter IS, et al. Sensory changes and loss of intraepidermal nerve fibers in painful unilateral nerve injury. Clin J Pain 2009;25(8):683–90.

168. Yamashita T, Ishii S, Usui M. Pain relief after nerve resection for post-postsur neuralgia. J Bone Joint Surg Br 1998;80(3):499–503.

169. Watson J, Gonzalez M, Romero A, et al. Neuromas of the hand and upper extremity. J Hand Surg Am 2010;35(3):499–510.

170. Kakinoki R, Ikeguchi R, Atiyya AN, et al. Treatment of postpostsur painful neuromas at the digit tip using neurovascular island flaps. J Hand Surg Am 2008;33(3):348–52.

171. Bonilla G, Di Masi G, Battaglia D, et al. Pain and brachial plexus lesions: evaluation of initial outcomes after reconstructive microsurgery and validation of a new pain severity scale. Acta Neurochir (Wien) 2011;153(1):171–6.

172. Elliot D, Sierakowski A. The surgical management of painful nerves of the upper limb: a unit perspective. J Hand Surg Eur Vol 2011;36(9):760–70.

173. Dreval ON, Ogleznev K, Kandel EI. Destruction of the entry zone of the posterior roots combined with selective rhizotomy in pain syndromes due to a lesion of the brachial plexus. Zh Vopr Neirokhir Im N N Burdenko 1990;(1):19–22 [in Russian].

174. Waisbrod H, Panhans C, Hansen D, et al. Direct nerve stimulation for painful peripheral neuropathies. J Bone Joint Surg Br 1985;67(3):470–2.

175. Novak CB, Mackinnon SE. Outcome following implantation of a peripheral nerve stimulator in patients with chronic nerve pain. Plast Reconstr Surg 2000;105(6):1967–72.

176. Huntoon MA, Burgher AH. Ultrasound-guided permanent implantation of peripheral nerve stimulation (PNS) system for neuropathic pain of the extremities: original cases and outcomes. Pain Med 2009;10(8):1369–77.

177. Kent M, Upp J, Spevak C, et al. Ultrasound-guided peripheral nerve stimulator placement in two soldiers with acute battlefield neuropathic pain. Anesth Analg 2012;114(4):875–8.

178. McRoberts WP, Roche M. Novel approach for peripheral subcutaneous field stimulation for the treatment of severe, chronic knee joint pain after total knee arthroplasty. Neuromodulation 2010; 13(2):131–6.

179. Yakovlev AE, Resch BE. Treatment of chronic intractable hip pain after iliac crest bone graft harvest using peripheral nerve field stimulation. Neuromodulation 2011;14(2):156–9 [discussion: 159].

180. Fontaine D, Bruneto JL, El Fakir H, et al. Short-term restoration of facial sensory loss by motor cortex stimulation in peripheral post- neuropathic pain. J Headache Pain 2009;10(3):203–6.

181. Carroll D, Joint C, Maartens N, et al. Motor cortex stimulation for chronic neuropathic pain: a preliminary study of 10 cases. Pain 2000;84(2–3): 431–7.

182. Nguyen JP, Keravel Y, Feve A, et al. Treatment of deafferentation pain by chronic stimulation of the motor cortex: report of a series of 20 cases. Acta Neurochir Suppl 1997;68:54–60.

183. Lefaucheur JP, Drouot X, Cunin P, et al. Motor cortex stimulation for the treatment of refractory peripheral neuropathic pain. Brain 2009;132(Pt 6): 1463–71.

184. Meglio M, Cioni B, Rossi GF. Spinal cord stimulation in management of chronic pain. A 9-year experience. J Neurosurg 1989;70(4): 519–24.

185. Forrest JB. The response to epidural steroid injections in chronic dorsal root pain. Can Anaesth Soc J 1980;27(1):40–6.

186. Bertelli JA, Ghizoni MF. Pain after avulsion injuries and complete palsy of the brachial plexus: the possible role of nonavulsed roots in pain generation. Neurosurgery 2008;62(5):1104–13 [discussion: 1113–4].

187. Jabbari B, Machado D. Treatment of refractory pain with botulinum toxins–an evidence-based review. Pain Med 2011;12(11):1594–606.

188. Bittar RG, Otero S, Carter H, et al. Deep brain stimulation for phantom limb pain. J Clin Neurosci 2005;12(4):399–404.

189. Chan BL, Witt R, Charrow AP, et al. Mirror therapy for phantom limb pain. N Engl J Med 2007; 357(21):2206–7.

190. Ephraim PL, Wegener ST, MacKenzie EJ, et al. Phantom pain, residual limb pain, and back pain in amputees: results of a national survey. Arch Phys Med Rehabil 2005;86(10):1910–9.

191. Flor H. Phantom-limb pain: characteristics, causes, and treatment. Lancet Neurol 2002;1(3):182–9.

192. Flor H, Nikolajsen L, Staehelin Jensen T. Phantom limb pain: a case of maladaptive CNS plasticity? Nat Rev Neurosci 2006;7(11):873–81.

193. Kooijman CM, Dijkstra PU, Geertzen JH, et al. Phantom pain and phantom sensations in upper limb amputees: an epidemiological study. Pain 2000;87(1):33–41.

194. Subedi B, Grossberg GT. Phantom limb pain: mechanisms and treatment approaches. Pain Res Treat 2011;2011:864605.

195. Weeks SR, Anderson-Barnes VC, Tsao JW. Phantom limb pain: theories and therapies. Neurologist 2010;16(5):277–86.

196. Ahmed-Labib M, Golan JD, Jacques L. Functional outcome of brachial plexus reconstruction after trauma. Neurosurgery 2007;61(5):1016–22 [discussion: 1022–3].

197. Carlstedt T. Root repair review: basic science background and clinical outcome. Restor Neurol Neurosci 2008;26(2–3):225–41.

198. Carlstedt T. Nerve root replantation. Neurosurg Clin N Am 2009;20(1):39–50, vi.

199. Chen HJ, Tu YK. Long term follow-up results of dorsal root entry zone lesions for intractable pain after brachial plexus avulsion injuries. Acta Neurochir Suppl 2006;99:73–5.

200. Sindou MP, Blondet E, Emery E, et al. Microsurgical lesioning in the dorsal root entry zone for pain due to brachial plexus avulsion: a prospective series of 55 patients. J Neurosurg 2005;102(6):1018–28.

Intracranial Ablative Procedures for the Treatment of Chronic Pain

Jayant P. Menon, MD, MEng

KEYWORDS

- Thalamotomy • Mesencephalic tractotomy • Anterior cingulotomy

KEY POINTS

- Stereotactic ablative procedures have been in use for several years. Technique, efficacy, and side effects for each of these procedures have not changed significantly in the past several years. Central ablation can be considered for some patients with intractable pain, although these procedures are irreversible, unlike neuromodulatory procedures, which are generally both reversible and adjustable.
- Lesions of the centromedian and centrolateral nuclei of the thalamus are still used for the treatment of pain.
- Mesencephalic tractotomy of extralemniscal pathways lateral to the spinothalamic tract (STT) and medial leminiscus can result in relief of intractable pain without loss of sensation or dysesthesia.
- Cingulotomy can result in long-term pain relief, although it can be associated with impairments of attention and risk to other cognitive domains.

INTRODUCTION: NATURE OF THE PROBLEM

Pain is a multimodal subjective experience. The experience of pain is described as distributed in 3 dimensions: cognitive, affective, and sensory.[1] Frontal and limbic areas are believed to subserve the cognitive-evaluative component of pain. Limbic cortex, cingulum, hypothalamus, thalamus, and various midbrain regions are thought to contribute to the motivational-affective component of pain. Primary somatosensory cortex, thalamus, STT, and local nerve endings are involved in the sensory component of pain. When peripheral treatments fail, and modulatory procedures are not possible, central ablative procedures can be used for the treatment of pain,[2] even though the use of these procedures has declined in recent years with the advent of neuromodulatory techniques.

DIAGNOSIS

The characterization and diagnosis of pain is one of the most common tasks in medicine. The experience of pain has somatosensory, affective, and cognitive components.[3] From early attempts, including the McGill inventory,[4] to current taxonomies,[5] the accurate diagnosis and classification of chronic pain remains a challenging problem. The 3-component model of pain (sensory, affective, and cognitive), however, still forms the basis of most pain treatment regimens and is a good framework to study the role of central ablative surgical procedures for pain.

CLINICAL OUTCOMES AND TRENDS IN THE LITERATURE

An excellent review of destructive procedures for nonmalignant pain was conducted recently[6] and includes several of the most recent articles regarding ablative procedures for pain. Of the 146 articles, 131 constituted class III evidence. Most of the class I and class II evidence studies were for radiofrequency rhizotomy and did not include central procedures for pain. This

Disclosures: None.
Stanford Neurosurgery, 300 Pasteur Drive, Boswell Building, A301, Stanford, CA 94305-5327
E-mail address: jmenon16@stanford.edu

Neurosurg Clin N Am 25 (2014) 663–670
http://dx.doi.org/10.1016/j.nec.2014.06.003
1042-3680/14/$ – see front matter © 2014 Elsevier Inc. All rights reserved.

demonstrates a need for prospective trials to better describe the efficacy of these procedures and to compare them with more recent modulatory approaches (**Fig. 1**).

Thalamotomy

Thalamotomy has enjoyed the most attention recently, largely due to significant contributions by many investigators to identify the pathophysiological biomarkers of the manifestation of chronic pain in the thalamus and of their modulation by various ablative treatments. Patients with greater than 1 year of medically refractory neuropathic pain are reported the best candidates for contralateral thalamotomy.

The STT and spinoreticulothalamic tract terminate in the medial and lateral thalamus (ventral posterolateral nucleus [VPL]/ventral posteromedial nucleus [VPM]),[7] before projecting to the lateral prefrontal cortex. Destruction of the VPL/VPM interrupts these specific pain pathways, which project somatotopically to primary sensory cortex and are thought to subserve the discriminatory aspect of pain.

The medial, nonspecific thalamic nuclei include the centralis lateralis (CL) and centromedian (CM)/parafascicular (PF). The efferents from these thalamic nuclei to associative and paralimbic areas provides an additional target to modulate the affective component of pain. The lateral nuclei include the ventrocaudal nucleus, the medial posterior nucleus, and the posterior centrolateral nucleus (CLp). Bilateral receptive fields from spinal Rexed laminae V–VII travel via the STT to the CLp.[8] CLp has diffuse efferent projections to the primary somatosensory cortex, insula, and anterior cingulate cortex as well shorter projections to the thalamic reticular nucleus.[8,9]

Theories of imbalance between the medial (nonspecific) and lateral (specific) groups form the basis for some thalamic procedures for pain. In one theory, the medial thalamus overinhibits the lateral thalamus.[10] A second theory states that uninhibited output of heat and burning signals from the medial thalamus result from the loss of cold inputs from the lateral thalamus.[11] Finally, diffuse low-threshold calcium bursts from around the CLp implicate the reticular thalamic nuclei as well.[12] Taken together, it is possible to postulate that the STT has excitatory inputs to the medial and lateral thalamus. The thalamic reticular nucleus has inhibitory inputs to the medial and lateral thalamus. These are in turn driven by excitatory outputs from the medial and lateral thalamus in a feedback loop. In the central pain condition, often characterized by anesthesia dolorosa, it is proposed that the lateral thalamus no longer receives STT excitatory input and is further inhibited by the reticular nucleus, resulting in loss of information to the thalamus and loss of modulation of thalamocortical networks by ascending pathways.[10–12] Support for these theories can be found in electrophysiological and imaging studies. Intraoperative recordings in patients with central pain demonstrate decreased spontaneous activity in the lateral versus medial thalamus.[13] Imaging studies of patients with neuropathic pain show decreased regional blood flow in the posterior-dorsal part of the thalamus corresponding to the dorsal CL posterior nucleus.

Centromedial Lesions

Medial thalamic lesions[14,15] have focused on the destruction of the CM/PF. The target is located approximately 8 to 10 mm lateral from midline, approximately 4 mm superior to the anterior commissure (AC)–posterior commissure (PC)

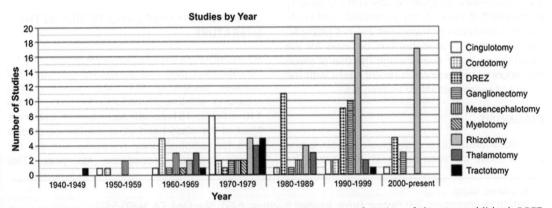

Fig. 1. Histogram showing the number of publications by category as a function of the year published. DREZ, Dorsal Root Entry Zone. (*From* Cetas JS, Saedi T, Burchiel KJ. Destructive procedures for the treatment of nonmalignant pain: a structured literature review. J Neurosurg 2008;109(3):389–404.)

plane, and approximately 5 mm anterior to the PC but exact stereotactic location can vary depending on patient anatomy and prior lesions, as for other thalamic targets. Intraoperative localization of the CM/PF can be aided by microelectrode recordings, which may identify characteristic bursting patterns elicited by intraoperative sensory evoked potentials. Intraoperative test macrostimulation of these nuclei may evoke a contralateral light tingling or painful burning sensation.[16]

In addition, 2 populations of nociceptive neurons with wide bilateral fields exist in the CM/PF.[15] One group is represented diffusely in the nucleus and is characterized by neurons that respond to noxious stimulus after a long latency and continue to respond after the stimulation ends. The other group is restricted to the medial basal CM/PF and is characterized by short latency response as well as short latency cessation after stimulus termination. Furthermore, Jeanmonod and colleagues[10] reported on spontaneously bursting cells unrelated to noxious stimulus and without receptive fields in the CM of the chronic pain patients.

Lenz has proposed that localization of the CM/PF complex can be aided by initially targeting the ventral caudal parvocellular pars internus, where a taste response can be elicited. This landmark can help define the inferior border and lateral third of the CM.[17] Stimulating other medial thalamic nuclei (medial dorsal and periventricular nuclei) causes a generalized uncomfortable sensation.

A recent clinical results study targeting the mesial thalamus shows that greater than 50% pain relief was achieved in 67% of patients, with 20% of patients achieving complete relief. The best results were in patients with deafferentation pain, where 71% experienced more than 50% pain relief. Complications of treatment did occur, including mixed somatosensory deficits in 9%, transient oculomotor deficits in 5%, and significant verbal deficits in 1 patient of 69 total patients treated. Dysesthesia was associated with inadvertent lesions of the lateral thalamus.[15]

Central Lateral Lesions

Lateral lesions focus on the posterior CLp. The approximate stereotactic coordinates for this nucleus are 2 mm posterior to the PC, 6 mm lateral to the lateral to the thalamoventricular border, at the AC-PC plane. As for other targets, these can vary—sometimes substantially—depending on patient anatomy and lesions. One of the proposed advantages for targeting the CLp is its distance from the somatosensory nuclei, which may reduce the risk for sensory deficits with lesioning. Additionally, there is strong evidence that the CLp has direct STT input.[18]

Lesions are placed 1 to 2 mm above the intercommisural plane to avoid inadvertent injury to the pretectum if the lesion is too posterior. The mediodorsal nucleus and putamen are directly posterior to the CLp. Inadvertent lesions to the putamen alleviate pain but only for a short time.[19,20] Inadvertent mediodorsal nucleus lesions may cause no obvious clinical effect.[21] Technical difficulties may arise when targeting the nucleus due to mechanical deflection at the ependyma, encountered in typical transventricular approaches to thermoablation of this area. The mechanical deflection can result in errors of 1 mm in the anteroposterior and medial-lateral direction and up to 1.9 mm in the dorsoventral.[22]

Intraoperative targeting of the CLp can also be refined by microelectrode physiology, which may show pathologic low-threshold spikes and low-frequency (4 Hz) oscillations.[10] The low-threshold spike activity has been found in a variety of diseases with so-called positive signs, including tinnitus, movement disorders, multifocal epilepsy, and central and peripheral neuropathic pain.[12] Normal cortical low-frequency oscillations occur during certain stages of sleep and cognitive activation.[23] Widespread, continuous, state-independent overproduction of low-frequency oscillations, however, is pathologic and associated with a pathologic state termed, thalamocortical dysrhythmia (TCD).[24]

In the largest trial of CL thalamotomy, in 96 patients, more than 50% of patients had greater than 50% pain relief whereas 20% had complete pain relief.[25] Mean duration of pain was decreased by 65% to 90%. Intermittent-type pain syndromes were improved in 54% of patients. Constant-type pain was decreased in 30% of patients and allodynia pain was alleviated in 60% of patients. Overall, 30% of patients decreased their drug intake postoperatively. Complications were also reported and included partial and partially reversible pretectal visual deficits. Serious complications, such as intraventricular hemorrhage, thalamic edema, and thalamic hemorrhage, were reported in 5% of patients.

Recent Advances

To avoid radiation, infection, and mechanical brain shift, Jeanmonod's group has been investigating the use of MR imaging–guided focused ultrasound CLp thalamotomy for chronic neuropathic pain.[26] Multiple sources of ultrasound are focused at a single point in the CLp, creating a thermal lesion comparable to those made with radiofrequency. MR imaging thermography allows for the accurate visualization of the lesion and estimation of temperature to ensure adequate lesion. In a study of 12 patients treated for chronic refractory neuropathic pain, the first patient had an inadequate lesion at maximum temperature of 42°C and was excluded from the study. Of the remaining 11, the next 2 patients received lesions that were too small on T2-weighted and diffusion tensor imaging (DTI) to have clinical effect; 9 patients had adequate lesioning with maximum temps of 51°C to 64°C and only data for these patients were included in analysis. The investigators reported mean pain relief of 49% (9 patients followed up) at 3 months and 57% at 1 year (8 patients followed up at 1 year) (Fig. 2).

Targeting of thalamic nuclei by diffusion-based white matter targeting has been used successfully for the treatment of tremor[27] and is being investigated for thalamotomy for pain as well.[28] Diffusion-based imaging allows for more accurate targeting based on individual white fiber tract patient anatomy rather than population-based studies.[29] In addition, to better understand those who do not respond to thalamic lesioning, investigators have created spiking neuron computation models of thalamic pain circuits to simulate TCD. Simulated lesions show decreased low-frequency bursting in simulated cortex.[30] EEG studies of TCD in nonresponders show these patients have persistent pathologic dysrhythmia after thalamotomy where responders have a decrement in low-frequency activity. This is proposed as a biomarker of treatment response.[31]

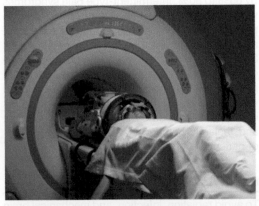

Fig. 2. Photograph of a patient ready for the sonication. (From Jeanmonod D, Werner B, Morel A, et al. Transcranial magnetic resonance imaging-guided focused ultrasound: noninvasive central lateral thalamotomy for chronic neuropathic pain. Neurosurg Focus 2012;32(1):E1.)

MESENCEPHALIC TRACTOTOMY

Mesencephalic tractotomy has been successfully used for the treatment of denervation pain, such as central dysesthesia, in the upper extremity, head, or neck. Potential candidate patients for mesencephalic tractotomy are those who fail medical management, neuromodulation, intrathecal infusions, and thoracic or cervical cordotomy, or those patients whose pain is from structures more superior than what cervical cordotomy can treat. In particular, neuropathic pain from head or neck malignancy could be a potential indication. Patients with chronic nonmalignant pain do not respond well to this technique.

The current targets are based on human electrophysiological mapping studies performed by Nashold and Wilson.[32] The approximate coordinates have been reported at 5 mm posterior to PC, 5 mm below the AC-PC plane, and 5 to 10 mm lateral from the midline. Amano[33] targets a point closer to the midline and within the reticular formation, approximately located at 14 mm posterior to the mid AC-PC point, 5 mm below AC-PC line, and 5 mm lateral from midline.[21] The typical trajectory intersects the AC-PC at 65° to 70°, 2° to 4° lateral from the sagittal plane. The starting point is from a coronal or just precoronal entry point to avoid oculomotor fibers just caudal to the target. Injuries in these fibers cause disturbances in extraocular motion and decreased to 0% by moving the target to the level of the inferior colliculus.[34] Nashold described a 3-mm long and 1.2-mm diameter extraleminscal mesencephalotomy lesion closer to the midline and away from the spinothalamic and medial leminscal paths, resulting in relief of intractable pain without loss of sensation or dysesthesia.[35]

In addition to stereotactic targeting, intraoperative physiology can be useful to confirm or refine the site for neuroablation. Mapping studies with mesencephalic electrodes done by Nashold found that stimulation of the STT at the level of the PC produced burning, numbness, or cold sensations in the contralateral face, arm, and chest.[32] Stimulation of the STT at the level of the superior colliculus produced similar sensations in the trunk, chest, arm, and face. Stimulation of the medial lemniscus produced contralateral hemibody extremity tremor. If stimulation was applied more laterally into the reticular formation or periaqueductal gray, it produced a diffuse and nonspecific sensation, including a sense of vibration, blushing, fear, or panic.

Walker first performed the open lateral surgical approach to lesion the STT at the level of the midbrain in 1942.[36,37] A lateral approach to the

STT at the level of the inferior colliculus passed through the medial lemniscus and resulted in significant hemianesthesia and severe dysesthesia. Speigel pioneered the stereotactic approach with a spinoquintothalamic tractotomy for facial dysesthesia. The quintothalamic tract is synonymous with the trigeminothalamic tract; it carries pain and temperature sensations from the face to the VPM.[38]

Mesencephalic tractotomies are better applied to control malignant pain than noncancer pain. Of 13 patients with pain of central origin, mesencephalotomy at the level of the inferior colliculus resulted in 58% long-term pain relief and 23% nonsymptomatic ocular problems, with 0% mortality.[39]

A recent case study[40] highlights the successful use of 3-T MR imaging preoperative imaging and intraoperative mapping with a monopolar 2-mm diameter electrode that has an additional, 0.5-mm angled extruding electrode at the tip. In this case report, the investigators treat malignant neuropathic left face and neck pain. A 1-mm straight bipolar electrode 5 mm to the right of midline at the level of the superior colliculus produced heat sensation in the left face. A 2-mm monopolar electrode with a 0.5-mm noninsulated extruding tip was used to map lateral targets without multiple linear passes through the brain. The tip can extrude a maximum of 8.5 mm at a 30° angle from the main electrode (**Fig. 3**). Stimulating 9 mm to the right of midline caused tingling and warm sensations in the left arm more than left face. Stimulating 8 mm from midline produced contralateral cool vibratory sensations in the left arm and face and at 7 mm right of midline produced a warm sensation in the left face. Standard 1-mm straight electrodes were placed at 8 mm, then 5 mm and right of midline to create thermal ablations at 70°C, 75°C, 80°C, 85°C, and 90°C each for 90 seconds. Postoperative left face, body, and upper extremity analgesia resulted in adequate pain control for 17 months before the

patient expired at 18 months postoperative from extensive metastatic burden.

CINGULOTOMY

During performance of their notable series of frontal leucotomy procedures, Freeman and Watts[41] noted a marked relief of intractable pain in psychiatric patients. Because the motivational-affective component of pain contributes to the fear, suffering, and anxiety of pain, cingulectomy and cingulotomy were proposed to treat this component of chronic pain.[2]

Recent neuroimaging studies agree with prior investigations that cingulate cortex activity is significantly altered in the setting of chronic pain compared with control.[42] Patients with chronic low back pain from lumbar disk herniation were found to have multiple frontal white and gray matter changes, including increased gray matter volume in the dorsal anterior cingulate compared with controls.[43] The anterior midcingulate cortex is implicated as an area of overlap between negative affect, pain, and cognitive control based on functional MR imaging and DTI studies.[44] Newer studies suggest that long-term potentiation of glutaminergic synaptic transmission in the anterior cingulate contributes to the centralization of chronic pain.[45] Chronic non-neuropathic pain has been associated with increases in blood flow in the anterior cingulate and dorsolateral prefrontal cortex.[46]

In 1954 Le Beau[47] performed the first open resection of 4 cm of the anterior cingulate gyrus for intractable pain, called cingulectomy. Unilateral and bilateral cingulotomies that affect a large volume of the cingulate fasciculus were subsequently developed. In addition to relieving pain, symptoms of withdrawal from narcotics or alcohol were blunted after these procedures.[48] Malignant pain of the head and neck with associated sensations

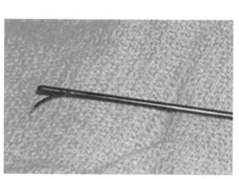
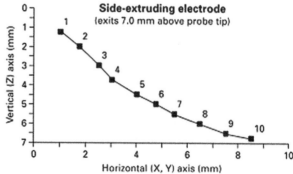

Fig. 3. The electrode tip can extrude a maximum of 8.5 mm at a 30° angle from the main electrode. (*From* Fountas KN, Lane FJ, Jenkins PD, et al. MR-based stereotactic mesencephalic tractotomy. Stereotact Funct Neurosurg 2004;82(5–6):230–4.)

of respiratory distress was successfully treated in humans by cingulotomy.[49] Cingulotomy for the discomfort of chronic dyspnea in a patient with malignant mesothelioma has also been reported.[50] Patients with significant preexisting brain disease, sociopathic personalities, or advanced age are generally not thought good candidates for cingulotomy.[51]

Stereotactic targeting of the cingulum was described in 1962 by Foltz and White.[52] The original technique was based on the ventriculographic identification of the most anterior point of the frontal horn of the lateral ventricle and then measuring 7 mm laterally from midline and 20 to 25 mm posteriorly. The lesions are placed 1 to 2 mm above the roof of the lateral ventricle in the anterior cingulate gyrus. A planned trajectory starting near the coronal suture guides radiofrequency electrode in an appropriate trajectory. The investigators created a first lesion with 85° of ablating heat for 90 seconds. The electrode is then withdrawn 10 mm and a second ablation is repeated to create an elliptical lesion. Bilateral lesions are often pursued to treat chronic pain. Patients are discharged in 1 to 2 days after monitoring for decreased narcotic requirements and cognitive complications.

A recent review of stereotactic cingulotomy for cancer pain found only 8 unique studies demonstrating 32% to 83% of patients with meaningful pain relief. Mild cognitive decline, including decreased attentional focus, apathy, and decreased activity, were seen as side effects of the procedure.[53] Detailed and specific testing for cognitive impacts after bilateral cingulotomy was also reviewed recently.[54] In this study of patients with intractable cancer pain due to metastatic disease, 71% of patients had long-term pain relief whereas most cognitive domains measured by a 120-minute battery of tests remained unchanged except for subtle impairments in attention.

SUMMARY

Three main techniques, described previously, delineate a possible role for intracranial ablative procedures in patients with chronic pain. Recent studies demonstrate a continued need for clinical investigation into central mechanisms of neuroablation to best define its role in the care of patients with otherwise intractable and severe pain syndromes.

REFERENCES

1. Melzack R. Phantom limbs, the self and the brain (the D. O. Hebb Memorial Lecture). Canadian Psychology/Psychologie canadienne. Canadian Psychological Association 1989;30(1):1–16.
2. Melzack R, Torgerson WS. On the language of pain. Anesthesiology 1971;34(1):50–9.
3. Price DD. Psychological and neural mechanisms of the affective dimension of pain. Science 2000; 288(5472):1769–72.
4. Melzack R. Pain measurement and assessment. New york (NY): Raven Press; 1983.
5. Fillingim RB, Bruehl S, Dworkin RH, et al. The ACTTION-American Pain Society Pain Taxonomy (AAPT): an evidence-based and multidimensional approach to classifying chronic pain conditions. J Pain 2014;15(3):241–9.
6. Cetas JS, Saedi T, Burchiel KJ. Destructive procedures for the treatment of nonmalignant pain: a structured literature review. J Neurosurg 2008; 109(3):389–404.
7. Bowsher D. Termination of the central pain pathway in man: the conscious appreciation of pain. Brain 1957;80(4):606–22.
8. Craig AD, Burton H. Spinal and medullary lamina I projection to nucleus submedius in medial thalamus: a possible pain center. J Neurophysiol 1981;45(3):443–66.
9. Moruzzi G, Magoun HW. Brain stem reticular formation and activation of the EEG. Electroencephalogr Clin Neurophysiol 1949;1(1–4):455–73.
10. Jeanmonod D, Magnin M, Morel A. Thalamus and neurogenic pain: physiological, anatomical and clinical data. Neuroreport 1993;4(5):475–8.
11. Craig AD. A new version of the thalamic disinhibition hypothesis of central pain. Pain Forum 2011; 7(1):1–14. American Pain Society.
12. Jeanmonod D, Magnin M, Morel A. Low-threshold calcium spike bursts in the human thalamus. Common physiopathology for sensory, motor and limbic positive symptoms. Brain 1996; 119(Pt 2):363–75.
13. Hirato M, Kawashima Y, Shibazaki T, et al. Pathophysiology of central (thalamic) pain: a possible role of the intralaminar nuclei in superficial pain. Acta Neurochir Suppl (Wien) 1991;52:133–6.
14. Hitchcock ER, Teixeira MJ. A comparison of results from center-median and basal thalamotomies for pain. Surg Neurol 1981;15(5):341–51.
15. Burchiel KJ. Surgical management of pain. Thieme; 2011.
16. Fairman D. Evaluation of results in stereotactic thalamotomy for the treatment of intractable pain. Confin Neurol 1966;27(1):67–70.
17. Lenz FA, Kwan HC, Dostrovsky JO, et al. Characteristics of the bursting pattern of action potentials that occurs in the thalamus of patients with central pain. Brain Res 1989;496(1–2):357–60.
18. Mehler WR. The posterior thalamic region in man. Confin Neurol 1966;27(1):18–29.

19. Richardson DE. Thalamotomy for control of chronic pain. Advances in stereotactic and functional neurosurgery Chapter 11. Vienna (Austria): Springer; 1974. p. 77–88.

20. Richardson DE. Thalamotomy for intractable pain. Stereotact funct neurosurg 1967;29(2–5):139–45.

21. Lozano AM, Gildenberg PL, Tasker RR. Textbook of stereotactic and functional neurosurgery + ereference. New York (Philadelphia): Springer Science & Business Media; 2012.

22. Bourgeois G, Magnin M, Morel A, et al. Accuracy of MRI-guided stereotactic thalamic functional neurosurgery. Neuroradiology 1999;41(9):636–45.

23. Klimesch W. EEG alpha and theta oscillations reflect cognitive and memory performance: a review and analysis. Brain Res Brain Res Rev 1999; 29(2–3):169–95.

24. Llinás RR, Ribary U, Jeanmonod D, et al. Thalamocortical dysrhythmia: a neurological and neuropsychiatric syndrome characterized by magnetoencephalography. Proc Natl Acad Sci U S A 1999;96(26):15222–7. PMCID: PMC24801.

25. Jeanmonod D, Magnin M, Morel A, et al. Surgical control of the human thalamocortical dysrhythmia: I. Central lateral thalamotomy in neurogenic pain. Thalamus & related systems. Cambridge University Press; 2001;1(01):71–9.

26. Jeanmonod D, Werner B, Morel A, et al. Transcranial magnetic resonance imaging-guided focused ultrasound: noninvasive central lateral thalamotomy for chronic neuropathic pain. Neurosurg Focus 2012;32(1):E1.

27. Coenen VA, Allert N, Mädler B. A role of diffusion tensor imaging fiber tracking in deep brain stimulation surgery: DBS of the dentato-rubro-thalamic tract (drt) for the treatment of therapy-refractory tremor. Acta Neurochir (Wien) 2011;153(8): 1579–85 [discussion: 1585].

28. Kincses ZT, Szabó N, Valálik I, et al. Target identification for stereotactic thalamotomy using diffusion tractography. PLoS One 2012;7(1):e29969. PMCID: PMC3251609.

29. Henderson JM. "Connectomic surgery": diffusion tensor imaging (DTI) tractography as a targeting modality for surgical modulation of neural networks. Front Integr Neurosci 2012;6:15. PMCID: PMC3334531.

30. Henning Proske J, Jeanmonod D, Verschure PF. A computational model of thalamocortical dysrhythmia. Eur J Neurosci 2011;33(7):1281–90.

31. Michels L, Moazami-Goudarzi M, Jeanmonod D. Correlations between EEG and clinical outcome in chronic neuropathic pain: surgical effects and treatment resistance. Brain Imaging Behav 2011; 5(4):329–48.

32. Nashold BS, Wilson WP. Central pain. Observations in man with chronic implanted electrodes in the midbrain tegmentum. Confin Neurol 1966;27(1): 30–44.

33. Amano K, Iseki H, Notani M. Rostral mesencephalic reticulotomy for pain relief. Report of 15 cases. Acta Neurochir (Wien) (1980) [Suppl] 30:391–3.

34. Nashold BS Jr. Extensive cephalic and oral pain relieved by midbrain tractotomy. Confin Neurol 1972;34:382–8.

35. Shieff C, Nashold BS. Stereotactic mesencephalic tractotomy for thalamic pain. Neurol Res 1987; 9(2):101–4.

36. Walker AE. Relief of Pain by Mesencephalic Tractotomy. Arch. Neurol. & Psychiat 1942;48:865.

37. Walker AE. Somatotopic Localization of Spinothalamic and Secondary Trigeminal Tracts in Mesencephalon, ibid. 1942;48:884.

38. Spiegel EA, Wycis HT. Mesencephalotomy in intractable facial pain. Trans Am Neurol Assoc 1952;56(77th Meeting):186–9.

39. Shieff C, Nashold BS. Thalamic pain and stereotactic mesencephalotomy. Acta Neurochir Suppl (Wien) 1988;42:239–42.

40. Fountas KN, Lane FJ, Jenkins PD, et al. MR-based stereotactic mesencephalic tractotomy. Stereotact Funct Neurosurg 2004;82(5–6):230–4.

41. Freeman W, Watts JW. Pain of organic disease relieved by prefrontal lobotomy. Lancet 1946; 1(6409):953–5.

42. Buckalew N, Haut MW, Aizenstein H, et al. White matter hyperintensity burden and disability in older adults: is chronic pain a contributor? PMR 2013; 5(6):471–80.

43. Luchtmann M, Steinecke Y, Baecke S, et al. Structural brain alterations in patients with lumbar disc herniation: a preliminary study. PLoS One 2014; 9(3):e90816.

44. Shackman AJ, Salomons TV, Slagter HA, et al. The integration of negative affect, pain and cognitive control in thecingulate cortex. Nature Reviews Neuroscience; 12:154–67.

45. Zhuo M. Long-term potentiation in the anterior cingulate cortex and chronic pain. Philos Trans R Soc Lond B Biol Sci 2013;369(1633):20130146.

46. Youssef AM, Gustin SM, Nash PG, et al. Differential brain activity in subjects with painful trigeminal neuropathy and painful temporomandibular disorder. Pain 2014;155(3):467–75.

47. Le Beau J. Anterior cingulectomy in man. J Neurosurg 1954;11(3):268–76.

48. Meyer M. A study of efferent connexions of the frontal lobe in the human brain after leucotomy. Brain 1949;72(3):265–96, 3pl.

49. Foltz EL. Current status and use of rostral cingulumotomy. South Med J 1968;61(9):899–908.

50. Pereira EA, Paranathala M, Hyam JA, et al. Anterior cingulotomy improves malignant mesothelioma

pain and dyspnoea. Br J Neurosurg 2014;28(4): 471–4.

51. Hurt RW, Ballantine HT. Stereotactic anterior cingulate lesions for persistent pain: a report on 68 cases. Clin Neurosurg 1974;21:334–51.

52. Foltz EL, White LE. Pain "relief" by frontal cingulumotomy. J Neurosurg 1962;19(2):89–100.

53. Viswanathan A, Harsh V, Pereira EA, et al. Cingulotomy for medically refractory cancer pain. Neurosurg Focus 2013;35(3):E1.

54. Yen CP, Kuan CY, Sheehan J, et al. Impact of bilateral anterior cingulotomy on neurocognitive function in patients with intractable pain. J Clin Neurosci 2009;16(2):214–9.

Deep Brain Stimulation for Chronic Pain

Intracranial Targets, Clinical Outcomes, and Trial Design Considerations

Orion Paul Keifer Jr, PhD[a], Jonathan P. Riley, MD, MS[b], Nicholas M. Boulis, MD[b],*

KEYWORDS

- Deep brain stimulation • Surgery • Chronic pain • Clinical trial design • Sensory thalamus
- Intracranial stimulation • Anterior cingulate cortex • Periventricular and periaqueductal gray

KEY POINTS

- For more than half a century, neurosurgeons have attempted to treat pain from a diversity of causes using acute and chronic intracranial stimulation.
- Targets of stimulation have included the sensory thalamus, periventricular and periaqueductal gray, the septum, the internal capsule, the motor cortex, posterior hypothalamus, and more recently, the anterior cingulate cortex.
- The current work focuses on presenting and evaluating the evidence for the efficacy of these targets in a historical context while also highlighting the major challenges to having a double-blind placebo-controlled clinical trial.
- Considerations for pain research in general and use of intracranial targets specifically are included.

INTRODUCTION

The use of electrical stimulation as a neurosurgical tool is rooted firmly in the history of treating hypokinetic and hyperkinetic disorders. Its emergence was directly related to the use of neurosurgical interventions that included lesions to the thalamus and fibers projecting to and from the thalamus as a treatment of motor signs like rigidity, bradykinesia, and tremor.[1–6] Although promising, these results were overshadowed by the introduction of L-Dopa as a method for treating Parkinson disease.[7] The use of chronic intracranial stimulation for the treatment of neurologic disorders would remain nearly quiescent for nearly 2 decades until 1987, when Benabid and colleagues[8] reintroduced thalamic stimulation for Parkinson patients who had emerging symptoms after a unilateral thalamotomy. The renaissance of intracranial chronic stimulation further flourished after Parkinson patients on chronic L-Dopa developed adverse side effects.[9,10] From there, the 1990s through the present would see a strong reemergence of the use of chronic stimulation in hyperkinetic and hypokinetic disorders with targets including the subthalamic nucleus, globus pallidus internus, and ventral intermediate thalamus (Vim).[11–14]

Embedded within the success story of deep brain stimulation (DBS) for movement disorders

Funding Sources: No related funding sources.
Conflict of Interest: No related conflicts of interest.
[a] MD/PhD Program, School of Medicine, Emory University, Suite 375-B, 1648 Pierce Drive, Atlanta, GA 30322, USA; [b] Department of Neurosurgery, Emory University, 1365-B Clifton Road Northeast, Suite 2200, Atlanta, GA 30322, USA
* Corresponding author.
E-mail address: nboulis@emory.edu

Neurosurg Clin N Am 25 (2014) 671–692
http://dx.doi.org/10.1016/j.nec.2014.07.009
1042-3680/14/$ – see front matter © 2014 Elsevier Inc. All rights reserved.

is the use of chronic intracranial stimulation as an intervention for pain. The work of Heath and Mickle in the 1950s is often thought of as the birth of intracranial stimulation for pain control. Their observation that septal stimulation acutely alleviated intractable pain would lead to the birth of the field. From there, DBS targets for pain control would expand to include the internal capsule (IC), the ventral posterolateral nucleus (VPLP) and the ventral posteromedial nucleus (VPM) of the sensory thalamus (STH), the centro-median parafasicular region (CM-Pf) of the thalamus, the periaqueductal/paraventricular gray (PAG/PVG), the posterior hypothalamus (PH), the motor cortex, the nucleus accumbens (NAcc), and the anterior cingulate cortex. The following sections highlight the past, present, and future DBS targets used to treat various types of pain.

INTRACRANIAL TARGETS

Within each target section is a brief review of the history behind stimulating the area for pain, the current literature surrounding its use as a target, and the current clinical standing of that area. Tables present a summarized account for the literature on each region. Each entry is based on the information reported in the article with no attempts to standardize terminology across studies. In other words, independent criteria for "successful treatment" (most reports will define this as >50% improvement of their outcome measure), "side effects" (listed side effects only pertain to stimulation, not due to the surgery or postoperative care), or "pain type" (details of patients conditions and source of pain) have not been defined. Several

reports included stimulation to multiple targets for pain (eg, a patient will have electrodes placed in the VPLP/VPM and PVG/PAG). These articles are listed once in the table corresponding to the target used for most patients but are noted in the charts for the other brain areas. The notes section of the table contains an abbreviated accounting of other areas stimulated and any additional aspects of the article that should be considered.

Septal Interventions

The stimulation of the septal region of the human brain (**Table 1**) was first initiated by Heath and Mickle[15] likely based on the rewarding (or "pleasurable") effects seen in rats.[20] In their work, Heath and Mickle noted that most patients with septal stimulation were more alert and spoke more rapidly. In addition, a few patients were also acutely relieved of their chronic pain (pain due to either rheumatoid arthritis or advanced carcinoma). Later work stimulating the medial forebrain bundle in patients with terminal carcinoma also echoed these results.[16] In particular, Ervin and colleagues[16] stimulated the medial forebrain bundle, among many other areas, and noted an amelioration of the pain reported in their patients with cancer. Because the medial forebrain bundle is part of the mesolimbic pathway, including ventral tegmentum, and NAcc, and also connects to septal nuclei, it is not clear what part of the "pleasure system" could be generating these results. More directly, Gol[17] attempted to study the effects of septal stimulation on pain further and showed some success in a few patients but not the majority (2 of 6 patients). Given these early challenges and only moderate success, it appears that the

Table 1
Review of the studies investigating the clinical role for septal stimulation for the treatment of pain

Study, Year	Study Type	Pain Type	Total- (Implanted)- Success	Electrode and Stimulation Parameters	Side Effects
Heath & Mickle,[15] 1960	CS	RA/ CP	6-NFS	4 Strand, silver-plated copper wire, plastic insulation, silver ball tip	Rapid speech, alert, acute relief of pain
Ervin et al,[16] 1969	CS	CP	NFS	NFS	Mild euphoria, acute relief of pain
Gol,[17] 1967	CS	CP/BP	6-1	Heavy, single-lead electrode, 6 terminal, silver ball tip, 2000–5000 c/s, 0–12 V	More cheerful, alert
Schvarcz,[18] 1985	CS	CP/DP	10-10-6	Standard DBS electrode	Feeling of warmth, well-being, relaxation
Schvarcz,[19] 1993	CS	CP/DP	19-19-12	Bipolar or tetrapolar electrode	Feeling of warmth, well-being

Abbreviations: BP, back pain; CP, cancer pain; CS, case series; NFS, not further specified; RA, rheumatoid arthritis; V, volts.

septum has fallen out of favor. However, it should be noted that 2 works have been published by Schvarcz[18,19] that suggest a nearly 60% success rate of intractable pain relief with septal stimulation. Currently, septal targeting is not common and there is not a double-blind, randomized, placebo-controlled trial to evaluate it efficacy.

IC Interventions

The idea of stimulating the internal capsule as a therapeutic option for treating intractable pain (**Table 2**) started in 1974 when Fields and Adams reported efficacy in a case report.[21] Their results would later expand to a case series.[22] These results would be further bolstered by other groups in the late 1970s to mid-1980s.[23,28,29] Interestingly, the notion of stimulating the IC for pain would remain dormant for more than 2 decades until Franzini and colleagues[32] reported a case study in 2008. As of late, Plow and colleagues[33] have published their clinical trial design for stimulation of the ventral striatum and anterior limb of the internal capsule. Although the proposal by Plow and colleagues[33] is not the first clinical trial for the treatment of pain with DBS, it does hold a great deal of promise because it improves several limitations of older clinical trials (discussed later in the Consideration for Trial Design Section).

STH, VPM/Lateral Nucleus Interventions

Primary literature focusing on the treatment of intractable pain with STH stimulation (**Table 3**) dates to the early 1970s. Inspired by the results of VPM lesions,[73] the gate control theory of pain,[74] and the paresthesias noted by Ervin,[16] the often cited paper by Hosobuchi and colleagues[34] would involve the treatment of facial anesthesia dolorosa with stimulation of the VPM nucleus of the thalamus. They noted success in 4 of 5 patients. That year and a year later, Mazars and colleagues[35,36] published their work (started in the early 1960s) on treating intractable pain with thalamic stimulation with 13 of 17 patients showing benefit. Expanding more broadly to chronic neuropathic pain in general, Turnbull and colleagues[39] showed complete or partial success in 14 of 18 patients (including cases of complex regional pain syndrome, lumbar arachnoiditis, phantom limb pain, and plexus avulsion) when stimulating the ventral posterior portion of the thalamus. During these early studies, it was noted that some patients showed an acute relief of pain with VPM/VPLP stimulation, but that the pain would recur gradually. Several attempts would be made to prevent stimulation tolerance. In the peri(aqueductal)ventricular gray (PV[A]G) literature, Hosobuchi[75] would propose the use of L-tryptophan, and Meyerson and colleagues[76] would propose the use L-Dopa to prevent the reduction of the DBS effect. Tsubokawa[26,27] would pay particular attention to this phenomenon as he further explored VPLP stimulation over several studies. He would introduce the use of L-Dopa and L-Tryptophan supplements in thalamic stimulation to help mitigate the appearance of "stimulation tolerance," although this practice would not continue because of the lack of evidence for efficacy. Interestingly, stimulation tolerance is still a very real concern and is only further compounded with current work that has suggested that there is also an insertional effect (benefit with electrode insertion but no stimulation, as opposed to a developing tolerance to stimulation[66]).

The late 1980s and early 1990s would show the first attempts by neurosurgeons to summarize their cases with DBS of the VPLP/VPM and PVG/PAG.[47,50] These results would, for the first time, cast some doubt on the efficacy of DBS for pain (eg, previous reports had success rates in the 60%–80% range, and reports in this era would document long-term success in the 30%–40% range). They would also come at a time when the US Food and Drug Administration (FDA) ruled that DBS devices must be undergo evaluation for safety and efficacy with chronic pain.[77] To add further complication, this ruling would come out at nearly the same time as the retirement of older-generation Medtronic 4 contact platinum electrodes (3380); hence, the appearance of a newer model (thinner diameter and more narrowly spaced contacts) in the literature (3387). Therefore, 2 clinical trials were conducted to evaluate the use of DBS electrodes for the treatment of chronic, intractable pain (1993 was the final report on model 3380, 1999 for 3387). Summarized years later in 2001, Coffey and colleagues[77] would evaluate the new and older electrodes (3380 and 3387) across 2 centers with 246 patients in a prospective clinical trial. The results for VPLP/VPM and PVG/PAG stimulation were disappointing. In the case of the model 3380 electrode trial, only 46.1% of patients showed greater than 50% improvement at 12 months, which dropped to 17.8% at 24 months. The 3387 numbers were even more disheartening with only 16.2% showing greater than 50% pain relief at 12 months and only 13.5% at 24 months (note that withdrawals were counted as failures with these calculations).

Fortunately, despite Medtronic not pursuing FDA approval for DBS electrode use for intractable pain patients, several studies have been published in the interim showing some efficacy of STH stimulation in specific situations.[61,65,78] Currently, the

Table 2
Review of the studies investigating the clinical role for internal capsule stimulation for the treatment of pain

Study, Year	Study Type	Pain Type	Total- (Implanted)- Success	Electrode and Stimulation Parameters	Side Effects	Notes
Fields & Adams,[21] 1974	CR	SH	1-1-1	Medtronic, 30–150 Hz, 0.25–0.45 ms, 0.7 mA	Paresthesias	F-U: 12 mo
Adams et al,[22] 1974	CS	SH, PSP, SCI	6-5-5	Medtronic, 30–150 Hz, 0.25–0.45 ms, 0.7 mA	Paresthesias	STH electrodes; bilateral pain, patient shifted electrode position = lost unilateral therapeutic effect. VPLP stimulation led to worse pain
Hosobuchi et al,[23] 1975	Please see entry in the STH Section					
Boethius et al,[24] 1976	CS	AD, TPS, PI, PLP	5-5-4	Medtronic, 10–100 Hz, 0.1–0.3 ms, 0.15–7 mA	Motor responses, visual phenomena	Pulvinar, CM-Pf, STH, PAG electrodes; Pulvinar, STH, IC successful
Hosobuchi et al,[25] 1979	Please see entry in the PV(A)G Section					
Tsubokawa et al,[26] 1982	Please see entry in the STH Section					
Tsubokawa et al,[27] 1984	Please see entry in the STH Section					
Namba et al,[28] 1984	CS	PSP, TPS	7-6-5	Medtronic, 50 Hz, 0.2–1.0 ms, 2–8 V	Feeling of warmth	F-U: 9–31 mo
Namba et al,[29] 1985	CS	PSP, TPS, MS	11-11-8	Medtronic, 50 Hz, 0.6 ms, 2–3 V	Paresthesias; muscle contraction (putamen involvement)	STH electrodes; most medial/posterior IC past the posterior commissure level
Young et al,[30] 1985	Please see entry in the PV(A)G Section					
Kumar et al,[31] 1997	Please see entry in the PV(A)G Section					
Farnzini et al,[32] 2008	CR	TS	1-1-1	Medtronic, 3389, 100 Hz, 60 ms, 1 V	Paresthesias, contralateral motor responses	Pain/spasticity reduction; F-U 60+ mo
Plow et al,[33] 2013	Write up of design of clinical trial NCT01072656					

Abbreviations: AD, anesthesia dolorosa; CR, case report; CS, case series; F-U, follow-up; Hz, Hertz; mA, milliampere; ms, millisecond; PI, plexus injury; PLP, phantom limb pain; PSP, poststroke pain; SCI, spinal cord injury; SH, subdural hematoma; TPS, thalamic pain syndrome; TS, V, volts.

STH is often co-targeted with the PVG/PAG areas as first studied by Hosobuchi.[44] The most recent work for DBS stimulation of the STH for pain control suggests that the VPLP/VPM should be considered a second-line treatment target if PAG/PVG stimulation should fail.[71] A well-powered, double-blind, randomized, placebo-controlled trial has yet to occur.

CM-Pf Interventions

The CM-Pf intralaminar complex of the thalamus has a small history of stimulation for the control of pain (**Table 4**). A comprehensive review of the potential for the CM-Pf is provided by Weigel and Krauss,[83] while the evidence in patients was mostly driven by Andy,[79,80] with a more recent interest by Krauss and colleagues.[82] Given the recent resurgence of exploring different neurosurgical targets for intractable, chronic pain control, this area may be of future interest.

P(A)VG Interventions

Boethius and colleagues[24] and Richardson and Akil[84-86] used previous work in animals[87-89] as evidence to target the PAG and PVG (**Table 5**) for alleviation of chronic and acute pain.[99] For Richardson and Akil, of the 6 patients they tested, 5 patients had the electrode traversing the PVG alongside the medial aspect of the nucleus parafascicularis. Of these 5 patients, 3 patients (phantom limb pain, carcinoma-related pain, and thalamic pain syndrome) showed good-to-excellent reduction in pain.[84] In the course of their study, they noted that stimulation of the PAG also resulted in pain reduction, albeit at the cost of increased side effects, including nystagmus, vertigo, and nausea. Their follow-up work included chronic implantation of electrodes targeting the PVG for patients with chronic intractable pain. Of these 8 patients, 7 patients (lumber disc disease, carcinoma, brachial plexus avulsion, spine/back/hip injury, pancoast tumor) showed fair to good results (the eighth patient was addicted to narcotics and did not complete the study).[85] In complementary work, Hosobuchi and colleagues[90] showed that PAG stimulation was effective in 6 patients (3 carcinoma pains, 1 diabetic neuropathy, 1 sacral chordoma, and 1 facial anesthesia dolorosa, albeit the latter had more relief with fifth VPM stimulation).

Working toward a mechanism and building on the work of others,[76] Hosobuchi and colleagues[25] would show higher levels of β-endorphins during PAG stimulation. These results, in combination with studies, noted that the benefits of DBS for pain could be reversed by the opioid antagonist[76,90,100] naloxone, and an opioid-mediated mechanism was put forth. However, ultimately, further studies would not replicate the effect, changes in β-endorphin levels were attributed to contrast agents casting doubt on this as a mechanism.[27,51,101,102] Despite that lack of a cogent mechanism, PV(A)G stimulation use as a therapeutic tool for intractable chronic pain would continue to increase. As noted in the STH section, PV(A)G stimulation was often combined or compared with stimulation in other areas. This stimulation has led to the assertion that stimulation of the PAG/PVG is preferred in cases of somatogenic pain, and the STH is preferred in cases of neurogenic pain.[44] As a review of the PAG/PVG and STH charts clearly shows, this assertion is only partially consistent with the evidence.

Like the STH stimulation, PAG/PVG was evaluated in the clinical trials reported by Coffey,[77] although the data were not parsed by stimulation site, limiting any definitive conclusions. Importantly, since that time, many studies have attempted to address the efficacy of PAG/PVG stimulation better.[62,70,71,96-98] These studies include a randomized, placebo-controlled, N-of-1 series by Green and colleagues[96] and a meta-analysis by Bittar and colleagues,[97] both having favorable conclusions on the use of DBS for chronic intractable pain. A well-powered, double-blind, randomized, placebo-controlled trial has yet to be done.

PH Interventions

In the following section, reports on stimulation of the PH and surrounding area for the treatment of cluster headaches are briefly reviewed (**Table 6**; for a more comprehensive review of the specific topic, see Magis and Schoenen, 2012[116]). In expanding on the conventional targets of DBS for pain, Leone and colleagues[103,104] and Franzini and colleagues[105] reported that stimulation of the PH (targeted based on the circadian and hormonal findings with cluster headaches[117]) helped ameliorate cluster headache–related pain. Of the 5 patients reported, 2 were able to receive stimulation only and 3 were on lower doses of analgesic medication. They further expanded their findings a year later to 8 patients: 3 requiring no medication and 5 requiring low doses of methysergide and verapamil.[106] They would provide further evidence of the success of the treatment of a rare disorder known as short-lasting unilateral neuralgiform headache attacks with conjunctival injection and tearing, which would be corroborated by another case report.[118] **Table 6** documents their growing cohort of patients,[109] including attempts to treat

Table 3
Review of the studies investigating the clinical role for STH stimulation for the treatment of pain

Study, Year	Study Type	Pain Type	Total-(Implanted)-Success	Electrode and Stimulation (F, PW, V)	Side Effects	Notes
Hosobuchi et al,[34] 1973	CS	AD	5-4	7 Intertwined, insulated, platinum wires. 0–4.5 V, 0.4-ms pulse, 60–125 Hz	Paresthesias	F-U: 3–24 mo
Mazars et al,[35] 1973	CS	PLP, PHP, AD, DP	14-13	Monopolar or bipolar gold/copper electrodes, 0.6–1.8 V, 20–50 Hz, 2-ms pulse	NFS	NFS
Mazars et al,[36] 1974	CS	PLP, AD, TPS, PHP	25-18	Monopolar or bipolar gold/copper electrodes, 0.6–1.8 V, 20–50 Hz, 2-ms pulse	NFS	First cohort of 17 patients: external stimulators; second cohort of 8 patients: implantable stimulators
Adams et al,[22] 1974	Please see entry in the IC Section					
Hosobuchi et al,[23] 1975	CS	AD, TPS, PP	11-9	7 Intertwined, insulated, platinum wires. 0–4.5 V, 0.4-ms pulse, 60–125 Hz	NFS	IC electrodes; 2 patients who failed, medullary syndrome
Mazars,[37] 1975	CS	PLP, AD, TPS, PHP, PP, PI, CP	44-29	Monopolar or bipolar gold/copper electrodes, 0.6–1.8 V, 20–50 Hz, 2 ms	NFS	NFS
Boethius et al,[24] 1976	Please see entry in the IC Section					
Schvarcz,[38] 1980	CS	TPS, PCD, SCI	6-6-4	Medtronic, 20 Hz, 0.25 ms, 0.5 mA	Sensation of well-being and relaxation	Medial posterior inferior thalamic stimulation, F-U: 6–42 mo
Turnbull et al,[39] 1980	CS	LA, PI, CRPS	18-14-12	Medtronic, 75–100 Hz, NFS	Paresthesias	PV(A)G electrodes

Study						
Plotkin,[40] 1982	Please see entry in the PV(A)G Section					
Siegfried,[41] 1982	CS	PHP	10-8	Platinum electrode, monopolar, 33–195 Hz, NFS	NFS	F-U: 8–17 mo
Roldan et al,[42] 1982	CS	AD	2-2-2	Medtronic, 80–120 Hz, NFS	NFS	F-U: 5–11 mo
Tsubokawa et al,[26] 1982	CS	CP, TPS, PP	5-5-4	Medtronic, 50 Hz, 200 μs, 0.1–2.0 V	Stimulation tolerance	PV(A)G, IC electrodes; L-Dopa supplement
Tsubokawa et al,[43] 1982	CS	SCI, STP, PLP	6-6-5	Medtronic, 25–100 Hz, NFS	Rapid stimulation tolerance noted	Used L-Dopa and L-Tryptophan for stimulation tolerance, F-U: 12 mo
Hosobuchi,[44] 1983	Please see entry in the PV(A)G Section					
Tsubokawa et al,[27] 1984	CS	CP, PLP	14-14-13	Platinum electrode, NFS	Stimulation tolerance noted	PV(A)G, IC electrodes; no clear relationship between STH stimulation and β-Endorphin/pain levels
Tsubokawa et al,[45] 1985	CS	PLP, PHP, CP	24-24-24	Medtronic, NFS		PV(A)G electrodes
Namba et al,[29] 1985	Please see entry in the IC Section					
Schvarcz,[18] 1985	Please see entry in Septal Section					
Young et al,[30] 1985	Please see entry in the PV(A)G Section					
Kumar & Wyant,[46] 1985	Please see entry in the PV(A)G Section					
Hosobuchi,[47] 1986	Please see entry in the PV(A)G Section					
Young & Brechner,[48] 1986	Please see entry in the PV(A)G Section					
Siegfried,[49] 1987	CS	PHP, AD, TSP, PI, PLP, STP, PP, DP	112-112-89	Medtronic, 33–100 Hz, 0.5–2 ms, 0.5–3 V	Paresthesias	F-U: 6–72 mo

(continued on next page)

Table 3
(continued)

Study, Year	Study Type	Pain Type	Total-(Implanted)-Success	Electrode and Stimulation (F, PW, V)	Side Effects	Notes
Levy et al,[50] 1987	CS	TPS, PN, AD, PP, PCD, PLP, CP, BP	141-141-84l, 42LT	Medtronic, STH, 20–100 Hz, 3–8 V; PV(A)G, 5–15 Hz, 1–5 V	PV(A)G: diplopia, nausea, vertical gaze palsies, blurred vision, horizontal nystagmus, persistent oscillopsia; STH, paresthesias, local pain	PV(A)G electrodes; review of literature, differentiated deafferentation and nociceptive pain, F-U: 24–169 mo
Young & Chambi,[51] 1987	Please see entry in the PV(A)G Section					
Kumar et al,[52] 1990	Please see entry in the PV(A)G Section					
Gybels & Kupers,[53] 1990	CS	PHP, TPS, PLP, FBS, PI, AD, SCI	36-36-22l, 11LT	NFS	NFS	F-U: up to 120 mo, 48 mo avg
Kuroda et al,[54] 1991	CR	CM	1-1-1	Medtronic, NFS	NFS	Histologic analysis of placement medial lemniscus and VIM
Schvarcz,[19] 1993	Please see entry in the Septal Section					
Hariz & Bergenheim,[55] 1995	CS	PLP, DP, TPS, CP	14-9	Monopolar ISSAL, NFS	Paresthesias	Comparison to ablative procedures, F-U: 1–72 mo
Taira et al,[56] 1998	CR	FP	1-1-1	Medtronic 3387, 200 Hz, 100 μs, NFS	NFS	Patient cotreated for pain/movement disorder, F-U: 10 mo
Katayama et al,[57] 2001	CS	PLP	19-10-6	Medtronic, NFS	NFS	10 STH electrodes after spinal cord stimulation failed
Katayama et al,[58] 2001	CS	PSP	45-12-7	Medtronic, NFS	NFS	12 STH electrodes after spinal cord stimulation failed

Study	Type	Pain condition	Number	Device/parameters	Effect	Comments
Coffey,[77] 2001	CT MC P	LBP, LP, TPS, PI, PHP, TMJ, AD, MS, FBS	194-169-90I, 30LT for the 3380 trial; 50-37-8I, 5LT for the 3387 trial	Medtronic, 3380/3387, NFS	NFS	Data not parsed for analysis of target location
Nandi et al,[59] 2002	Please see entry in the PV(A)G Section					
Nandi et al,[60] 2003	Please see entry in the PV(A)G Section					
Marchand et al,[61] 2003	CS PC Pseudo-DB	TN, FP, LP, PI	6-6-6	NFS	NFS	Small, significant effect of stimulation vs control
Green et al,[62] 2004	Please see entry in the PV(A)G Section					
Romanelli & Heit,[63] 2004	CR	PSP	1-1-1	Medtronic 3387, 31–130 Hz, 60 μs, 0–3.0 V	Stimulation tolerance	Patient tolerance at 29 mo, autonomous control of stimulation mitigated tolerance
Bittar et al,[64] 2005	Please see entry in the PV(A)G Section					
Yamamoto et al,[65] 2006	CS	PLP, STP	18-18-14	Medtronic 3387, 20–135 Hz, 0.15–0.21 ms, NFS	NFS	NFS
Hamani et al,[66] 2006	CS R	PSP, FP, PLP, MS, SCI	21-13-5	Medtronic 3387, 25–125 Hz, 60–250 μs, 0–10 V	Insertional effect of 45%	PV(A)G electrodes
Owen et al,[67] 2006	Please see entry in the PV(A)G Section					
Owen et al,[68] 2006	Please see entry in the PV(A)G Section					
Green et al,[62] 2006	Please see entry in the PV(A)G Section					
Rasche et al,[69] 2006	Please see entry in the PV(A)G Section					
Owen et al,[70] 2007	Please see entry in the PV(A)G Section					
Boccard et al,[71] 2013	Please see entry in the PV(A)G Section					
Pereira et al,[72] 2013	CS P	PLP, PI	12-11-11	Medtronic 3387, 5–50 Hz, 200–450 μs, 0.5–5 V	Unremarkable	F-U at 1, 3, 6, and 12 mo

Abbreviations: AD, anesthesia dolorosa; CP, cancer pain; CR, case report; CRPS, complex regional pain syndrome; CS, case series; CT, clinical trial; DB, double blind; F-U, follow-up; FBS, failed back syndrome; FP, facial pain; Hz, Hertz; LBP, lower back pain; LP, leg pain; mA, milliampere; MS, multiple sclerosis; ms, millisecond; NFS, not further specified; P, prospective; PHP, postherpetic pain; PI, plexus injury; PLP, phantom limb pain; PP, paraplegia pain; PSP, poststroke pain; R, retrospective; SCI, spinal cord injury; STP, stump pain; TMJ, temporomandibular joint; TN, trigeminal neuralgia; TPS, thalamic pain syndrome; V, volts.

Table 4
Review of the studies investigating the clinical role for centro-median parafascicular complex stimulation for the treatment of pain

Study, Year	Type of Study	Type of Patient	Total-(Implanted)-Success	Electrode and Stimulation Parameters	Side Effects	Notes
Boethius et al,[24] 1976	Please see the IC Section					
Ray & Burton,[126] 1980	CS	FBS, CP, SCI, PSP, TSP, PLP	28-26-23	Medtronic, NFS	Feeling of warmth, visual effects	F-U: 1–33 mo
Andy,[79] 1980	CS	PAD	4-4-4	Bipolar platinum electrode. 25–125 Hz, 0.1–0.5 ms, 6–20 V	NFS	4 Patients with dyskinesia, 1 without pain but stimulation treated dyskinesia
Andy,[80] 1983	CS	TPS, HA	5-5-5	Electrode NFS, 50 Hz, 200 ms, 0.1–5.0 V	NFS	Stimulation of the CM-Pf with concurrent EEG recordings
Krauss et al,[81] 2001	CS P	NFS	11-10-10	Quadripolar electrodes, NFS	NFS	CM-Pf was compared with STH stimulation and was found more efficacious
Krauss et al,[82] 2002	CS P	—	3-2-2	Medtronic 3387, NFS	NFS	Part of a larger case series, this paper focused on movement disorders

Abbreviations: CP, cancer pain; CS, case series; EEG, electroencephalogram; F-U, follow-up; FBS, failed back syndrome; HA, headache; Hz, Hertz; ms, millisecond; NFS, not further specified; P, prospective; PAD, pain associated with dyskinesia; PLP, phantom limb pain; PSP, poststroke pain; SCI, spinal cord injury; TPS, thalamic pain syndrome; V, volts.

atypical facial pain, where stimulation of the PH was unsuccessful in 3 patients.[110] In addition, other groups would publish their results for stimulating the posterior thalamus for cluster headaches, mostly showing positive results,[107,111,112] although there were also notable failures.[113]

Given the calls for a larger, well-controlled, double-blind clinical trials, Fontaine and colleagues[114] would report on 11 patients in a prospective crossover, double-blind, multicenter study assessing the efficacy and safety of unilateral hypothalamic DBS in cluster headaches. Interestingly, during the 1-month randomization phase, there were no differences in primary or secondary outcomes between those with and without stimulation. In the following open phase of the trial over the course of 10 months, however, there was notable success in 60% of the patients (in keeping with previous reports). Although the reasons for the discrepancy are not clear, the authors postulate that the rather short period (1 month) of randomization at the start of the trial may have been too brief because the effect is thought to take weeks to over a month. Second, the report stated that default stimulation parameters were used, whereas efficiency was only higher after highly individualized and exhaustive measures were taken to tune the stimulation parameters. Third, they noted higher variability than expected in their primary outcome measures, suggesting their study was underpowered. In an interesting follow-up using the same patients, Fontaine and colleagues[119] determined the anatomic localization of their placed electrodes using computed tomography and magnetic resonance imaging, determining that effective placements (using coordinates of studies listed in the chart) tended to be more posterior than the hypothalamus. In the 5 responders of the cohort of 10, structures located less than 2 mm from the centers of effective contacts were as follows: the mesencephalic gray substance, the red nucleus, the fascicle retroflexus, the fascicle longitudinal dorsal, the nucleus of ansa lenticularis, the fascicle longitudinal medial, and the thalamus superficialis medial. Revising their coordinates, Seijo and colleagues[115] modified their targeting to include the PH (additionally the stimulation area included the fasciculus mammillotegmentalis, the fasciculus mammillotegmentalis, and the fasciculus medialis telencephali). Using this targeting with 5 patients, an average of 54 days were used to optimize parameters, resulting in 2 patients becoming completely pain free, 2 having a reduction of more than 90%, and 1 having a reduction of attacks to half of the original value. In terms of long-term follow-up, Piacentino and colleagues[120] recently reported on 4 patients who had greater than a 50% decrease in pain intensity perception for more than 5 years. Clearly, the results are optimistic, although a better powered clinical trial is necessary to be conclusive.

Motor Cortex Interventions

Expanding beyond "deep brain" structures, Tsubokawa and colleagues[121] noted particular difficulty with VPLP and IC stimulation in thalamic syndrome patients and therefore pursued the stimulation of the cortex, particularly precentral and postcentral, to evaluate their potential for treatment of chronic pain. In a study of 11 patients with thalamic syndrome, they were able to show an improvement in the pain acutely in 8 of these patients, with 3 of those patients losing efficacy by 2 years. Since that time, research into motor cortex stimulation (MCS) has expanded drastically. This is addressed in the article by Ostergard and colleagues, "Motor Cortex Stimulation for Chronic pain" in this issue.

Other Areas

Along the course of DBS for chronic pain, a few other areas have been targeted for stimulation. In the mid-1980s, Katayama and colleagues[122] presented work on the successful stimulation of the pontomesencephalic parabrachial region for the alleviation of pain in 2 patients with cancer pain. Also, in the parabrachial region, in 1992, Young and colleagues[123] would stimulate the Kolliker Fuse nucleus, showing relief of pain in 3 of the 6 patients. However, there is no clear follow-up work on targeting the parabrachial region for DBS to alleviate chronic pain. More recently, Mallory and colleagues[124] targeted the NAcc ventral striatum in a case report of central poststroke pain, noting success when combining NAcc stimulation with commiserate PV(A)G stimulation (although they report stimulating the NAcc alone helps alleviate pain). Finally, targeting the affective components of pain, Boccard and colleagues[125] recently reported success when stimulating the anterior cingulate cortex of a patient with neuropathic pain.

CONSIDERATIONS FOR PATIENT SELECTION AND TRIAL DESIGN

Given that the evidence for the use of chronic intracranial stimulation for the control of pain is still controversial, there is a clear need for well-designed and executed clinical trials. The aforementioned studies have highlighted a large

Table 5
Review of the studies investigating the clinical role for PVG/PAG stimulation for the treatment of pain

Study, Year	Study Type	Pain Type	Total-(Implanted)-Success	Electrode and Stimulation Parameters	Side Effects	Notes
Boethius et al,[24] 1976	Please see entry in the IC Section					
Richardsen & Akil,[84] 1977	CS	PLP, CP, TPS	6-3	Radionics, Monopolar, stainless steel electrode, 25–75 Hz, 0.5–5 V	Nystagmus, vertigo, nausea	Five patients had an electrode over the PVG
Richardsen & Akil,[85] 1977	CS	SCI, CP, PI, BP	8-7-7	Medtronic, 0–250 Hz, 0.250 ms, 0–4 V	Paresthesias, relaxation, dizziness, anxiety	F-U: 2–18 mo
Hosobuchi et al,[90] 1977	CS PC	CP, PN, AD	6-6-5	Medtronic, 10–20 Hz, 0.2–1.2 ms, 3–4 V	Oscillopsia, ocular fluttering, nausea, hot feeling, stimulation tolerance	Patient developed tolerance, stopped stimulation, and tolerance decreased, F-U: 3–18 mo
Meyerson et al,[76] 1978	CS	CP	9-7	Custom, platinum-iridium, 4–6 contacts, NFS	Transient diplopia, pleasant warmth spreading to body	Used L-Dopa, F-U: average 3 mo
Hosobuchi et al,[25] 1979	CS	PCD, TPS, LA, CP	6-6	Medtronic, PV(A)G, 5–20 Hz, 3–10 V; IC, 50–75 Hz, 3–5 V		IC electrodes
Turnbull et al,[39] 1980	Please see entry in the STH Section					
Dieckmann & Witzmann,[91] 1982	CS	PI, PLP, AD, TPS, PP, PHP, PCD	52: 23 PVG/PAG & 23 STH-32	Multiple platinum electrode types, NFS		F-U: 6–30 mo
Plotkin,[40] 1982	CS	FBS, CP, PP, STP, BP	48-38	Medtronic, NFS	NFS	STH electrodes (12 reported, NFS); F-U: 6–42 mo
Boivie & Meyerson,[92] 1982	CS	CP	5-5-4	6-Pole, platinum iridium, 30 Hz, 0.2 ms, 0.2–0.4 mA	Pleasant feeling of warmth	Confirmed anatomic location; F-U 1–17 mo
Hosobuchi,[44] 1983	CS	BP, LP, CIP	11-11-11	Medtronic, 2–60 Hz, 0–10 V, 0.1–0.5 ms	Paresthesia with VPLP/VPM, headache with dual stimulation	Dual implant of PAG and STH, F-U: 12–36 mo
Tsubowkawa et al,[27] 1984	Please see entry in the STH Section					
Schvarcz,[18] 1985	Please see entry in Septal Section					

Study	Type	Indications	Numbers	Parameters	Side effects	Comments
Young et al,[30] 1985	CS	FBS, CP, SCI, PHP, PI	48-43-38	Medtronic, NFS	Eye movement disorders, motor responses	IC, STH electrodes; F-U: 2–60 mo, 20 avg
Kumar & Wyant,[46] 1985	CS	BP, CP	18-18-14	Medtronic, 50–100 Hz, 0.5 ms, 3–4 V	Transient blurred vision	Subthalamic nucleus electrodes; F-U: 6–48 mo
Tsubokawa et al,[45] 1985	Please see entry in the STH Section					
Young & Brechner,[48] 1986	CS	CP	17-16-15	NFS	NFS	STH electrodes; F-U: 1–21 mo 5.8 avg
Hosobuchi,[47] 1986	CS	TP, AD, PHP, PI, PP, PLP, PCD, BP, LP	65 PV(A)G, 76 STH: 64 PV(A)G, 252STH, 50 PV(A)G, 44 STH	Medtronic, PAG, 30–30 Hz, 0.2–0.3 ms, 2–4 V: VPLP/VPM, 50–100 Hz, 0.2–0.3 ms, 2–6 V	Dysconjugate vertical eye movements	Use of L-Dopa, L-Tryptophan, F-U: 24–168 mo
Baskins et al,[93] 1986	CS MC	CP, PN	7-7-7I, 6LT	Medtronic, 20 Hz, 1–4 V, NFS	Stimulation tolerance	Confirmed anatomic location; F-U: 1–7 mo
Hosobuchi,[94] 1987	CS	CP	7-2-2	Monopolar electrode, Pulse width 0.5 ms, 0.5–1.5 Amps, 30 Hz	5 Reported feelings of nausea, fright, piloerection, cold sensation	Stimulation of dorsal PAG
Young & Chambi,[51] 1987	CS	NFS	52-45-45I, 29LT	Medtronic, 60 Hz, 0.1–1 ms, NFS	High levels of stimulation tolerance, feeling of warmth, diplopia, oscillopsia	STH electrodes in separate cohort, no Naloxone reversal
Levy et al,[50] 1987	Please see entry in the STH Section					
Kumar et al,[52] 1990	CS R	BP, LP, TPS, PN, CP	48-39-30	Medtronic, PVG, 25–50 Hz, 0.1–0.5 ms, 1–5 V: VPM/VPLP, 50–100 Hz, 0.2–0.8 ms, 3–8 V	Blurred vision, stimulation tolerance	STH electrodes; F-U: 6–120 mo
Gybels & Kupers,[53] 1993	CS	TPS, PI, PLP, SCI, FBS	36-36-22I, 211LT	NFS		
Schvarcz,[19] 1993	Please see entry in the Septal Section					
Tasker & Vilela Filho,[95] 1995	CS	NFS	54-25-15	NFS	Warmth, pleasure	Ventrocaudal nucleus electrodes; compare PAG vs PVG

(continued on next page)

Table 5
(continued)

Study, Year	Study Type	Pain Type	Total-(Implanted)-Success	Electrode and Stimulation Parameters	Side Effects	Notes
Kumar et al,[31] 1997	CS R	FBS, PHP, TPS, TN, CP, PLP	68-53-42	Medtronic 3280 & 3387, PV(A)G, 25–50 Hz, 0.1–0.5 ms, 1–5 V; STH, 50–100 Hz, 0.2–0.8 ms, 2–8 V	Stimulation tolerance	IC and STH electrodes; F-U: 78 mo avg
Nandi et al,[59] 2002	CS	PSP	4-2-2	Medtronic 3387, 3389, 15 Hz, 0.45 ms, 5 V	Motor response	STH and MC electrodes; failure of MCS in 5/6
Nandi et al,[60] 2003	CS	PSP, TN, MS	8-6-6	Medtronic 3389, 3387, 5–35 Hz, 210 μs, 1.5–2.5 V	PV(A)AG >50 Hz elicited pain, STH elicited paresthesias	STH electrodes; noted a correlation of thalamic electrical activity and chronic pain, F-U: 3–30 mo, 9 mo avg
Green et al,[96] 2004	CT P PC RA	TPS, PLP, PHP	7-7-4	Medtronic 3387, NFS	Feeling of warmth	STH electrodes; F-U at 6 mo
Bittar et al,[64] 2005	CS	PLP	3-3-3	Medtronic 3387, NFS		STH electrodes; F-U: 8–20 mo
Bittar et al,[97] 2005	Meta-analysis: "DBS is frequently effective when used in well-selected patients"					
Hamani et al,[66] 2006	Please see entry in the STH Section					
Owen et al,[67] 2006	CS P	PSP, PLP, AD, SCI	34-26-14	Medtronic 3387, PVG, 5–30 Hz, 120–450 ms, 0.8–4.5 V; STH, 10–50 Hz, 60–400 ms, 0.7–4.4 V	NFS	STH electrodes

Study	Type	Indications	Numbers	Device/Settings	Side Effects	Electrodes/Follow-up
Owen et al,[68] 2006	CS R	PSP	15-12-12	Medtronic 3387, NFS	Eye bobbing	STH electrodes; F-U: 27 avg
Green et al,[62] 2006	CS P	AD, TN, POP	7-7-5	Medtronic 3387, 10–50 Hz, 120 μs, <3 V	Feeling of warmth, paresthesias, eye disorders	STH electrodes
Rasche et al,[69] 2006	CS	FBS, AD, PLP, SCI, PSP, PHP	56-32-22	Medtronic 3387, NFS	PVG: feeling of warmth, dizziness, floating, eye deviations, gaze paralysis; STH: paresthesias	STH electrodes; F-U: 12–96 mo
Owen et al,[70] 2007	CS	PSP, PLP, AD, SCI, MS, PHP, CP	47-38-32	Medtronic 3387, PV(A)G, 5–30 Hz, 120–450 ms, 0.8–4.5 V; STH, 10–50 Hz, 60–400 ms, 0.7–4.4 V	PVG: feeling of warmth; STH: paresthesias	STH electrodes; PV(A)G alone or with STH stimulation was most efficacious
Owen et al,[98] 2008	CS	PSP, PI, STP	4-3-3	Medtronic 3387, NFS	NFS	Surgical planning with diffusion tensor imaging
Boccard et al,[71] 2013	CSP	PLP, STP, PI, PSP, SCI, FP	85-74-39	Medtronic 3387, St. Jude 6143, 5–50 Hz, 200–450 μs, 0.5–5 V	NFS	STH electrodes; F-U: 28 mo avg

Abbreviations: AD, anesthesia dolorosa; BP, back pain; CP, cancer pain; CS, case series; CT, clinical trial; F-U, follow-up; FP, face pain; FBS, failed back syndrome; Hz, Hertz; LP, leg pain; mA, milliampere; MC, multicenter; MS, multiple sclerosis; ms, millisecond; NFS, not further specified; P, prospective; PHP, postherpetic pain; PI, plexus injury; PLP, phantom limb pain; POP, postoperative pain; PP, paraplegia pain; PSP, poststroke pain; R, retrospective; SCI, spinal cord injury; STP, stump pain; TN, trigeminal neuralgia; TPS, thalamic pain syndrome; V, volts.

Table 6
Review of the studies investigating the clinical role for PH stimulation for the treatment of pain

Study, Year	Study Type	Pain Type	Total-(Implanted)-Success	Electrode and Stimulation Parameters	Side Effects	Notes
Leone et al,[103] 2001 Leone et al,[104] 2004	CR	CH	1-1-1	Medtronic 3389, 180 Hz, 60 μs, 1–7 V	NFS	F-U: 42 mo
Franzini et al,[105] 2003	CS	CH	5-5-5	Medtronic 3389, 180 Hz, 60 μs, 1–7 V	>4 V: conjugated eye deviation, extreme verbal reports (eg, "near to death")	F-U: 2–22 mo
Franzini et al,[106] 2004	CS	CH	8-8-8	Medtronic 3389, 180 Hz, 60 μs, 1–3.8 V	NFS	F-U: 2–26 mo
Schoenen et al,[107] 2005	CS	CH	6-4-4	Medtronic 3389, 180 Hz, 60 μs, 1–3 V	Transient diplopia, dizziness	One patient died of intracerebral hemorrhage with ventricular inundation, F-U: 14.5 mo avg
Leone et al,[108] 2005	CR	SUNCT	1-1-1	Medtronic 3389, 180 Hz, 60 μs, 1–4 V	>4 V diplopia	Patient underwent blind stimulator deactivation and symptoms reappeared
Leone et al,[109] 2006	CS	CH	16-16-16	Medtronic 3389, 180 Hz, 60 μs, 1–7 V	Hemorrhage of the 3rd ventricle, diplopia	9 patients stimulators turned off, single blind, and recurrence of symptoms, F-U: 23 mo
Broggi et al,[110] 2007	CS	SUNCT, CH, FP	20-?-14	Medtronic 3389, 180 Hz, 60 μs, 1–7 V	NFS	4 Cases of stimulation cessation leading to attacks, F-U: 23 mo avg

Study	Type	Condition		Stimulation parameters	Adverse effects	Outcome
Starr et al,[111] 2007	CS	CH	4-2	Medtronic 3387, 180 Hz, 60 μs, 0–3 V	NFS	—
Bartsch et al,[112] 2008	CS	CH	6-3	Medtronic 3387, 3389, 130–185 Hz, 60 μs, 0–5.5 V	Vertigo and diplopia	F-U: 17-mo avg
Pinsker et al,[113] 2008	CS	CH	2-0	Medtronic, 180–185 Hz, 60 μs, 3–5.5 V	NFS	Patients showed an initial response, by 3 mo pain returned
Fontaine et al,[114] 2010	CT PC DB MC P	CH	11-6	Medtronic 3389, 185 Hz, 60 μs, set to 3 V or 80% of side effects	Transient visual disturbances, hemiparesis, micturition syncope	Reported successes in open arm of the trial
Seijo et al,[115] 2011	CS	CH	5-5	Medtronic 3389, 130 Hz, 60–12 μs, 2–3.5 V	Myosis, euphoria, diplopia	F-U: 33 mo avg

Abbreviations: avg, average; CH, chronic headache; CR, case report; CS, case series; CT, clinical trial; DB, double blind; F-U, follow-up; FP, face pain; Hz, Hertz; NFS, not further specified; P, prospective; SUNCT, short-lasting unilateral neuralgiform headache attacks with conjunctival injection and tearing; V, volts.

number of points about researching pain in general and the role of intracranial stimulation specifically.

General Consideration of Pain Research

- There is no well-validated classification scheme for pain; the current use of somato-genic and neurogenic or nociceptive versus neuropathic is helpful, but not necessarily divided along the lines of therapeutic options.
- There is no well-validated and objective method of evaluating pain; current methods rely heavily on subjective reports (see the Visual Analog Scale [VAS] and McGill Pain Questionnaire [MPQ]).

Specific Considerations to Chronic Stimulation for the Treatment of Pain

- The patients used for chronic intracranial stimulation research are already biased because they have failed nearly all other pain-control methods.
- There is no easy way to optimize DBS param-eters while also keeping double-blind and placebo-controlled requirements, especially if the stimulation results in a perceivable entity (paresthesias).
- Patients require adjustment of their parame-ters for optimal effect both in the operating room and during the long-term follow-up.
- Based on a limited pain classification scheme and lack of objective measures, it is hard to understand why patients have successful in-terventions while others fail.

Importantly, Plow and colleagues[33] have proposed an exciting clinical trial design (NCT01072656) for the use of intracranial stimulation, which includes a much needed control arm that has been absent in many past studies.

SUMMARY

The use of DBS for the control of intractable, chronic pain has a history stretching more than half a century. Within this literature, targets have varied from major white matter tracts like the inter-nal capsule to a specific gray matter island, like the Kolliker Fuse nucleus. Perhaps more impressive, the type and causes of the chronic pain in the pa-tients have been even more diverse from crush in-juries to poststroke pain. In lieu of all this variability, it is not surprising that the field still has inconsistent results on the efficacy of DBS for treating pain.

As noted, much of the literature is retrospective case reports that leave much to be desired in terms of blinding, controls, and pain measures. There have been only a few clinical trials, and those have had major limitations. Nevertheless, overall, the preponderance of evidence is in favor of DBS for specific patients. Although many would point to the clinical trials sponsored by Medtronic in the 1990s as a definitive challenge to the use of DBS for pain, it should be noted that those trials were hampered by a lack of enrollment, long-term follow-up, randomization, placebo control, and the inability to address the concerns listed in the gen-eral considerations on pain research and specific considerations to chronic stimulation for the treat-ment of pain sections. Thus, like the studies before those clinical trials, the results are hardly definitive. A major benefit of the publication of the Medtronic trials has been an increase in more rigorous studies being published on the use of DBS with pain. Furthermore, it has encouraged scientists and neurosurgeons to expand beyond the clas-sical brain targets and explore other options within known pain and affective circuits. Finally, and most importantly, more recent and ongoing clinical trials have the promise of being flexible, while rigorous, well-controlled, randomized, and blind, allowing for more definitive conclusions on DBS efficacy in chronic pain treatment.

REFERENCES

1. Spiegel EA, Wycis HT, Szekely EG, et al. Stimula-tion of Forel's field during stereotaxic operations in the human brain. Electroencephalogr Clin Neu-rophysiol 1964;16:537–48.
2. Hassler R, Riechert T. Indications and localization of stereotactic brain operations. Nervenarzt 1954; 25(11):441–7 [in German].
3. Cooper IS. Anterior chorodial artery ligation for involuntary movements. Science 1953;118(3059): 193.
4. Albe Fessard D, Arfel G, Guiot G, et al. Character-istic electric activities of some cerebral structures in man. Ann Chir 1963;17:1185–214 [in French].
5. Bekhtereva NP, Grachev KV, Orlova AN, et al. Utili-zation of multiple electrodes implanted in the subcortical structure of the human brain for the treatment of hyperkinesis. Zh Nevropatol Psikhiatr Im S S Korsakova 1963;63:3–8 [in Russian].
6. Sem-Jacobsen CW. Depth electrographic stimula-tion and treatment of patients with Parkinson's dis-ease including neurosurgical technique. Acta Neurol Scand Suppl 1965;13(Pt 1):365–77.
7. Cotzias GC, Papavasiliou PS, Gellene R. Modifica-tion of Parkinsonism–chronic treatment with L-dopa. N Engl J Med 1969;280(7):337–45.
8. Benabid AL, Pollak P, Louveau A, et al. Combined (thalamotomy and stimulation) stereotactic surgery

of the VIM thalamic nucleus for bilateral Parkinson disease. Appl Neurophysiol 1987;50(1–6):344–6.

9. Vingerhoets FJ, Villemure JG, Temperli P, et al. Subthalamic DBS replaces levodopa in Parkinson's disease: two-year follow-up. Neurology 2002;58(3): 396–401.

10. Marsden CD. Problems with long-term levodopa therapy for Parkinson's disease. Clin Neuropharmacol 1994;17(Suppl 2):S32–44.

11. Limousin P, Krack P, Pollak P, et al. Electrical stimulation of the subthalamic nucleus in advanced Parkinson's disease. N Engl J Med 1998;339(16): 1105–11.

12. Benabid AL, Pollak P, Gervason C, et al. Long-term suppression of tremor by chronic stimulation of the ventral intermediate thalamic nucleus. Lancet 1991;337(8738):403–6.

13. Siegfried J, Lippitz B. Bilateral chronic electrostimulation of ventroposterolateral pallidum: a new therapeutic approach for alleviating all parkinsonian symptoms. Neurosurgery 1994;35(6):1126–9 [discussion: 1129–30].

14. Kumar R, Lozano AM, Kim YJ, et al. Double-blind evaluation of subthalamic nucleus deep brain stimulation in advanced Parkinson's disease. Neurology 1998;51(3):850–5.

15. Heath RG, Mickle WA. Evaluation of seven years' experience with depth electrode studies in human patients. In: Re R, Odd C, editors. Electrical studies on the unanesthetized brain. New York: Harper & Brothers; 1960. p. 214–47.

16. Ervin FR, Mark VH, Stevens J. Behavioral and affective responses to brain stimulation in man. Proc Annu Meet Am Psychopathol Assoc 1969;58:54–65.

17. Gol A. Relief of pain by electrical stimulation of the septal area. J Neurol Sci 1967;5(1):115–20.

18. Schvarcz JR. Chronic stimulation of the septal area for the relief of intractable pain. Appl Neurophysiol 1985;48(1–6):191–4.

19. Schvarcz JR. Long-term results of stimulation of the septal area for relief of neurogenic pain. Acta Neurochir Suppl 1993;58:154–5.

20. Olds J, Milner P. Positive reinforcement produced by electrical stimulation of septal area and other regions of rat brain. J Comp Physiol Psychol 1954; 47(6):419–27.

21. Fields HL, Adams JE. Pain after cortical injury relieved by electrical stimulation of the internal capsule. Brain 1974;97(1):169–78.

22. Adams JE, Hosobuchi Y, Fields HL. Stimulation of internal capsule for relief of chronic pain. J Neurosurg 1974;41(6):740–4.

23. Hosobuchi Y, Adams JE, Rutkin B. Chronic thalamic and internal capsule stimulation for the control of central pain. Surg Neurol 1975;4(1):91–2.

24. Boethius J, Lindblom V, Meyerson BA, et al. Effects of multifocal stimulation on pain and somatosensory

functions. Sensory functions of the skin in primates, with special reference to man. Oxford (United Kingdom): Pergamon Press; 1976. p. 531–48.

25. Hosobuchi Y, Rossier J, Bloom FE, et al. Stimulation of human periaqueductal gray for pain relief increases immunoreactive beta-endorphin in ventricular fluid. Science 1979;203(4377):279–81.

26. Tsubokawa T, Yamamoto T, Katayama Y, et al. Deep brain stimulation for relief of intractable pain. Clinical results of thalamic relay stimulation (author's transl). Neurol Med Chir (Tokyo) 1982;22(3):211–8 [in Japanese].

27. Tsubokawa T, Yamamoto T, Katayama Y, et al. Thalamic relay nucleus stimulation for relief of intractable pain. Clinical results and beta-endorphin immunoreactivity in the cerebrospinal fluid. Pain 1984;18(2):115–26.

28. Namba S, Nakao Y, Matsumoto Y, et al. Electrical stimulation of the posterior limb of the internal capsule for treatment of thalamic pain. Appl Neurophysiol 1984;47(3):137–48.

29. Namba S, Wani T, Shimizu Y, et al. Sensory and motor responses to deep brain stimulation. Correlation with anatomical structures. J Neurosurg 1985; 63(2):224–34.

30. Young RF, Kroening R, Fulton W, et al. Electrical stimulation of the brain in treatment of chronic pain. Experience over 5 years. J Neurosurg 1985; 62(3):389–96.

31. Kumar K, Toth C, Nath RK. Deep brain stimulation for intractable pain: a 15-year experience. Neurosurgery 1997;40(4):736–46 [discussion: 746–7].

32. Franzini A, Cordella R, Nazzi V, et al. Long-term chronic stimulation of internal capsule in poststroke pain and spasticity. Case report, long-term results and review of the literature. Stereotact Funct Neurosurg 2008;86(3):179–83.

33. Plow EB, Malone DA Jr, Machado A. Deep brain stimulation of the ventral striatum/anterior limb of the internal capsule in thalamic pain syndrome: study protocol for a pilot randomized controlled trial. Trials 2013;14:241.

34. Hosobuchi Y, Adams JE, Rutkin B. Chronic thalamic stimulation for the control of facial anesthesia dolorosa. Arch Neurol 1973;29(3): 158–61.

35. Mazars G, Merienne L, Ciolocca C. Intermittent analgesic thalamic stimulation. Preliminary note. Rev Neurol 1973;128(4):273–9 [in French].

36. Mazars G, Merienne L, Cioloca C. Treatment of certain types of pain with implantable thalamic stimulators. Neurochirurgie 1974;20(2):117–24 [in French].

37. Mazars GJ. Intermittent stimulation of nucleus ventralis posterolateralis for intractable pain. Surg Neurol 1975;4(1):93–5.

38. Schvarcz JR. Chronic self-stimulation of the medial posterior inferior thalamus for the alleviation of

deafferentation pain. Acta Neurochir Suppl 1980; 30:295–301.

39. Turnbull IM, Shulman R, Woodhurst WB. Thalamic stimulation for neuropathic pain. J Neurosurg 1980;52(4):486–93.

40. Plotkin R. Results in 60 cases of deep brain stimulation for chronic intractable pain. Appl Neurophysiol 1982;45(1–2):173–8.

41. Siegfried J. Monopolar electrical stimulation of nucleus ventroposteromedialis thalami for postherpetic facial pain. Appl Neurophysiol 1982;45(1–2):179–84.

42. Roldan P, Broseta J, Barcia-Salorio JL. Chronic VPM stimulation for anesthesia dolorosa following trigeminal surgery. Appl Neurophysiol 1982;45(1–2): 112–3.

43. Tsubokawa T, Yamamoto T, Katayama Y, et al. Clinical results and physiological basis of thalamic relay nucleus stimulation for relief of intractable pain with morphine tolerance. Appl Neurophysiol 1982;45(1–2):143–55.

44. Hosobuchi Y. Combined electrical stimulation of the periaqueductal gray matter and sensory thalamus. Appl Neurophysiol 1983;46(1–4):112–5.

45. Tsubokawa T, Katayama Y, Yamamoto T, et al. Deafferentation pain and stimulation of the thalamic sensory relay nucleus: clinical and experimental study. Appl Neurophysiol 1985;48(1–6):166–71.

46. Kumar K, Wyant GM. Deep brain stimulation for alleviating chronic intractable pain. Can J Surg 1985;28(1):20–2.

47. Hosobuchi Y. Subcortical electrical stimulation for control of intractable pain in humans. Report of 122 cases (1970-1984). J Neurosurg 1986;64(4): 543–53.

48. Young RF, Brechner T. Electrical stimulation of the brain for relief of intractable pain due to cancer. Cancer 1986;57(6):1266–72.

49. Siegfried J. Sensory thalamic neurostimulation for chronic pain. Pacing Clin Electrophysiol 1987; 10(1 Pt 2):209–12.

50. Levy RM, Lamb S, Adams JE. Treatment of chronic pain by deep brain stimulation: long term follow-up and review of the literature. Neurosurgery 1987; 21(6):885–93.

51. Young RF, Chambi VI. Pain relief by electrical stimulation of the periaqueductal and periventricular gray matter. Evidence for a non-opioid mechanism. J Neurosurg 1987;66(3):364–71.

52. Kumar K, Wyant GM, Nath R. Deep brain stimulation for control of intractable pain in humans, present and future: a ten-year follow-up. Neurosurgery 1990; 26(5):774–81 [discussion: 781–2].

53. Gybels J, Kupers R. Deep brain stimulation in the treatment of chronic pain in man: where and why? Neurophysiol Clin 1990;20(5):389–98.

54. Kuroda R, Nakatani J, Yamada Y, et al. Location of a DBS-electrode in lateral thalamus for

deafferentation pain. An autopsy case report. Acta Neurochir Suppl 1991;52:140–2.

55. Hariz MI, Bergenheim AT. Thalamic stereotaxis for chronic pain: ablative lesion or stimulation? Stereotact Funct Neurosurg 1995;64(1):47–55.

56. Taira T, Kawamura H, Takakura K. Posterior occipital approach in deep brain stimulation for both pain and involuntary movement. A case report. Stereotact Funct Neurosurg 1998;70(1):52–6.

57. Katayama Y, Yamamoto T, Kobayashi K, et al. Motor cortex stimulation for phantom limb pain: comprehensive therapy with spinal cord and thalamic stimulation. Stereotact Funct Neurosurg 2001;77(1–4):159–62.

58. Katayama Y, Yamamoto T, Kobayashi K, et al. Motor cortex stimulation for post-stroke pain: comparison of spinal cord and thalamic stimulation. Stereotact Funct Neurosurg 2001;77(1–4): 183–6.

59. Nandi D, Smith H, Owen S, et al. Peri-ventricular grey stimulation versus motor cortex stimulation for post stroke neuropathic pain. J Clin Neurosci 2002;9(5):557–61.

60. Nandi D, Aziz T, Carter H, et al. Thalamic field potentials in chronic central pain treated by periventricular gray stimulation – a series of eight cases. Pain 2003;101(1–2):97–107.

61. Marchand S, Kupers RC, Bushnell MC, et al. Analgesic and placebo effects of thalamic stimulation. Pain 2003;105(3):481–8.

62. Green AL, Owen SL, Davies P, et al. Deep brain stimulation for neuropathic cephalalgia. Cephalalgia 2006;26(5):561–7.

63. Romanelli P, Heit G. Patient-controlled deep brain stimulation can overcome analgesic tolerance. Stereotact Funct Neurosurg 2004;82(2–3): 77–9.

64. Bittar RG, Otero S, Carter H, et al. Deep brain stimulation for phantom limb pain. J Clin Neurosci 2005;12(4):399–404.

65. Yamamoto T, Katayama Y, Obuchi T, et al. Thalamic sensory relay nucleus stimulation for the treatment of peripheral deafferentation pain. Stereotact Funct Neurosurg 2006;84(4):180–3.

66. Hamani C, Schwalb JM, Rezai AR, et al. Deep brain stimulation for chronic neuropathic pain: long-term outcome and the incidence of insertional effect. Pain 2006;125(1–2):188–96.

67. Owen SL, Green AL, Nandi D, et al. Deep brain stimulation for neuropathic pain. Neuromodulation 2006;9(2):100–6.

68. Owen SL, Green AL, Stein JF, et al. Deep brain stimulation for the alleviation of post-stroke neuropathic pain. Pain 2006;120(1–2):202–6.

69. Rasche D, Rinaldi PC, Young RF, et al. Deep brain stimulation for the treatment of various chronic pain syndromes. Neurosurg Focus 2006;21(6):E8.

70. Owen SL, Green AL, Nandi DD, et al. Deep brain stimulation for neuropathic pain. Acta Neurochir Suppl 2007;97(Pt 2):111–6.

71. Boccard SG, Pereira EA, Moir L, et al. Long-term outcomes of deep brain stimulation for neuropathic pain. Neurosurgery 2013;72(2):221–30 [discussion: 231].

72. Pereira EA, Boccard SG, Linhares P, et al. Thalamic deep brain stimulation for neuropathic pain after amputation or brachial plexus avulsion. Neurosurg Focus 2013;35(3):E7.

73. Obrador S, Bravo G. Thalamic lesions for the treatment of facial neuralgias. J Neurol Neurosurg Psychiatry 1960;23:351–2.

74. Melzack R, Wall PD. Pain mechanisms: a new theory. Science 1965;150(3699):971–9.

75. Hosobuchi Y. Tryptophan reversal of tolerance to analgesia induced by central grey stimulation. Lancet 1978;2(8079):47.

76. Meyerson BA, Boethius J, Carlsson AM. Percutaneous central gray stimulation for cancer pain. Appl Neurophysiol 1978;41(1–4):57–65.

77. Coffey RJ. Deep brain stimulation for chronic pain: results of two multicenter trials and a structured review. Pain Med 2001;2(3):183–92.

78. Katayama Y, Yamamoto T, Kobayashi K, et al. Deep brain and motor cortex stimulation for post-stroke movement disorders and post-stroke pain. Acta Neurochir Suppl 2003;87:121–3.

79. Andy OJ. Parafascicular-center median nuclei stimulation for intractable pain and dyskinesia (painful-dyskinesia). Appl Neurophysiol 1980; 43(3–5):133–44.

80. Andy OJ. Thalamic stimulation for chronic pain. Appl Neurophysiol 1983;46(1–4):116–23.

81. Krauss JK, Pohle T, Weigel R, et al. Somatosensory thalamic stimulation versus center median-parafasicular complex stimulation in 11 patients with neuropathic pain. Stereotact Funct Neurosurg 2001;77:194.

82. Krauss JK, Pohle T, Weigel R, et al. Deep brain stimulation of the centre median-parafascicular complex in patients with movement disorders. J Neurol Neurosurg Psychiatry 2002;72(4): 546–8.

83. Weigel R, Krauss JK. Center median-parafascicular complex and pain control. Review from a neurosurgical perspective. Stereotact Funct Neurosurg 2004;82(2–3):115–26.

84. Richardson DE, Akil H. Pain reduction by electrical brain stimulation in man. Part 1: acute administration in periaqueductal and periventricular sites. J Neurosurg 1977;47(2):178–83.

85. Richardson DE, Akil H. Pain reduction by electrical brain stimulation in man. Part 2: chronic self-administration in the periventricular gray matter. J Neurosurg 1977;47(2):184–94.

86. Richardson DE, Akil H. Chronic Self-Administered brain stimulation for the relief of intractable pain. Paper presented at: 7th Annual Meeting of Neuro Electric. Soc. 1974. Louisiana. November 21, 1974.

87. Reynolds DV. Surgery in the rat during electrical analgesia induced by focal brain stimulation. Science 1969;164(3878):444–5.

88. Mayer DJ, Wolfle TL, Akil H, et al. Analgesia from electrical stimulation in the brainstem of the rat. Science 1971;174(4016):1351–4.

89. Cox VC, Valenstein ES. Attenuation of aversive properties of peripheral shock by hypothalamic stimulation. Science 1965;149(3681):323–5.

90. Hosobuchi Y, Adams JE, Linchitz R. Pain relief by electrical stimulation of the central gray matter in humans and its reversal by naloxone. Science 1977;197(4299):183–6.

91. Dieckmann G, Witzmann A. Initial and long-term results of deep brain stimulation for chronic intractable pain. Appl Neurophysiol 1982;45(1–2):167–72.

92. Boivie J, Meyerson BA. A correlative anatomical and clinical study of pain suppression by deep brain stimulation. Pain 1982;13(2):113–26.

93. Baskin DS, Mehler WR, Hosobuchi Y, et al. Autopsy analysis of the safety, efficacy and cartography of electrical stimulation of the central gray in humans. Brain Res 1986;371(2):231–6.

94. Hosobuchi Y. Dorsal periaqueductal gray-matter stimulation in humans. Pacing Clin Electrophysiol 1987;10(1 Pt 2):213–6.

95. Tasker RR, Vilela Filho O. Deep brain stimulation for neuropathic pain. Stereotact Funct Neurosurg 1995;65(1–4):122–4.

96. Green AL, Shad A, Watson R, et al. N-of-1 trials for assessing the efficacy of deep brain stimulation in neuropathic pain. Neuromodulation 2004;7(2): 76–81.

97. Bittar RG, Kar-Purkayastha I, Owen SL, et al. Deep brain stimulation for pain relief: a meta-analysis. J Clin Neurosci 2005;12(5):515–9.

98. Owen SL, Heath J, Kringelbach M, et al. Pre-operative DTI and probabilistic tractography in four patients with deep brain stimulation for chronic pain. J Clin Neurosci 2008;15(7):801–5.

99. Akil H, Liebeskind JC. Monoaminergic mechanisms of stimulation-produced analgesia. Brain Res 1975;94(2):279–96.

100. Adams JE. Naloxone reversal of analgesia produced by brain stimulation in the human. Pain 1976;2(2):161–6.

101. Dionne RA, Mueller GP, Young RF, et al. Contrast medium causes the apparent increase in beta-endorphin levels in human cerebrospinal fluid following brain stimulation. Pain 1984;20(4): 313–21.

102. Fessler RG, Brown FD, Rachlin JR, et al. Elevated beta-endorphin in cerebrospinal fluid after

electrical brain stimulation: artifact of contrast infusion? Science 1984;224(4652):1017–9.

103. Leone M, Franzini A, Bussone G. Stereotactic stimulation of posterior hypothalamic gray matter in a patient with intractable cluster headache. N Engl J Med 2001;345(19):1428–9.

104. Leone M, Franzini A, Broggi G, et al. Long-term follow-up of bilateral hypothalamic stimulation for intractable cluster headache. Brain 2004; 127(Pt 10):2259–64.

105. Franzini A, Ferroli P, Leone M, et al. Stimulation of the posterior hypothalamus for treatment of chronic intractable cluster headaches: first reported series. Neurosurgery 2003;52(5):1095–9 [discussion: 1099–101].

106. Franzini A, Ferroli P, Leone M, et al. Hypothalamic deep brain stimulation for the treatment of chronic cluster headaches: a series report. Neuromodulation 2004;7(1):1–8.

107. Schoenen J, Di Clemente L, Vandenheede M, et al. Hypothalamic stimulation in chronic cluster headache: a pilot study of efficacy and mode of action. Brain 2005;128(Pt 4):940–7.

108. Leone M, Franzini A, D'Andrea G, et al. Deep brain stimulation to relieve drug-resistant SUNCT. Ann Neurol 2005;57(6):924–7.

109. Leone M, Franzini A, Broggi G, et al. Hypothalamic stimulation for intractable cluster headache: long-term experience. Neurology 2006; 67(1):150–2.

110. Broggi G, Franzini A, Leone M, et al. Update on neurosurgical treatment of chronic trigeminal autonomic cephalalgias and atypical facial pain with deep brain stimulation of posterior hypothalamus: results and comments. Neurol Sci 2007; 28(Suppl 2):S138–45.

111. Starr PA, Barbaro NM, Raskin NH, et al. Chronic stimulation of the posterior hypothalamic region for cluster headache: technique and 1-year results in four patients. J Neurosurg 2007;106(6): 999–1005.

112. Bartsch T, Pinsker MO, Rasche D, et al. Hypothalamic deep brain stimulation for cluster headache: experience from a new multicase series. Cephalalgia 2008;28(3):285–95.

113. Pinsker MO, Bartsch T, Falk D, et al. Failure of deep brain stimulation of the posterior inferior hypothalamus in chronic cluster headache - report of two cases and review of the literature. Zentralbl Neurochir 2008;69(2):76–9.

114. Fontaine D, Lazorthes Y, Mertens P, et al. Safety and efficacy of deep brain stimulation in refractory cluster headache: a randomized placebo-controlled double-blind trial followed by a 1-year open extension. J Headache Pain 2010; 11(1):23–31.

115. Seijo F, Saiz A, Lozano B, et al. Neuromodulation of the posterolateral hypothalamus for the treatment of chronic refractory cluster headache: experience in five patients with a modified anatomical target. Cephalalgia 2011;31(16):1634–41.

116. Magis D, Schoenen J. Advances and challenges in neurostimulation for headaches. Lancet Neurol 2012;11(8):708–19.

117. Leone M, Bussone G. A review of hormonal findings in cluster headache. Evidence for hypothalamic involvement. Cephalalgia 1993;13(5): 309–17.

118. Bartsch T, Falk D, Knudsen K, et al. Deep brain stimulation of the posterior hypothalamic area in intractable short-lasting unilateral neuralgiform headache with conjunctival injection and tearing (SUNCT). Cephalalgia 2011;31(13):1405–8.

119. Fontaine D, Lanteri-Minet M, Ouchchane L, et al. Anatomical location of effective deep brain stimulation electrodes in chronic cluster headache. Brain 2010;133(Pt 4):1214–23.

120. Piacentino M, D'Andrea G, Perini F, et al. Drug-resistant cluster headache: long-term evaluation of pain control by posterior hypothalamic deep-brain stimulation. World Neurosurg 2014;81(2): 442.e11–5.

121. Tsubokawa T, Katayama Y, Yamamoto T, et al. Treatment of thalamic pain by chronic motor cortex stimulation. Pacing Clin Electrophysiol 1991;14(1): 131–4.

122. Katayama Y, Tsubokawa T, Hirayama T, et al. Pain relief following stimulation of the pontomesencephalic parabrachial region in humans: brain sites for nonopiate-mediated pain control. Appl Neurophysiol 1985;48(1–6):195–200.

123. Young RF, Tronnier V, Rinaldi PC. Chronic stimulation of the Kolliker-Fuse nucleus region for relief of intractable pain in humans. J Neurosurg 1992; 76(6):979–85.

124. Mallory GW, Abulseoud O, Hwang SC, et al. The nucleus accumbens as a potential target for central poststroke pain. Mayo Clin Proc 2012; 87(10):1025–31.

125. Boccard SG, Pereira EA, Moir L, et al. Deep brain stimulation of the anterior cingulate cortex: targeting the affective component of chronic pain. Neuroreport 2014;25(2):83–8.

126. Ray CD, Burton CV. Deep brain stimulation for severe, chronic pain. Acta Neurochir Suppl (Wien) 1980;30:289–93.

Motor Cortex Stimulation for Chronic Pain

Thomas Ostergard, MD, MS, Charles Munyon, MD, Jonathan P. Miller, MD*

KEYWORDS

- Motor cortex stimulation • Chronic pain • Central pain • Post-stroke pain • Anesthesia dolorosa
- Trigeminal neuropathy • Trigeminal deafferentation pain • Trigeminal neuropathic pain

KEY POINTS

- Motor cortex stimulation (MCS) provides relief of many chronic pain syndromes that have been refractory to multiple treatment modalities.
- MCS has been used successfully to treat pain in patients with central post-stroke pain, anesthesia dolorosa, post-herpetic neuralgia, multiple sclerosis, phantom limb pain, and spinal cord injury.
- Patients undergo a craniotomy for implantation, followed by a trial period of stimulation. Patients who are considered to be responders then undergo implantation of the pulse generator for chronic stimulation.
- Multiple techniques are available for localizing the precentral gyrus: Frameless stereotaxy with or without functional magnetic resonance imaging, somatosensory evoked potentials, and facial electromyography.
- Stimulation parameters vary widely, and patients often require multiple programming sessions. Some patients that experience return of their symptoms can be "recaptured" through programming changes.

INTRODUCTION

The relationship between the motor cortex and certain types of pain has been known for many years, but the nature of that relationship remains obscure. In 1954, Penfield and Japser reported relief of severe pain after resection of the primary motor cortex; previous resection of the sensory cortex had not been effective.[1] The obvious morbidity of this approach prevented its widespread adoption. Subcortical neurostimulation for pain primarily focused on sensory pathways.[2] However, stimulation of the primary sensory area was not found to be effective.[3] In 1991, Tsubokawa made the serendipitous observation that chronic stimulation of the precentral gyrus below the threshold to produce a motor response was able to alleviate certain types of deafferentation pain.[4] Subsequently, Meyerson and associates observed that the technique was particularly effective for trigeminal neuropathic pain.[5] Since that time, a number of reports have confirmed efficacy for a number of deafferentation pain syndromes.[6–13]

The mechanism of action for motor cortex stimulation (MCS) has been attributed to modulation of pathologic hyperactivity in thalamic relay nuclei that results from deafferentation, possibly because sensory neurons below a deafferenting lesion cannot exert physiologic inhibition of nociceptive neurons.[3] Higher order neurons within the sensory pathway are known to exhibit enhanced sensitivity when afferent signals are lost.[14–17] Thalamic hyperactivity has been identified as a correlate of deafferentation pain in a feline

Disclosures: None.

Department of Neurological Surgery, University Hospitals Case Medical Center, 11100 Euclid Avenue, Cleveland, OH 44106, USA

* Corresponding author.

E-mail address: jonathan.miller@uhhospitals.org

model, and MCS has been shown to normalize this to a greater degree than stimulation of the primary somatosensory cortex.[3] However, the precise pathway involved remains elusive.

INDICATIONS AND PATIENT SELECTION

Most reports of successful pain control using MCS involve deafferentation owing to some form of neurologic injury. This includes post-stroke pain,[3] trigeminal neuropathic pain/anesthesia dolorosa,[5] post-herpetic neuralgia,[18] multiple sclerosis,[19] phantom limb pain,[20,21] spinal cord injury,[22,23] brachial plexus lesions,[24] pelvic pain,[25] and complex regional pain syndrome.[10] As with any invasive treatment, patients should have failed maximal medical management before MCS is considered. Before surgery, patients should undergo a pain psychology screening.

MCS has proven to be an effective treatment option in many refractory pain syndromes. However, when counseling patients, it should be remembered that the percentage of patients who achieve good long-term pain control remains suboptimal with current techniques, and it is difficult to predict who will respond well. In addition to a standard discussion regarding the risks and benefits of the procedure, patients should also be counseled regarding the frequent need for reprogramming sessions.

OPERATIVE TECHNIQUE

1. Positioning. Patients are placed under general anesthesia with intubation and positioned supine in a Mayfield head holder with the head turned contralateral (**Fig. 1**). A shoulder roll is used if the patient's habitus requires it.
2. Preoperative medications. Routine surgical antibiotic prophylaxis is administered before incision.

3. Incision. Preoperative magnetic resonance imaging (MRI) is used with frameless stereotaxy for intraoperative navigation, allowing the surgeon to create a small incision overlying the relevant portion of the precentral gyrus.
4. Craniotomy. Two burr holes are created and connected to create a small crantiotomy over the precentral gyrus.
5. Localization and Implantation. The central sulcus is localized by the presence of N20-P20 phase reversal on median nerve somatosensory evoked potentials. A 2 × 4, 8-contact paddle electrode is placed in the epidural space overlying the facial or upper extremity region of the motor cortex. The electrode is then used for motor evoked potentials with electromyography to confirm motor activity. Iced saline is prepared for irrigation if a seizure is induced. The minimum thresholds for motor activity and any seizure activity are noted. After confirmation, a paddle electrode is sutured to the dura over the precentral gyrus over the motor area that corresponds to the patient's pain distribution.
6. Closure. Leads are tunneled and externalized using percutaneous extensions. The inner table of the bone flap is thinned to allow for the increased mass effect from the paddle electrode as well as an exiting site for the electrode leads. The incision is closed in layers, and a sterile dressing is applied to the externalized leads.
7. Stimulation parameters and trial. Optimal pain relief is usually noted with fairly low frequency and high pulse width. Initial stimulation parameters are 50 Hz with 450 μsec pulse width. If any intraoperative after discharges are noted, maximal voltage is set at 70% of the after discharge threshold. Otherwise, maximal voltage is set at 70% of the voltage required for

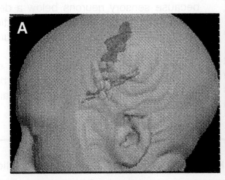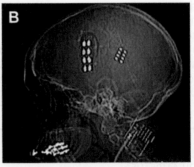

Fig. 1. (*A*) Surface rendering of preoperative magnetic resonance imaging showing central sulcus (*pink*), sylvian fissure (*blue*), and planned electrode (*green*) and contact (*yellow*) positions. (*B*) Postoperative lateral scout view of a computed tomography of the head. Metallic artifact from the implanted electrode shows good correlation with preoperative planning.

motor unit action potentials on electromyography. Our current practice is to perform electrode implantation at the start of the week and allow the patient to the end of the week to detect a significant difference in symptomatology. Given the high rate of programming changes and the wide variance of interpatient stimulation parameters, implantation of the IPG is performed at the end of the week if the patient has any improvement in his or her symptoms.

LOCALIZATION OF THE PRIMARY MOTOR CORTEX

Accurate localization of the primary motor cortex (Brodmann area 4) can be performed with a multitude of techniques. Anatomically, the central sulcus is easily identifiable because it does not connect to any other sulcus. The postcentral sulcus lies posteriorly and is identified by its connection with the intraparietal sulcus, which runs perpendicularly toward the occipital lobe. The precentral sulcus lies anteriorly, which is frequently bisected into the inferior precentral sulcus and superior precentral sulcus. The central sulcus can be visualized on MRI as the superficial sulcus just anterior to the prominent cingulate sulcus. The precentral sulcus can be visualized on MRI by observing its connection with the superior frontal sulcus on an high axial image and the inferior frontal sulcus on a lateral sagittal image. Landmarks can assist in estimating the somatotopic organization of the precentral gyrus. When viewed on axial images, the "omega sign" describes the appearance of a knoblike structure that maps to the hand region of the precentral gyrus.[26] The upper extremity is usually represented posterior to the middle frontal gyrus, the face is represented in an area between the inferior frontal sulcus and the sylvian fissure, and the lower extremity is represented medially from the convexity onto the paracentral lobule. When these landmarks are combined with modern MRI techniques, frameless stereotaxy can allow the surgeon to plan the incision and craniotomy locations precisely.

There are multiple functional techniques to confirm the location of the central sulcus and precentral gyrus as well as the somatotopy of the precentral gyrus. Somatosensory evoked potentials, generated by stimulation of the median or ulnar nerves, are well known to neurosurgeons. Observation of the N20–P20 phase reversal confirms the location of the central sulcus. Motor evoked potentials allow for identification of the somatotopic organization of the precentral gyrus. The location with the lowest motor threshold for a given anatomic region is considered to be the somatotopic localization of that region. Identification of the motor threshold also assists with determination of programming parameters to maximize pain control while minimizing seizures from exceeding motor thresholds.

Functional MRI (fMRI) has been used to confirm somatotopy of the motor cortex, and it can be useful in cases of severe motor deficit or amputation where the often partially remapped motor cortex can be established by fMRI.[20] Mogilner and Rezai described a multimodality technique that utilizes frameless MRI with fiducials, fMRI, somatosensory evoked potentials, motor evoked potentials, and magnetoencephalography.[27] Pirotte reported a case series comparing preoperative fMRI localization with intraoperative functional localization and showed excellent concordance between the techniques.[28,29] However, intraoperative functional localization with stimulation remains the gold standard. In modern neurosurgery, frameless stereotaxy is ubiquitous, easy to perform, and allows for accurate planning of a minimal incision and craniotomy.

VARIATIONS IN TECHNIQUE

The first descriptions of MCS were performed by placing epidural electrodes through a burr hole with only local anesthesia,[4,5] but more recent series report the use of small craniotomies to allow for improved intraoperative monitoring.[9,30,31] Both local anesthesia[9,22,32–35] and general anesthesia[6,8,20,23,28,36,37] have been described. Use of facial electromyography allows for confirmation of proper location. The stimulation amplitude necessary for clinical facial twitching can be determined postoperatively during the trial period.

Subdural electrode placement has been described by a few authors.[12,18,38] Initially, there was concern that individuals with increased spaces in cerebrospinal fluid, such as the elderly, would not have a good response to epidural stimulation, although evidence for this concern is lacking. Subdural placement is associated with greater energy efficiency, but also an increased rate of complications, including subdural hematomas and a higher reported rate of seizures with subdural placement.[39] Overall response rates between subdural and epidural placements are similar, although opening of the dura may be necessary for coverage of lower extremity pain, which requires placement of an electrode along the medial part of the hemisphere, with about one half of cases reporting lower extremity coverage used subdural electrodes. The overall efficacy of pain control was similar to the efficacy of electrodes positioned in the upper extremity or facial regions.[39]

A multitude of stimulation parameters have been reported for MCS. Most authors report using an empiric starting voltage or starting at a set percentage of the seizure threshold recorded during intraoperative testing. Pain relief has been reported with frequencies from 5 to 130 Hz, pulse widths from 60 to 450 μsec, and amplitudes from 0.5 to 10 V, so considerable trial and error may be necessary to identify empirically the ideal stimulation parameters.[40] In 1 study of intensive reprogramming for recapturing, the average amplitude giving pain relief was 5 V. Three of the 6 patients had seizures during programming sessions with a mean seizure threshold of 8.9 V.[40]

CLINICAL OUTCOMES

In 1 metaanalysis of the over 200 reported cases of MCS for chronic neuropathic pain,[41] 56.7% of all implanted patients were found to have a good postoperative outcome, defined as greater than 50% reduction in pain. Overall success rates are somewhat higher for facial pain (68%) than for central pain (54%),[41] although individual reports for trigeminal neuropathic pain report successful pain relief in as many as 85%.[39] Although most patients do not perceive stimulation, there is frequently a significant placebo effect; as many as 35% of patients obtain relief during the trial period without stimulation, and sometimes patients are unaware that the device is turned off or malfunctioning.[8,23]

Duration of treatment response is always a concern in the treatment of chronic pain. In 1 series of MCS for neuropathic facial pain, only 5 of 8 patients who had immediate relief continued to do well at 6 months, but those 5 continued to experience relief at a mean of 33 months of follow-up.[32] Patients who achieved long-term relief were more likely to have idiopathic trigeminal neuropathic pain rather than trigeminal deafferentation pain owing to intentional nerve injury and were more likely to require multiple programming sessions.[32] Other reports have identified similar proportions of immediate and long-term responders.[5,9]

PREDICTORS OF OUTCOME

Multiple authors have searched for prognostic factors to improve patient selection, but this topic remains controversial. Several series have suggested that there is a direct correlation between MCS efficacy and the degree of remaining motor function[8,42] or sensory function.[43] However, other studies have not confirmed these findings. Some studies have also suggested improved outcomes in patients whose pain responds to thiopental and poor improvement with opiates,[44] whereas others have suggested ketamine sensitivity may be predictive of MCS efficacy.[12]

Emerging data suggest that repetitive transcranial magnetic stimulation may provide a noninvasive way to screen patients. A recent study retrospectively analyzed 59 patients who underwent active or sham repetitive transcranial magnetic stimulation before MCS implantation.[45] Repetitive transcranial magnetic stimulation showed a very good positive predictive value (79%) but a poor negative predictive value (35%). As a result, it is uncertain whether this screening test would be able to exclude patients as appropriate candidates for MCS.

COMPLICATIONS AND CONCERNS

Reports of MCS have demonstrated favorable complication rates, with an overall complication rate of about 5%. The majority of reported complications consist of common perioperative issues seen in functional neurosurgery, such as wound breakdown or infection (5.1%),[41] hardware breakage from trauma,[8] and seizures (12%).[41]

Stimulation of the motor cortex is known to be associated with the potential to induce seizures, and most seizures observed during MCS occur during programming sessions. In 1 report, a patient was noted to have a very low stimulation-induced seizure threshold associated with a perioperative cortical venous infarct that also produced resulting right hemiparesis and aphasia.[46] The risk of developing epilepsy after MCS is very low, although it has been reported.[47]

As with most functional neurosurgery procedures, the most serious complications of MCS involve intracranial hemorrhage in the epidural or subdural spaces, depending on the implantation site. Epidural hematomas can produce speech difficulties and require evacuation when large.[5,30,48] Subdural hemorrhages can produce significant morbidity; in 2 such cases, 1 patient's function was reduced to a persistent vegetative state and the other died.[11]

SUMMARY

MCS is well tolerated and can be an effective treatment option in patients with deafferentation pain syndromes. It has been used successfully in pain disorders that are otherwise extraordinarily difficult to treat. More than 200 cases have been reported in the literature, with about a general efficacy of about 50%. The majority of treated patients have central pain syndrome; however, patients with neuropathic facial pain have reported the greatest benefit. After localization of the precentral gyrus, the electrode is implanted and patients undergo a stimulation trial. If the trial is successful, a pulse generator is implanted. Rare serious events have been reported, but most complications consist of well-known issues with chronically implanted hardware in functional neurosurgery.

REFERENCES

1. Penfield W, Jasper HH. Epilepsy and the functional anatomy of the human brain. New York: Little Brown & Company; 1954.
2. Hosobuchi Y. Subcortical electrical stimulation for control of intractable pain in humans. Report of 122 cases (1970-1984). J Neurosurg 1986;64:543–53.
3. Tsubokawa T, Katayama Y, Yamamoto T, et al. Chronic motor cortex stimulation in patients with thalamic pain. Neuroscience 1993;55:643–51.
4. Tsubokawa T, Katayama Y, Yamamoto T, et al. Chronic motor cortex stimulation for the treatment of central pain. Acta Neurochir Suppl (Wien) 1991; 52:137–9.
5. Meyerson BA, Lindblom U, Linderoth B, et al. Motor cortex stimulation as treatment of trigeminal neuropathic pain. Acta Neurochir Suppl (Wien) 1993;58: 150–3.
6. Brown JA, Pilitsis JG. Motor cortex stimulation for central and neuropathic facial pain: a prospective study of 10 patients and observations of enhanced sensory and motor function during stimulation. Neurosurgery 2005;56:290–7 [discussion: 290–7].
7. Burchiel KJ. A new classification for facial pain. Neurosurgery 2003;53:1164–6 [discussion: 1166–7].
8. Carroll D, Joint C, Maartens N, et al. Motor cortex stimulation for chronic neuropathic pain: a preliminary study of 10 cases. Pain 2000;84:431–7.
9. Ebel H, Rust D, Tronnier V, et al. Chronic precentral stimulation in trigeminal neuropathic pain. Acta Neurochir (Wien) 1996;138:1300–6.
10. Fonoff ET, Hamani C, Ciampi de Andrade D, et al. Pain relief and functional recovery in patients with complex regional pain syndrome after motor cortex stimulation. Stereotact Funct Neurosurg 2011;89: 167–72.
11. Saitoh Y, Yoshimine T. Stimulation of primary motor cortex for intractable deafferentation pain. Acta Neurochir Suppl (Wien) 2007;97:51–6.
12. Saitoh Y, Kato A, Ninomiya H, et al. Primary motor cortex stimulation within the central sulcus for treating deafferentation pain. Acta Neurochir Suppl (Wien) 2003;87:149–52.
13. Saitoh Y, Shibata M, Hirano S, et al. Motor cortex stimulation for central and peripheral deafferentation pain. Report of eight cases. J Neurosurg 2000;92: 150–5.
14. Guenot M, Bullier J, Rospars JP, et al. Single-unit analysis of the spinal dorsal horn in patients with neuropathic pain. J Clin Neurophysiol 2003;20(2): 143–50.
15. Jeanmonod D, Sindou M, Mauguière F. Intraoperative electrophysiological recordings during microsurgical DREZ-tomies in man. Stereotact Funct Neurosurg 1990;54–55:80–5.
16. Ovelmen-Levitt J, Johnson B, Bedenbaugh P, et al. Dorsal root rhizotomy and avulsion in the cat: a comparison of long term effects on dorsal horn neuronal activity. Neurosurgery 1984;15(6):921–7.
17. Davis KD, Kiss ZH, Tasker RR, et al. Thalamic stimulation-evoked sensations in chronic pain patients and in nonpain (movement disorder) patients. J Neurophysiol 1996;75(3):1026–37.
18. Esfahani DR, Pisansky MT, Dafer RM, et al. Motor cortex stimulation: functional magnetic resonance imaging–localized treatment for three sources of intractable facial pain. J Neurosurg 2011;114:189–95.
19. Tanei T, Kajita Y, Wakabayashi T. Motor cortex stimulation for intractable neuropathic facial pain related to multiple sclerosis. Neurol Med Chir (Tokyo) 2010; 50:604–7.
20. Roux FE, Ibarrola D, Lazorthes Y, et al. Chronic motor cortex stimulation for phantom limb pain: a functional magnetic resonance imaging study: technical case report. Neurosurgery 2001;48:681–7 [discussion: 687–8].
21. Saitoh Y, Shibata M, Sanada Y, et al. Motor cortex stimulation for phantom limb pain. Lancet 1999;353:212.
22. Nguyen JP, Lefaucheur JP, Decq P, et al. Chronic motor cortex stimulation in the treatment of central and neuropathic pain. Correlations between clinical, electrophysiological and anatomical data. Pain 1999;82:245–51.
23. Nuti C, Peyron R, Garcia-Larrea L, et al. Motor cortex stimulation for refractory neuropathic pain: four year outcome and predictors of efficacy. Pain 2005;118: 43–52.
24. Ali M, Saitoh Y, Oshino S, et al. Differential efficacy of electric motor cortex stimulation and lesioning of the dorsal root entry zone for continuous vs paroxysmal pain after brachial plexus avulsion. Neurosurgery 2011;68(5):1252–7 [discussion: 1257–8].
25. Louppe JM, Nguyen JP, Robert R, et al. Motor cortex stimulation in refractory pelvic and perineal pain: report of two successful cases. Neurourol Urodyn 2013;32:53–7.
26. Yousry TA, Schmid UD, Alkadhi H, et al. Localization of the motor hand area to a knob on the precentral gyrus. A new landmark. Brain 1997;120(Pt 1):141–57.
27. Mogilner AY, Rezai AR. Epidural motor cortex stimulation with functional imaging guidance. Neurosurg Focus 2001;11:E4.

28. Pirotte B, Neugroschl C, Metens T, et al. Comparison of functional MR imaging guidance to electrical cortical mapping for targeting selective motor cortex areas in neuropathic pain: a study based on intraoperative stereotactic navigation. AJNR Am J Neuroradiol 2005;26:2256–66.

29. Rainov NG, Fels C, Heidecke V, et al. Epidural electrical stimulation of the motor cortex in patients with facial neuralgia. Clin Neurol Neurosurg 1997;99:205–9.

30. Nguyen JP, Keravel Y, Feve A, et al. Treatment of deafferentation pain by chronic stimulation of the motor cortex: report of a series of 20 cases. Acta Neurochir Suppl (Wien) 1997;68:54–60.

31. Nguyen JP, Lefaucheur JP, Le Guerinel C, et al. Motor cortex stimulation in the treatment of central and neuropathic pain. Arch Med Res 2000;31:263–5.

32. Raslan AM, Nasseri M, Bahgat D, et al. Motor cortex stimulation for trigeminal neuropathic or deafferentation pain: an institutional case series experience. Stereotact Funct Neurosurg 2011;89:83–8.

33. Rainov NG, Heidecke V. Motor cortex stimulation for neuropathic facial pain. Neurol Res 2003;25:157–61.

34. Sharan AD, Rosenow JM, Turbay M, et al. Precentral stimulation for chronic pain. Neurosurg Clin N Am 2003;14:437–44.

35. Son UC, Kim MC, Moon DE, et al. Motor cortex stimulation in a patient with intractable complex regional pain syndrome type II with hemibody involvement. Case report. J Neurosurg 2003;98:175–9.

36. Saitoh Y, Hirano S, Kato A, et al. Motor cortex stimulation for deafferentation pain. Neurosurg Focus 2001;11:E1.

37. Velasco M, Velasco F, Brito F, et al. Motor cortex stimulation in the treatment of deafferentation pain. I. Localization of the motor cortex. Stereotact Funct Neurosurg 2002;79:146–67.

38. Delavallée M, Abu-Serieh B, de Tourchaninoff M, et al. Subdural motor cortex stimulation for central and peripheral neuropathic pain: a long-term follow-up study in a series of eight patients. Neurosurgery 2008;63:101–5 [discussion: 105–8].

39. Monsalve G. Motor cortex stimulation for facial chronic neuropathic pain: a review of the literature. Surg Neurol Int 2012;3:290.

40. Henderson JM, Boongird A, Rosenow JM, et al. Recovery of pain control by intensive reprogramming after loss of benefit from motor cortex stimulation for neuropathic pain. Stereotact Funct Neurosurg 2004;82:207–13.

41. Fontaine D, Hamani C, Lozano A. Efficacy and safety of motor cortex stimulation for chronic neuropathic pain: critical review of the literature. J Neurosurg 2009;110:251–6.

42. Katayama Y, Fukaya C, Yamamoto T. Poststroke pain control by chronic motor cortex stimulation: neurological characteristics predicting a favorable response. J Neurosurg 1998;89:585–91.

43. Drouot X, Nguyen JP, Peschanski M, et al. The antalgic efficacy of chronic motor cortex stimulation is related to sensory changes in the painful zone. Brain 2002;125:1660–4.

44. Yamamoto T, Katayama Y, Hirayama T, et al. Pharmacological classification of central post-stroke pain: comparison with the results of chronic motor cortex stimulation therapy. Pain 1997;72:5–12.

45. Lefaucheur JP, Ménard-Lefaucheur I, Goujon C, et al. Predictive value of rTMS in the identification of responders to epidural motor cortex stimulation therapy for pain. J Pain 2011;12:1102–11.

46. Moro E, Schwalb JM, Piboolnurak P, et al. Unilateral subdural motor cortex stimulation improves essential tremor but not Parkinson's disease. Brain 2011;134:2096–105.

47. Bezard E, Boraud T, Nguyen JP, et al. Cortical stimulation and epileptic seizure: a study of the potential risk in primates. Neurosurgery 1999;45:346–50.

48. Messina G, Cordella R, Dones I, et al. Improvement of secondary fixed dystonia of the upper limb after chronic extradural motor cortex stimulation in 10 patients: first reported series. Neurosurgery 2012;70:1169–75 [discussion: 1175].

Dorsal Root Entry Zone Lesion, Midline Myelotomy and Anterolateral Cordotomy

Peter Konrad, MD, PhD

KEYWORDS

- DREZ • Spinal cord • Cordotomy • Myelotomy • Pain

KEY POINTS

- Dorsal root entry zone lesioning is excellent for brachial plexus avulsion pain (54%–91% pain relief), "end-zone" spinal cord injury pain, and inoperable upper thoracic tumors that compress the brachial plexus.
- Open cordotomy is excellent for unilateral lower extremity pain due to malignancies, such as sarcoma of the hip and legs. Poor results for chronic, nonmalignant pain (such as spinal cord injury–related pain).
- Percutaneous cordotomy is excellent for pain related to malignancy in the lower quadrant, including abdominal wall, pelvic bone, and lower extremity (such as carcinomas and sarcomas invading the lower quadrant).
- Patients with visceral pain due to abdominal or pelvic malignancies are ideal candidates for midline myelotomy.

INTRODUCTION: NATURE OF THE PROBLEM

The goal of this article was to summarize the relevant anatomy and physiology of pain transmission into the spinal cord through the dorsal root entry zone (DREZ) and subsequently in the spinal cord, and in using this knowledge, to select appropriate patients for appropriate lesioning of the DREZ or spinal cord in the treatment of a variety of pain syndromes. Furthermore, details regarding operative technique from the author's experience should aid the reader in optimizing the outcomes and minimizing complications in appropriately selected patients for such procedures.

Clinical Anatomy of Pain Conduction in the Spinal Cord

Details regarding the anatomy and physiology of pain perception and transmission in the nervous system are discussed elsewhere in this text. The following section is a summary of the pertinent concepts when considering whether lesioning of the spinal cord would be appropriate in treating a painful condition. In our experience, the treatment of chronic pain is best optimized when the physician first understands the etiology of the pain and then arrives at an anatomic localization of the generator for the pain. Through understanding the exact character of the pain and its location, the

Disclosure Statement: The author has no disclosures related to this article.
Portions of this article appeared as Konrad P, Caputi F, El-Naggar AO. Radiofrequency dorsal root entry zone lesions for pain. Textbook of stereotactic and functional neurosurgery. 2009. p. 2251–68.
Functional Neurosurgery, Neurological Surgery and Biomedical Engineering, Vanderbilt University, Nashville, TN, USA
E-mail address: peter.konrad@vanderbilt.edu

surgeon can then make a thoughtful judgment as to whether the pain is, first of all, accessible, and second, where to make the lesion or pursue other forms of treatment, such as neuromodulation or pharmacotherapy. Furthermore, experienced surgeons then are able to weigh the accessibility of whether spinal cord lesions would have a reasonable chance of producing significant pain relief versus the potential complications that might be encountered with this procedure.

Spinal cord lesioning procedures are particularly suited for management of *somatic pain*, that is, painful sensation mediated through the spinothalamic tract. This is due to the discrete anatomy associated with pain mediated through the somatosensory pathways of the spinal cord. Although visceral pathways are also mediated through the spinal cord, alternate pathways through the autonomic nervous system and cranial nerves make it difficult to provide significant pain relief only through spinal cord–based procedures. Understanding the differences in the functional anatomy of these 2 types of pain is essential to success with patient selection and surgical outcomes.

Anatomy of pain pathways in the spinal cord

Several methods of classification of pain pathways in the spinal cord have been published.[1–5] One classification process is based on the physiologic understanding of the modality of pain transmission, namely nociceptive versus non-nociceptive pain fibers.[4,5] This classification distinguishes the pathways mediating pain generated by noxious stimuli (nociception) or non-noxious stimuli. This differentiation allows the surgeon to (1) differentiate whether transmission of painful sensation occurs primarily through somatic pain pathways mediated by the dorsal horn or whether alternate pain-enhancing pathways (for example mechanical or temperature sensitivity) are also involved, (2) whether appropriate medical therapy or other interventional therapy has been tried, and (3) what the potential prognosis for lesioning such pain pathways will be for a given patient. **Fig. 1** illustrates the nociceptive and other pain pathways as they enter the DREZ on cross-section of the spinal cord. This anatomy holds true for cervical, thoracic, and lumbar segments, but with different proportions.[3,6–10] Several anatomic features are worth noting from a surgical standpoint: (1) as fibers enter the dorsal horn, large fibers of proprioception are located medially, large myotactic fibers are located in the middle of the dorsal root, and smaller (C) fibers associated with nociception, autonomic function, and light touch are located on the lateral edge of the entry zone; (2) the Lissauer

tract is located immediately lateral to the DREZ and is responsible for longitudinal transmission of nociceptive information at least 2 segments superior and inferior to the point of entry into the cord; (3) the corticospinal tract, responsible for voluntary control motor function, is located in the white matter immediately lateral to the DREZ and dorsal to the dentate ligament; and (4) most nociceptive and other small diameter fibers synapse within Rexed lamina I to V of the dorsal horn of the spinal cord.

The lateral spinothalamic tract (STT) is the primary conductor of nociceptive information to the contralateral thalamus. Although the second-order neurons are mostly located in the dorsal horn of the cord, most projections of these neurons cross the midline just anterior to the central canal and then collect in the white matter tract of the SST located near the anterior, lateral spinal cord surface (**Fig. 2**). Understanding the exact location of where lesions should be performed depends on whether interruption of somatic pain pathways needs to be limited to a unilateral extremity or bilaterally.

Transmission of nociceptive information crosses the midline in the anterior commissure, and therefore represents a location by which bilateral conduction of painful sensation can be addressed in a single location in the spinal cord (see **Figs. 1** and **2**). The anterior commissure of the spinal cord is located just anterior to the central canal, deep within the interior of the spinal cord. Within a few millimeters and abutting the anterior surface of the spinal cord is the anterior spinal artery, an important anatomic landmark to respect when making lesions in the anterior spinal cord region.

Some additional anatomic concepts are unique to each lesioning procedure and worth mentioning next.

Unilateral limb pain and the DREZ

Success with DREZ lesioning is typically thought of for unilateral limb pain. Although bilateral DREZ procedures can be performed successfully, the anatomic concepts relate to pathology of the first-order neuron due to either deafferentation or miscommunication of nociceptive information in each DREZ as a separate pathologic entity. For conceptual simplicity, DREZ lesioning can be thought of as a treatment for pain that is believed to be confined to a unilateral limb. Understanding how and where pain is mediated on immediate entry into the dorsal aspect of the spinal cord helps the surgeon to know exactly how to place the lesion precisely with the most efficacy and least morbidity.

A

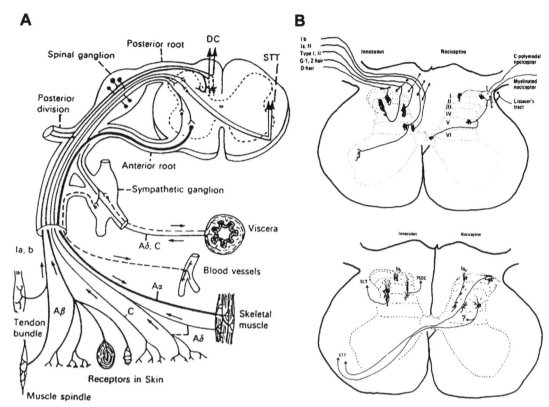

B

Fig. 1. Cross-sectional diagram of the spinal cord, illustrating the relevant histologic components related to the DREZ. (*A*) Nociceptive information is carried in C-type fibers along with other pain-related phenomena, such as thermal and cutaneous mechanoreceptive information, which typically enter the dorsal root entry zone in the lateral aspect of the rootlet. First-order neurons in the dorsal ganglion mediating nociceptive information synapse ipsilaterally with second-order neurons in Rexed lamina I to V. Large A-type fibers, which carry proprioceptive information from Golgi tendon organs or intrafuscal stretch receptors, are located in the medial aspect of the root entry zone and project up the cord ipsilaterally to their respective cervical nuclei (n. cuneatus and n. gracilus). (*B*) Nociceptive information associated with first-order neurons located in the dorsal root ganglion project to Rexed lamina I to V either in the same segment of entry or adjacent spinal cord segments in the Lissauer tract, located immediately lateral to lamina I to II. ([*A*] *From* Bonica JJ. Anatomic and physiologic basis of nociception and pain. In: Bonica JJ, editor. The management of pain. 2nd edition. vol. 1. Philadelphia: Lea and Febiger; 1990. p. 28–94; and [*B*] *Modified from* Light AR. Normal anatomy and physiology of the spinal cord dorsal horn. Appl Neurophysiol 1988;51(2–5):78–88.)

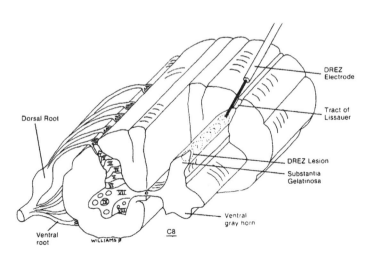

Fig. 2. Longitudinal diagram of the spinal cord, illustrating the relevant tract anatomy and relationship of the gray matter to tract location and blood supply. Angle of approach to DREZ lesions is slightly greater in the cervical (35° 106) than thoracic or lumbar-sacral segments. Also, note the proximity and somatotopic arrangement of the corticospinal tract and dorsal columns to the DREZ. The Lissauer tract is thought to mediate nociception into adjacent spinal segments as much as 2 segments from the point of entry into the DREZ. (*Modified from* Nashold B, Pearlstein R. The DREZ operation. Park Ridge (IL): The American Association of Neurological Surgeons; 1996.)

The arrival of nociceptive information into the spinal cord splits and either synapses in the dorsal horn (Rexed lamina I to V) or projects along the longitudinal axis of the spinal cord via the Lissauer tract. The Lissauer tract is a key pathway that conducts nociceptive information at least 2 segments above and below the DREZ (see **Fig. 2**A). Through this tract, the first-order neurons synapse with multiple segments of the spinal cord and distribute nociceptive information to nearby somatic zones that are involved in reflexive behavior.[11] However, it blurs the margin of nociceptive information, leading to a less distinct border of a painful zone described by the patient.[12–15] It is important, thus, for surgeons who contemplate the extent of DREZ lesioning to understand that up to 2 segments above and below a specific dermatomal segment may be involved in nociceptive transmission.

Another important anatomic concept to keep in mind is the relationship of the dorsal horn to adjacent white matter tracts (**Fig. 3**), and that these dimensions change throughout the spinal cord.[7,16–18] The following are important concepts: (1) the angle of the dorsal horn with respect to the sagittal axis is greater in the cervical enlargement (35°[7]) of the cord than in the lumbar-sacral enlargement (approximately 20°); (2) lateral to the dorsal horn is the corticospinal tract organized somatopically, with cervical, thoracic, and lumbar fibers arranged in a medial-to-lateral direction; and (3) the dorsal columns that are medial to the dorsal horn are organized with converse somatotopy, namely cervical proprioceptive fibers are lateral to lower extremity fibers. These relationships mean the following to the surgeon contemplating a lesion of the DREZ. If dorsal root fibers are

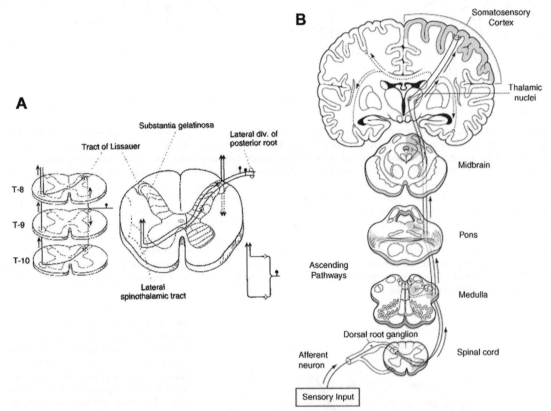

Fig. 3. (*A*) Divergence of cutaneous nociceptive information. Some projections of the first-order neuron (dorsal root ganglion) ascend or descend 1 or 2 segments ipsilaterally in the spinal cord via the Lissauer tract. The remaining projections usually synapse in the dorsal horn on Rexed lamina I to IV at the same segmental level. The second-order neurons then project typically to the contralateral spinothalamic tract located in the anterior lateral cord via the anterior commissure. (*B*) Schematic diagram of third-order neuron model of nociception transmission of somatic pain to the cortex. Note that the decussation of pain information occurs at the spinal segmental levels that innervate the cutaneous region. Therefore, treatment through either DREZ or myelotomy occurs at the same segmental level of peripheral innervation, but cordotomy must be performed contralaterally to the side of innervation and at least several segments superior. (*From* [*A*] Bonica J. Then management of pain. 2nd edition. Philadelphia: Lea and Febiger; 1990; and [*B*] Schuenke, et al. THIEME atlas of anatomy. Head and neuroanatomy. New York: Thieme Medical Publishers; 2007.)

avulsed, as commonly seen in pain associated with brachial or lumbar-sacral plexus trauma, then deviating laterally from the DREZ may result in ipsilateral hemiparesis below the level of the lesion.[19–22] Alternatively, if lesions deviate too medially from the DREZ, loss of proprioception may occur. These risks should be included in the consideration of this procedure.[23]

Unilateral limb/truncal pain and cordotomy

The advantage to lesioning the STT by cordotomy is to address the collective transmission of nociception entirely below the level of the lesion.[24,25] Cordotomy is most useful in addressing malignant pain; however, success for other types of nonmalignant pain also has been reported.[26] Consequently, the surgeon needs to decide whether the pain involves more than a specific region of the plexus in a limb. For example, although DREZ lesioning may address severe pain in the upper extremity (whether due to trauma or cancer) as high as the shoulder area, a cordotomy performed in the contralateral upper cervical STT will create significant numbness and dysesthesia in the arm and entire trunk and leg. This may be the desired outcome in a patient with cancer of the upper limb and trunk, but not in someone with a brachial plexus avulsion. *In general, patients who experience severe pain that originates from cancer involving the pelvis, leg, hip, and lower trunk are ideal candidates for a cordotomy procedure (whether open or percutaneous).*

The relevant anatomy to performing an open or percutaneous cordotomy lies in understanding the discrete somatotopy of the STT as it ascends the spinal cord. Several important concepts are evident:

- The STT lies just anterior to the dentate ligament and near the anterolateral surface of the cord.
- The anterior spinal artery is a significant vascular structure whose midline position must be appreciated and avoided during open transection of the STT.
- The corticospinal tract lies dorsal to the dentate ligament and should not be injured by either approach to the anterior half of the cord.
- The sacral fibers lie closest to the surface and posterior in the STT, followed by lumbar, thoracic, and cervical fibers located progressively more anterior and deeply.
- The levels of adequate pain control are several levels below the lesion; C1/2 percutaneous cordotomy can reach as high as C5, a T4 open cordotomy will result in T10 analgesia.[27]

These concepts are used to identify the location of the STT in the cervical region by either injecting contrast or performing high-resolution computed tomography (CT) scans to locate the dentate ligament and subsequently define the anterior quadrant of the intended lesion. It is imperative to know that the lesion is made anterior to the dentate ligament so as to avoid damaging the corticospinal tract. Also, the lower extremity pain fibers are located more closely to the dentate ligament and superficially. Hence, when performing awake test stimulation before radiofrequency lesioning of the cervical STT, insertion of the lesioning electrode just anterior to the dentate ligament will first produce paresthesia in the contralateral lower extremity first and advances rostral as the electrode is inserted deeper and more anterior into the STT.

Percutaneous cordotomy procedures are performed at the C1/2 interspace typically due to the ease of access to the anterior half of the spinal cord through a direct lateral approach with image guidance.[28] However, the anatomy must be visualized through either contrast injection with fluoroscopic guidance or CT guidance. Test stimuli confirm the location of the STT to the surgeon, and therefore the patient needs to be awake at least for this confirmatory test before lesioning. Other critical anatomic structures are nearby in the upper cervical region that can create serious or fatal complications, including respiratory interneurons near the intermediate gray matter, cardiovascular and sympathetic tracts, and the vertebral artery and its branches. Nonetheless, many neurosurgeons have learned this anatomy well and the overall complication rates for experienced surgeons performing cordotomies was well under 5% in large series.[29–31]

Open cordotomy requires being aware of additional anatomic structures that may be encountered while creating the anterolateral quadrant lesion. In particular, the lesion will usually extend medially into the interior of the gray matter and then anterior to encompass the spinocerebellar tracts. Sectioning the anterior gray matter will result in segmental loss of motor neuron innervation, which is well tolerated in the thoracic region but not in the cervical region.

Special attention must be given to any bilateral high cervical lesions for pain because of the presence of the respiratory drive neurons located immediately medial to the lateral spinothalamic tract (**Fig. 4**).[32,33] Although unilateral lesions at C1/2 are well tolerated and associated with a low frequency of respiratory complications, bilateral high cervical cordotomy lesions escalate the risk for respiratory complications significantly.[33]

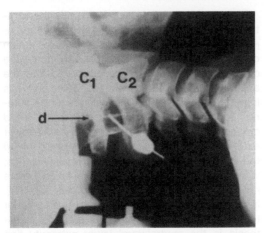

Fig. 4. Lateral radiograph showing percutaneous needle in position just anterior to the dentate ligament after dural puncture. Notice radiopaque contrast layering on top of the dentate ligament and the position of the needle just anterior to this in the C1-2 interspace. (*From* Lahuerta J, Lipton S, Wells JC. Percutaneous cervical cordotomy: results and complications in a recent series of 100 patients. Ann R Coll Surg Engl 1985;67(1):41–4.)

Abdominal/pelvic and bilateral lower extremity pain and midline myelotomy

The term midline myelotomy has evolved to encompass a midline lesion that may or may not involve the anterior commissure. Consequently, for discussion sake, commissurotomy will be used to discuss lesions involving the anterior commissure, and limited midline myelotomy will be used to discuss lesions involving just the dorsal columns.

Complete midline myelotomy (commissurotomy) is an attractive alternative to bilateral cordotomy because it addresses bilateral nociceptive pathways through a single midline incision (see **Fig. 1**). Projection of dorsal horn neurons to the contralateral spinothalamic tract cross anterior to the spinal canal either within the same segment or obliquely across several segments. Therefore, disruption of the anterior commissure should extend at least 2 to 3 levels surrounding the primary segmental level mediating the pain. For abdominal and pelvic pain, this would include the spinal cord segments from T10 to the conus.[34] When dividing the commissure from a posterior approach through the midline, it is necessary to divide the dorsal columns and should be done as close to the midline as possible so as to minimize deficits associated with loss of proprioception from dorsal column damage.

Neurosurgeons discovered that visceral pain relief was excellent in these patients in addition to the intended bilateral somatic pain reduction.

Some, like Mansuy and colleagues,[35] noted this effect despite poor coverage of the anterior commissure. Speculation began to emerge discussing the existence of a dorsal column visceral pain pathway. Willis and colleagues[36,37] eventually described the anatomic existence of a visceral pain pathway in the deep midline of the dorsal columns in animals, leading to the notion that interruption of this pathway alone would have an effect on visceral pain. A limited midline myelotomy that just lesions the dorsal columns and avoids cutting the anterior commissure was then described by Gildenberg and Hirshberg[38] in 1981 and then further reduced to a small transverse lesion by Nauta and colleagues[39] in 1997. This limited lesion only interrupts ascending pathways in the dorsal columns thought to mediate visceral pain. A nice personal perspective on the evolution of midline myelotomy procedures is provided by Gildenberg himself in 2001.[40]

Furthermore, on reaching the anterior sulcus of the cord, the commissure is divided and care must be exercised to avoid damaging the anterior spinal artery, which lies a few millimeters anterior.

Selection and Workup of Patients

Patients who are being considered for surgical lesioning for the treatment of pain, in general, should have failed more conservative management with medications. However, in cases of severe, debilitating pain that is poorly responsive to opioids or other forms of localized pain medication delivery (eg, neurolytic blocks), lesioning represents a highly effective neurosurgical therapy that returns significant quality of life to the patient. Ideally, the candidate who benefits most from a lesioning procedure versus medical management has *pain that is well localized to an accessible anatomic pathway for neurosurgical ablation or lesion*. Hence, understanding the spinal cord pathways of pain transmission, discussed previously, is requisite to proper patient selection and a desirable outcome. Many patients with severe pain related to cancer or trauma are willing to accept sensory deficits in exchange for significant pain relief; however, the skill of a neurosurgeon who selects a lesioning procedure for pain control is most evident when the loss of function is minimized as well as the pain. The following discussion reflects general principles and examples of appropriate patient selection for the 3 spinal cord lesioning procedures reviewed in this article: DREZ lesion, STT lesion (cordotomy), and midline myelotomy (commissurotomy).

Unilateral limb and plexus pain

Pain described in a unilateral limb or suggesting confinement to the plexus usually is best suited for DREZ lesioning. The pain needs to be primarily localized to the first-order neuron or the entry zone of the cord. Three types of patients are ideal candidates to consider for DREZ lesioning: traumatic brachial plexus injury, patients with segmental pain at the level of their spinal cord injury, and apical thoracic tumors (Pancoast tumor).[41] Additional details for each kind of patient are given in multiple other reviews.[20,41–44] However, the following are usually consistent findings that indicate candidacy for DREZ:

- Prickly or electric, shooting pain limited to the region of the plexus; or
- Partial or complete loss of sensation in the affected limb that may or may not be associated with motor loss in the same limb due to trauma; or
- Presence of pseudomeningocele seen on magnetic resonance imaging (MRI) or myelography of the affected spinal cord region associated with the trauma; or
- Presence of compressive lesion in the thoracic apex in proximity to or involving the inferior brachial plexus region; or
- Hyperpathia of the zone of transition between normal sensation and loss of sensation associated with spinal cord injury.

Findings that would indicate poor outcomes with DREZ include the following:

- Constant burning pain in the limb; or
- Presence of herpetic neuropathy; or
- Pain that extends outside the region of the limb, such as the shoulder, trunk, or pelvis; or
- Burning pain in the lower extremities that is well below the level of a spinal cord injury.

The anatomy of the spine as well as spinal cord should be known in patients before recommending a DREZ procedure. Typically an MRI or myelogram/CT of the region should be obtained to review spinal cord anatomy as well as bony defects that may be associated with previous surgeries or injury. Other extrinsic factors that contribute to the pain should be ruled out. Patients who describe pain that is worse with mechanical movement, slowly progressive sensory or motor deficits, "electric, shocklike" sensation with movement, or Lhermitte phenomenon have noncharacteristic neuropathic pain complaints. A thorough workup before offering a DREZ lesion would include determining the presence of mechanical instability, syringomyelia, compressive lesions (such as a herniated disc, hypertrophied ligamentum flavum,

or arachnoid cyst), or arachnoiditis. Even if the history suggests central neuropathic pain (burning, deep, steady pain at or below the level of the injury), an MRI of the affected region of the spine routinely obtained before surgery may prepare the surgeon for distorted anatomy that may be encountered with the planned exposure.

Unilateral lower quadrant pain

When pain extends beyond the leg and involves the hemipelvis and lower abdominal quadrant, a cordotomy is an excellent choice for surgical pain management. These patients are typically patients with cancer who have musculoskeletal involvement of the pelvis, hip joint, or thigh that creates pain well beyond the location of the lower extremity. Many times these patients have exhausted opioid analgesics, localized blocks or injections, or mechanical bracing. The neurosurgeon can make a significant impact on the comfort of these patients who are typically in the terminal phases of their disease with limited life expectancy.

Patients who have nonmalignant pain syndromes are not ideal candidates for either open or percutaneous cordotomy because of the recurrence rate of pain within a few years or the emergence of new central neuropathic pain (burning dysesthesias below the level of the lesion).[28] Patients with truncal herpetic neuropathy or lower extremity central neuropathic pain due to spinal cord injury, for instance, are better suited for more long-term neuromodulation therapies, such as intrathecal drug therapy or perhaps a neurostimulator implant (discussed elsewhere in this text).

Bilateral lower extremity pain or lower abdominal/pelvic pain

In patients with bilateral lower extremity pain and, in particular, with involvement of the pelvis and lower abdominal organs, a single lesion disconnecting the anterior commissure through a lower thoracic approach has been quite effective in relieving severe refractory pain. The typical patient is one with pelvic cancer or sarcoma that invades bilateral structures in the pelvis and lower extremities.[34] These patients can undergo a myelotomy with significant preservation of motor function, but may have reduced or lost bowel and bladder function. The lesion is elegant and effective in this population of patients and the loss of proprioception and potential bowel and bladder control may be acceptable to these patients who are otherwise bedridden with severe pain.

Most cases discussed for midline myelotomy are for patients with lower abdominal, pelvic, and lower extremity pain. However, patients who experience severe abdominal or pelvic pain due to malignancy appear to be ideal candidates for a limited division of only the dorsal columns so as to lesion the visceral pain pathways without interruption of the anterior commissure. Some patients with celiac region pain, associated with gastric or pancreatic cancer for example, undergo a limited high thoracic myelotomy with reasonably good outcomes.[45] Uterine and colorectal cancer pain also has been relieved by a limited dorsal myelotomy.[38,39] However, there is little literature discussing the value of this technique for thoracic cancer or mediastinal disease causing severe pain. The risks of respiratory and sympathetic damage (fibers located near the central gray matter) in creating a mid to upper cervical midline myelotomy are likely the reasons why this technique has not been used much for upper trunk and arm pain.

Surgical Technique

In general, one first must understand how many levels in particular should be involved in the lesion. **Fig. 5** illustrates the relationship between spinal nerve roots and vertebral levels. For DREZ lesioning, lesioning should encompass at least 2 levels above and below the involved segments. For cordotomy, effective analgesia occurs 3 to 4 levels contralateral to the lesion site. The same is true for midline myelotomy, namely the effect of the analgesia essentially begins 3 to 4 levels caudal to the lesioning site. Consequently, it is difficult to obtain adequate analgesia even with a C1 to percutaneous cordotomy above the level of C5.

Preoperative measures
Preoperative MRI or myelography and postmyelography CT scan can provide essential anatomic details regarding pseudomeningoceles, adhesions of the spinal cord, distorted spinal cord anatomy, or spinal deformities.[3,46–48] The value of such studies for each group of patients was highlighted previously. Steroids are commonly given at the beginning of the procedure to reduce postoperative spinal cord edema (eg, dexamethasone 6–10 mg intravenously [IV] every 6 hours tapered over a few days).

Approach laminectomy and durotomy for open procedures
Patients are positioned prone, under general anesthesia, and usually on a radiolucent table for fluoroscopic confirmation of vertebral levels. A hemilaminectomy that is performed for unilateral DREZ or open cordotomy lesions may reduce the likelihood of postlaminectomy kyphosis. This approach is appropriate for most cases in which no previous laminectomy has been performed; yet, it is much wiser to perform a standard

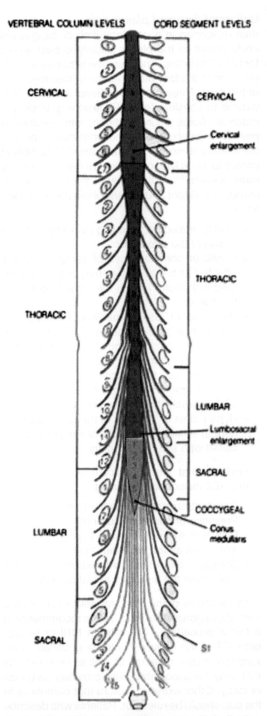

Fig. 5. Schematic of vertebral body versus spinal nerve root relationships. Notice the farther caudal one goes along the spinal axis, the greater the mismatch between spinal cord segment and vertebral body segment. Lesions placed in the cord should take into account the more rostral presence of spinal cord segments versus vertebral body segments.

laminectomy when intradural adhesions, syringomyelia, or distorted spinal cord anatomy are seen on preoperative imaging. For a unilateral DREZ or open cordotomy lesions, one can perform a hemilaminectomy with a high-speed drill exposing the dorsolateral spinal canal. For a bilateral DREZ lesion, a more standard laminectomy can be performed. The end result of the exposure needs to ensure that the appropriate spinal cord segments are exposed with an adequate opening to allow the dura to be reflected and the spinal cord visualized. Although the spinal cord segments align with vertebral segments in the cervical spine, inferiorly in the spine this relationship becomes discordant, and surgeons must make adjustments, as seen in **Fig. 5**.

If significant spinal cord injury has occurred, or if a midline myelotomy is planned, it is advisable to perform a bilateral laminectomy to ensure a view of both normal and abnormal anatomy. Use of the operating microscope with moderate to high-powered magnification is essential. Orientation of the midline, dorsal columns, vascular structures, dorsal rootlets, and dentate ligament all provide the neurosurgeon with appropriate entry landmarks and estimates of the location of the dorsal horn and corticospinal tract.[7] If the dura and arachnoid are opened separately, blood from decompression of the dura can be removed and controlled before it enters the subarachnoid space, reducing the potential for postoperative adhesions. Once the arachnoid is opened, an assistant who can continue to aspirate blood and cerebrospinal fluid (CSF) from the field is very helpful because it allows the neurosurgeon to maintain attention on the exact location and extent of the lesion as it occurs.

Closure of the arachnoid and dura can be accomplished in 1 layer with a fine suture (4-0 or 5-0). The use of dural sealants, such as thrombogenic derivatives (eg, Tisseel; Baxter, Deerfield, IL) or synthetic derivatives (eg, DuraSeal; Confluent Surgical, Waltham, MA) may reduce the incidence of CSF leak. Fascia and cutaneous closure are performed in routine fashion.

Postoperative care

Patients are typically observed closely in the intensive care unit for the first 24 hours for any new neurologic deficits, such as mild weakness or diminished proprioception inferior to the lesion. If new postoperative deficits emerge, urgent imaging with MRI or CT myelography is appropriate to rule out hematoma or other anatomic complications. Most patients, however, can be mobilized by the first postoperative day after an open cord lesioning procedure. To reduce likelihood for CSF leak, patients who underwent cervical or upper thoracic lesions are instructed to keep the head of the bed elevated at least 30°, whereas those who underwent thoracolumbar exposures are kept flat for 24 hours. Most patients are encourage to get out of bed by the first postoperative day and encouraged to mobilize. Dexamethasone in tapering amounts is usually administered over the course of several days, but may be prolonged if new deficits are encountered that may result from edema secondary to the lesion. Patients are mobilized typically on the first postoperative day. Pain management is converted from IV to oral medications in anticipation of discharge within 3 days postoperatively. Most patients who benefit from cord lesioning will notice significant pain reduction by the second postoperative day, and may require very little pain medication at the time of discharge.

Even though close attention is paid to reducing risk from intradural spinal cord surgery, complications, such as bowel and bladder dysfunction, CSF leak, infection, and hematoma formation, are rare. These complications are typical of surgery related to exposure of the spinal cord and closure of the wound. In addition, postlaminectomy kyphosis is more likely to occur in patients with multiple-level laminectomies that extend laterally into the facet joint or pars interarticularis and in patients with significant preexisting spondylosis.[49]

The following discussion is divided into each specific surgical technique for DREZ, cordotomy, and myelotomy.

DREZ Lesioning

The goal of DREZ lesioning is to create a selective destruction of neurons and fibers that enter the dorsal root entry zone. In 1979, Nashold and coworkers[50,51] first described DREZ microcoagulation for brachial plexus avulsion pain and soon thereafter for other conditions, such as spinal cord injury. **Fig. 6** illustrates the typical findings of a spinal cord injury in the lumbar region and the associated loss of innervation by the sensory rootlets in the dorsal part of the spinal cord. This figure illustrates the complexity of the anatomy typically involved in root avulsion and pain. Notice that the DREZ lesions follow along the dorsal lateral sulcus and an imaginary line from the T12 nerve root to the L2 nerve root seemed more caudally. Care should be taken to insert the DREZ electrode just lateral to the entry of the nerve root to be most effective in producing a lesion for both the segmental level of pain fibers as well as capturing the Lissauer tract. In this particular patient, who had spinal cord

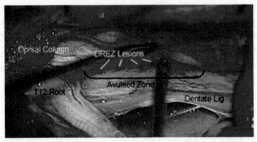

Fig. 6. Photograph of DREZ lesioning in the region of T12 to L2. Notice the avulsed nerve root segments extending throughout the L1 region of the spinal cord. The normal insertion of the T12 nerve root just rostral to the lesioning area indicates the general location of the dorsal lateral sulcus. Notice also the presence of the dentate ligament with respect to the midpoint of the cord. DREZ lesioning is carried out just lateral to the entry zone of the sensory nerve root, as seen by the probes present just lateral to the nerve root around L2.

injury, the pain was most noticeable in the L3 to 4 region of the thigh. Hence, the lesions are started just at the T12 nerve root level and extend caudal to the level of the injury below.

Fig. 5 illustrates the relationship of spinal nerve roots with vertebral segments. Notice that for the typical brachial plexus DREZ lesion, an exposure of the dorsal spinal cord from C4 to T1 will allow a view of the related dorsal roots (C5–T1).[3,7,52] For DREZ lesioning of the lower spinal cord related to spinal cord injury, it is advisable to expose at least 2 vertebral segments above the superior aspect of the painful zone. Typically, a bilateral laminectomy from T10 to L2 is performed for treatment of pain related to conus medullaris and cauda equina lesions.

Lesion location and technique

Fig. 7 shows the typical Nashold DREZ lesioning electrode and dimensions. Piercing the pia usually requires a sharp push, so as to minimize the deformation of the cord and minimize unwanted injury. The ideal location for the lesion should be at the lateral edge of the spinal rootlet as it enters the cord, where the nociceptive fibers are gathered (see preceding discussion of Clinical Anatomy of Pain Conduction in the Spinal Cord). The electrode should be inserted to the full depth of the exposed tip (2 mm), and in so doing, impedance measurements can be made to identify zones of injury.[53] Nashold and colleagues described low impedance values (approximately 500–1000 Ω) associated with areas of injury, versus 1200 to 2000 Ω for normal gray and white matter of the spinal cord, respectively. This may be useful in delineating the DREZ area and

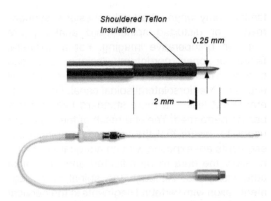

Fig. 7. The Nashold DREZ lesioning electrode for spinal lesioning procedures (Model NTCD; Cosman Medical, Burlington, MA). Note that the exposed tip measures 0.25 mm × 2 mm, thereby matching the appropriate depth necessary for most spinal cord applications. The electrode also contains a thermocouple, which allows for temperature measurement and feedback control for precise thermal lesioning when used with the Cosman lesion generator (RFG-1A; Cosman Medical). (*Courtesy of* Cosman Medical, Inc, Burlington, MA.)

avoiding deviating into adjacent spinal tracts. Somatosensory evoked potentials[54–56] and motor evoked potentials[57–59] may also aid in the identification of these adjacent tracts when there is significant anatomic distortion from previous injury. For cervical regions, the angle of the electrode is approximately 30° from midline, whereas in the lower thoracic region it is approximately 20°. The weight of the lesioning electrode is usually adequate to hold the electrode still without inadvertent dislodgement or movement during the brief lesion.

Lesions are made with the radiofrequency generator set to 75°C for 15 to 20 seconds.[52,60] This usually results in a 1 × 2-mm lesion.[61,62] The lesion is repeated down the length of the DREZ spaced approximately 1.0 to 1.5 mm apart, or essentially the width of the insulated end of the electrode. A typical unilateral DREZ procedure may result in a total of 40 to 60 lesions spanning 4 or more spinal cord segments.[19] Thus, an efficient DREZ lesioning technique requires a coordinated effort among the neurosurgeon, the surgical assistant, and the individual running the lesion generator. Once a lesion is created, a small tan discolored area is left or a small puncture is seen where the needle penetrated the cord (see **Fig. 6**). It is important to continually reevaluate that DREZ lesions are following the dorsal lateral sulcus if no dorsal rootlets are seen. Once lesioning starts, staying focused on the orientation and direction of the DREZ minimizes deviation from the intended zone for lesioning, and the location of the previous lesion is not lost.

If avulsed rootlets are seen throughout the intended lesioning zone, the neurosurgeon may find it useful to begin rostral or caudal to the avulsed segments in the region containing spinal rootlets to identify the dorsolateral sulcus and progress into the avulsed region. Finally, it is unusual to see significant arteries cross the dorsolateral sulcus, as it is a watershed zone between the dorsal spinal arteries and the anterior spinal artery.[8,9] However, a prudent neurosurgeon should always avoid injuring any significant arterial supply to the spinal cord.

The DREZ lesions are completed when either the lesions encompass 1 or 2 spinal cord segments above the painful zone or the impedances of the cord have normalized.

Complications for DREZ

Several reviews have been published regarding complications and outcomes of the DREZ procedure for RFL,[23,63] laser,[44] and microcoagulation.[64] **Table 1** summarizes the potential complications associated with radiofrequency DREZ lesioning for spinal cord procedures. In general, the most serious complications are usually associated with lesions that inadvertently are placed too far laterally and injure the corticospinal tract, resulting in permanent ipsilateral weakness below the lesion. This occurred in 3% to 14% of patients reported since 1990. It is most frequent with thoracic DREZ lesions where the dorsal horn is the thinnest and the margin for error is the least. Permanent sensory loss, namely ipsilateral loss of proprioception and light touch below the DREZ site, is tolerated better by patients, but is reported at a higher rate (2%–70% in reports since 1990). It appears that the smaller electrode[65] and experience with the technique has resulted in a lower complication rate.

Prognosis of pain relief

Table 2 summarizes a review of the literature reporting outcomes in 10 or more patients undergoing radiofrequency DREZ lesioning for various neuropathic conditions other than postamputation pain. Very few reports on the outcome for postamputation pain exist and these results from small studies of radiofrequency DREZ lesioning are also included.

Overall, the success of radiofrequency DREZ lesioning has improved over the years. It continues to remain true that the best results are obtained with patients who have brachial plexus avulsion. Patients can expect good to excellent reduction in brachial plexus avulsion pain 54% to 91% of the time, and it appears to last in at

least 50% of patients over 5 years. Patients who had end-zone pain rather than diffuse distal pain related to spinal cord injury (SCI) had better outcomes (78% vs 20%). Although follow-up studies for SCI pain are not nearly as long, the results also appear to hold for more than 3 years.[23] Both Tomas and Haninec[55] and Falci and colleagues[66] indicated that intraoperative electrophysiology of the dorsal horn during these procedures is likely to enhance the outcomes and reduce complications. Both of these groups suggest that tailoring the lesioning procedure to include areas of hyperactivity in the DREZ region will capture additional levels mediating pain not normally anticipated in the preoperative plan. Patients on the other hand who have a "dull, aching, burning pain" distal to the region of spinal cord injury are similar to those who complain of phantom-limb stump pain, and less optimal results are seen. These data suggest that lesioning of the DREZ will not encompass the pain pathways mediating this type of pain. In fact, autonomic pathways extrinsic to the spinal cord may mediate the refractory portions of the pain not treated by DREZ lesioning.[14,23,42]

DREZ lesioning for postherpetic neuralgia pain is associated with poor outcomes and increased morbidity. Although initial pain relief was seen in 29 of 32 patients in the first several months, Friedman and Bullitt[42] found that only 8 of these patients had good pain relief by a year. Considering the increased risk for motor deficits following thoracic DREZ lesioning (see **Table 1**), one should be cautious in offering good results in the long run in patients with this type of pain.

Laser or microsurgical DREZotomy lesioning has been extensively described by Sindou since 1972.[67] When others have compared the results with radiofrequency lesions, similar results were found[23] in a few reports. The advantage of radiofrequency lesioning is that the lesions are usually approximately 1 mm round and are highly reproducible.[60] Furthermore, insertion of the Nashold DREZ electrode will ensure a lesion depth of 2.5 mm with equal spacing around the electrode tip (see **Figs. 6** and **7**). Stimulation can easily be performed just before each lesion in areas in which the anatomy is obscure. These are advantageous over an open lesioning technique of the DREZ in which the spinal cord is visually disrupted. A disadvantage of the radiofrequency technique is the lack of visualization of the actual lesion within the spinal cord. There may be skip areas when lesions are not spaced tightly,[23,68] which may result in less optimal outcomes and potential for increased morbidity due to wandering from the DREZ line.

Table 1
Complications that potentially can occur with radiofrequency DREZ lesioning of the spinal cord reported in studies with 10 or more patients

Author, Year	Reason for DREZ	No. Patients	Permanent Sensory or Motor Loss	Transient Motor or Sensory Loss	Other, %
Samii & Moringlane,[21] 1984	BP, SCI	35	0	3% M, 25% M, 23% both	0
Richter & Seitz,[93] 1984	BP, SCI	10	30% S, 10% both	10% M	20
Thomas & Jones,[94] 1984	BP	34	12% M/S	50% M/S	
Garcia-March et al,[95] 1987	BP	11		9% M	
Friedman & Bullitt,[42] 1988	BP SCI PHN	39 56 32	60% M/S 5% M, 5% minor 69% M		16
Campbell et al,[96] 1988	BP	10	20% hyperreflexia		10
Ishijima et al,[97] 1988	BP, SCI, PHN	30	62% S		14
Saris et al,[98] 1988	Post-amputation	22	41% mild M/S		1
Saris et al,[99] 1988	Peripheral	12	>50% S, 8% M	17% M, 8% sphincter, 74% mild dysmetria	7
Young,[65] 1990	Various – l g electrode	21	24% S, 19% M, 5% both		
	Various – sm electrode	37	3% S, 5% M		1
Kumagai et al,[100] 1992	Various	17	71% S, 41% M		35
Edgar et al,[68] 1993	SCI	102	2% S, 3% M		5
Sampson et al,[17] 1995	Conus	29	3% S, 14% M, 10% sphincter	3% M	7
	Cauda equina	10		10% M	
Rath et al,[20] 1997	Various	73			
Samii et al,[101] 2001	BP	47	4% M	10% M	2
Falci et al,[66] 2002	SCI	41	70% S, 14% M		9
Tomas & Haninec,[55] 2005	BP	21	14% S/M		
Chen & Tu,[102] 2006	BP	60		25% S	
Awad et al,[103] 2013	BP, SCI, Cancer	19		11% M	

Abbreviations: BP, brachial plexus; DREZ, dorsal root entry zone; M, motor; PHN, postherpetic neuralgia; S, sensory; SCI, spinal cord injury.

Modified from Konrad P, Caputi F, El-Naggar AO. Radiofrequency dorsal root entry zone lesions for Pain. In: Lozano AM, Gildenberg PL, Tasker RR, editors. Textbook of stereotactic and functional neurosurgery. 2nd edition. Berlin: Springer; 2009. p. 2251–68.

Summary for DREZ

Radiofrequency DREZ lesioning is an excellent procedure to offer patients with medically refractory pain due to a variety of syndromes. In particular, patients with pain due to brachial plexus avulsion and end-zone pain related to traumatic spinal cord injury are to be considered for this procedure. The neurosurgeon contemplating this procedure should have a solid understanding of the microanatomy in the DREZ region of the spinal cord and be familiar with contemporary intraoperative physiologic testing

Table 2
Outcomes of pain relief in patients who underwent radiofrequency DREZ lesioning for the treatment of various painful conditions

Author, Year	No. Patients	Good Results (%)	Follow-up Period, mo
Brachial Plexus Avulsion Pain			
Thomas & Jones,[94] 1984	34	21 (62)	4–44
Samii & Moringlane,[21] 1984	22	20 (91)	
Garcia-March et al,[95] 1987	11	6 (54)	8–58 (mean, 17)
Campbell et al,[96] 1988	10	8 (80)	7–52
Ishijima et al,[97] 1988	17	14 (82)	6–57
Young,[65] 1990	18	13 (72)	
Freidman et al,[104] 1990	56	33 (59)	12–156
Samii et al,[101] 2001	47	30 (64)	24–216 (mean 168)
Tomas & Haninec,[55] 2005	21	13 (62)	4–96
Chen & Tu,[102] 2006	40	32 (80)	36–120
Awad et al,[103] 2013	10	6 (60)	2–144 (mean 78)
SCI Pain			
Weigand & Winkelmuller,[105] 1985	20	10 (50)	1–28
Friedman & Nashold,[12] 1986	31	23 (78) – end-zone pain	6–72
	25	5 (20) – diffuse pain	6–72
Young,[65] 1990	14	8 (57)	
Edgar et al,[68] 1993	46	42 (92)	2–96 (mean, 44)
Sampson et al,[17] 1995	39	21 (54)	(mean 36)
Falci et al,[66] 2002	41	33 (80)	12–72
Awad et al,[103] 2013	6	5 (83)	6–60 (mean 24)
Postherpetic Pain			
Friedman & Bullitt,[42] 1988	32	8 (25)	6–72
Young,[65] 1990	11	6 (54)	
Phantom-limb Pain			
Weigand & Winkelmuller,[105] 1985	7	1 (14)	1–28
Saris et al,[98] 1988	9	6 (67)	6–60

Pain relief is reported as either good (some medications needed postlesioning for pain control) or excellent (no pain medications needed for pre-operative pain control).

Abbreviations: DREZ, dorsal root entry zone; SCI, spinal cord injury.

Modified from Konrad P, Caputi F, El-Naggar AO. Radiofrequency dorsal root entry zone lesions for pain. In: Lozano AM, Gildenberg PL, Tasker RR, editors. Textbook of stereotactic and functional neurosurgery. 2nd edition. Berlin: Springer; 2009. p. 2251–68.

to optimize the outcomes from this surgical procedure.

Open Cordotomy

Initial description of the open cordotomy procedure for severe debilitating pain was written by Spiller and Martin in 1912.[69] It was in fact the most common surgical procedure for pain in the early part of the twentieth century.[70,71] Since then, the surgical procedure has not changed significantly. Exposure of the spinal cord for open cordotomy involves being able to adequately visualize and manipulate the lateral aspect of the spinal cord via the dentate ligament.

Lesioning technique

For unilateral cordotomy, a hemilaminectomy exposing the spinal canal from the midline to the facet joint is necessary. A durotomy was then made so as to easily visualize the dentate ligament and allow pop rotation of the spinal cord posteriorly. Once the dentate ligament is identified, it is disconnected from the dura and gently elevated, revealing the anterolateral part of the spinal cord (**Fig. 8**).

An improvised cordotomy instrument was created by snapping a Weck blade to a length of 4 to 8 mm and placing it at a right angle in Ryder forceps. The blade was inserted to a depth of 3 to 4 mm just underneath the dentate ligament and swept anteriorly. An angled microdissector was then used to reinforce the lesion by sweeping the instrument in the subpial space to ensure complete transection of the anterolateral spinal cord. Minimal bleeding would sometimes ensue, and this could typically be managed with conventional hemostatic techniques. Closure of the spinal cord dura and superficial layers is performed with the goal of reducing likelihood of spinal fluid leak.

Cordotomy can be expected to create a lesion with adequate analgesia several segments below on the contralateral side. For example, it is not uncommon to find a loss of pain and temperature below T8 after technically adequate open cordotomy at T4 to 5. This usually is sufficient to provide significant relief of lower quadrant pain that includes the pelvis, hip, thigh, and lower limb contralateral to the lesion.[27] In patients with bilateral leg pain and pelvic pain (for instance, a patient with osteosarcoma involving both hips), bilateral cordotomy has been successful.[25] **Table 3** provides a list of investigators who report on the technique and outcomes of open cordotomy. Although the literature contains few reports of large case series, this technique is still performed at selected medical centers in the treatment of cancer pain.[24,25,27]

Complications of open cordotomy

Table 3 includes a summary of complications seen with open cordotomy. The 2 most common complications are urinary retention or incontinence (11%–33%), permanent dysesthesias that may be bothersome (7%–11%), transient hemiparesis (3.5%–22%), and respiratory distress or suppression in cervical cordotomies (3.5%–4%). Mirror pain also has been an unusual complication of open thoracic cordotomies in patients with cancer (7%–11%) in which a similar pain is experienced in the opposite side of the original painful region within weeks to months after the cordotomy.[72]

Other complications that are shared with open dural procedures and laminectomies include possible mechanical spinal instability, CSF leak, and meningitis.

Prognosis of pain relief

Few long-term studies (longer than 2 years) exist for open cordotomy for cancer pain, likely because of short-term survival of the patient population usually indicated for this procedure.

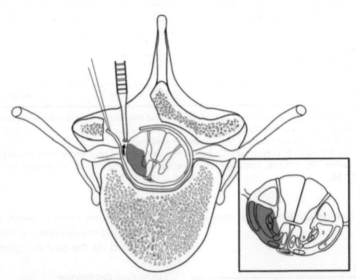

Fig. 8. Cross-section illustration of open cordotomy lesion. The gray shading illustrates the region that is lesioned after pial opening. The dentate ligament is used as a guide for identification of the posterior margin of the lesion. Various spinal cord tracts of interest are illustrated in the figure inset (1: corticospinal tract, 2: spinothalamic, 3: descending sympathetic fibers responsible for distal vasomotor and sudomotor innervation, 4: descending parasympathetic fibers responsible for innervation of distal bowel/bladder, 5: reticulospinal, 6: ventral spinocerebellar, 7: vestibulospinal, and 8: anterior corticospinal). (*From* Tomycz L, Forbes J, Ladner T, et al. Open thoracic cordotomy as a treatment option for severe, debilitating pain. J Neurol Surg A Cent Eur Neurosurg 2014;75(2):126–32.)

Table 3
Literature that reports significant experience with open cordotomy

Author, Year	No. Patients	Lesion Level	Good Results	Complications	Follow-up Period (mo)
Cowie & Hitchcock,[74] 1982	43 Cancer pain 13 Nonmalignant	C, T	93% immediate 55% at 1 y	Transient urinary retention (11%) Transient hemiparesis (3.5%) Permanent dysesthesia (7%) Death from respiratory failure – cervical (3.5%)	<18
Piscol,[75] 1975		C, T	Cancer: 65% long term Chronic pain: 20%–63% long term		>12
Tomycz et al et al,[24] 2014	4 Cancer pain 5 Nonmalignant	T	33% good 33% some improved	Mirror pain/dysesthesia (11%) Transient leg weakness (22%) Urinary incontinence (33%)	2–72 (31 median)
White et al,[72] 1950 White & Sweet,[76] 1969	145 Cancer pain 65 Nonmalignant	C T	54% longer than 1 y 77% by 6 mo 56% longer than 1 y	Urinary incontinence (13%) Leg weakness (5%) Mortality (4%–20%)	2–132

Studies containing follow-up of longer than 6 months are included.
Abbreviations: C, Cervical; T, Thoracic.

However, the best follow-up appears in reviews by White and colleagues,[72,73] Cowie and Hitchcock[74] and Piscol.[75] This is summarized in **Table 3**. A few facts need to be understood about the long-term prognosis of this procedure. More than half (77% reported by White and Sweet[76]) of the patients typically will have total immediate relief from their cancer pain, and one-fourth will have partial relief. However, the remaining patients may experience no benefit and unfortunately sustain some likelihood of neurologic decline. By the end of 6 months, more than half the patients will have a return of the pain and otherwise initially successful results. In Cowie and Hitchcock's[74] review of the literature, case series by Piscol[75] (1385 patients) and then Mansuy and colleagues[77] (124 patients) reported similar results of diminishing success after 1 year after open cordotomy from either cervical or thoracic lesions. It is also rare to consider re-lesioning the patient at a higher level.

These results, however, are appropriate for patients with severe medically refractory pain associated with metastatic cancer or high-grade lesions. It is not clear in the previously mentioned reviews whether the return of pain in patients with cancer who underwent cordotomy is due to failure of the lesion to hold, versus spread of the cancer to areas that are not encompassed by the lesion. The immediate pain relief following cordotomy is seen within moments of the lesion when done percutaneously (see later in this article) and within a day when the patient awakens from surgery for open cordotomy. Many of these patients actually need to be watched carefully postoperative because of the significant reduction in pain medications after successful cordotomy. It is gratifying to offer this focal neurosurgical procedure to patients who have minimal benefit from more generalized medical management. It many times will allow terminal patients to enjoy quality time with family while in their terminal phases of disease. Open thoracic cordotomy is an appropriate consideration in patients who have lower quadrant cancer pain and either cannot undergo an awake percutaneous cordotomy procedure or have significant risk of respiratory complications.

Percutaneous Cordotomy

Percutaneous cordotomy deserves separate discussion on technique, outcomes, and complications when compared with open cordotomy. Many excellent detailed reviews and discussions are present in the literature.[29,71–73,78,79] Tasker's discussion recently in 2009[28] is most useful for those who wish to understand the initial description, evolution of techniques, and successful strategies for this procedure. Today percutaneous cordotomy is performed using radiofrequency ablation reported first by Rosomoff and colleagues in 1965.[79] However, the initial use of a percutaneous ablation for pain in the cervical cord was performed a few years earlier in 1963 by Mullan and colleagues[80] using a strontium needle inserted into the STT. The use of radiofrequency techniques has significant advantages to lesion creation and, therefore, is still the most commonly used lesioning technique. The ability to test the effect of the attempted lesion, the ability to control the size of the lesion by adjusting time and temperature, and the ability to perform this in awake patients without the risk of general anesthesia continue to be significant advantages to this method of cordotomy over the open procedure.

Lesioning technique

Percutaneous cordotomy is normally performed through an orthogonal, transcutaneous approach to the C1/2 interspace. The goal is to initially identify the STT via stimulation and physiologic confirmation, and then to create a lesion that encompasses the contralateral pain and sensory perception usually from the trunk pelvis and leg. **Fig. 4** illustrates the anatomic relationships of successful passage of the percutaneous lesioning electrode into the STT at C1/2. As mentioned previously, a few key anatomic concepts must be remembered:

1. Entry into the spinothalamic tract occurs within 1 to 2 mm anterior to the dentate ligament
2. Sacral and lumbar fibers are initially encountered on penetration, with cervical and thoracic fibers lying more medial and anterior
3. The impedance of the electrode changes dramatically when passing from CSF into the parenchyma of the cord
4. Respiratory control lies immediately medial to the STT and is approximately 4 to 5 mm anterior into the cord.

With the patient supine and given intermittent light sedation, the identification of the approach to the C1 to 2 interspace is done with the assistance of fluoroscopy or x-ray in the past,[28] and more recently with CT guidance.[81,82] The patient's head must be immobilized to avoid sudden movement when the needle is placed into the spinal cord. Liberal use of local anesthetic will allow insertion of the needle percutaneously through an orthogonal approach into the dura with minimal patient discomfort, as long as no anesthetic is delivered intrathecally. With the patient in a supine position, the needle needs to be placed just anterior to the dentate ligament, so visualization of the dentate ligament is the requisite step in locating the needle correctly before insertion into the spinal cord. The unavailability of oil-based contrast agents (eg, Pantopaque) has been replaced by the use of water-soluble contrast (eg, Omnipaque) or a small amount of air, which can delineate the dentate ligament.

Once the needle is appropriately positioned just anterior to the dentate ligament, it can then be advanced into the spinal cord. Before doing so it is important to measure the impedance of the electrode and note the rise from approximately 300 to 400 Ω to more than 1000 Ω on entering the spinal cord white matter. Usually, penetration of the pia results in a brief increase in local pain reported by the patient. The location of the electrode can be seen at this point by imaging and confirmed many times by examination of the patient with electrical stimulation.[28,83]

Stimulation using low frequency (2–5 Hz) is used to create a motor response twitching in the ipsilateral neck muscles with low stimulus strength indicating presence of the needle to anterior or near the anterior roots. Twitching of the ipsilateral arm, shoulder, trunk, or leg muscles at low stimulus indicates that the tip is near the corticospinal tract and should be repositioned more anteriorly. Sensory stimulation is best done by switching the frequency to a higher rate (approximately 100 Hz). The patient should report contralateral sensory phenomena: usually a feeling of warmth or cold in the trunk or lower extremities contralateral to the stimulus. This should overlay the area of pain closely. If the patient reports ipsilateral arm or occipital paresthesias, the electrode is too posterior and lies, in fact, dorsal to the dentate ligament. Evoked sensory phenomena in the contralateral hand generally implies a good location for the electrode.

The electrode with a 2-mm exposed tip is typically used for creating the lesion following stimulation. Several versions of these electrodes are now available commercially and the reader is encouraged to review the articles by Kanpolat.[84,85] Once the lesioning electrode is physiologically confirmed to be located in the STT, then the lesion is performed. This is usually created at 70 to 80°C for approximately 60 seconds (30–40 mA for 30–60 seconds). The patient is examined during and after the lesioning procedure for any signs of motor weakness. Extent of analgesia can be documented once the lesion is completed. Ideally, documentation of decreased pinprick sensation should cover the entire painful area. If the extent of analgesia is not adequate,

the electrode can be slightly repositioned and an additional lesion can be created by using the same parameters. When bilateral cordotomies are needed, they should be separated by at least a week to minimize the unwanted side effects of this procedure.[83]

Complications of percutaneous cordotomy

Similar to open cordotomy, inadvertent damage to the spinal cord beyond the STT is the reason complications are seen. **Table 4** lists the complications seen in one of the largest reported series of percutaneous cordotomy (2616 patients; Lorenz and colleagues[28]). Mortality reported with this procedure (3% on average) is likely related to respiratory suppression (Ondine curse)[86] and seen only with bilateral procedures. Other complications that are routinely reported in descending order are bladder dysfunction (7.6%), temporary ipsilateral weakness (7.6%), ataxia (4.0%), respiratory dysfunction (3.5%), and permanent ipsilateral weakness (1.0%).[28,87] Although many believe that medial extension of the lesion is keyed to successful dense analgesia in the contralateral painful region, this increases the risk of respiratory complications. Another poorly discussed risk factor for complications

Table 4 Summary of experience with percutaneous cordotomy		
Author, Year	**No. Patients**	**Comments**
Rosomoff et al,[79] 1965	789	Initial: 90% 3 mo: 84% 1 y: 60% 2 y: 40%
Meglio & Cioni,[106,107] 1981	1279	Early pain relief: 87% Leg pain relief: 72% Weakness: 4.8% Hypotension: 1.8% Mortality: 1.6%
Lorenz et al,[71,87] 1998	2616	Bladder dysfunction: 7.6% Ipsilateral temporary weakness: 7.6% Ataxia: 4% Respiratory dysfunction: 3.5% Hypotension: 2.2% Permanent ipsilateral weakness: 1% Mortality: 3%

Abbreviations: C, Cervical; T, Thoracic.

Modified from Hodge CJ Jr, Christensen MD. Anterolateral cordotomy. In: Burchiel K, editor. Surgical management of pain. New York: Thieme; 2002. p. 732–44.

with this procedure is the presence of terminal disease in the patients for whom this procedure is selected.

Prognosis of pain relief

Most patients experience immediate pain relief following the lesion 90% of the time.[29,79] **Table 4** provides more detail regarding the long-term relief of pain with percutaneous cordotomy. In general, note that by 1 year only 50% to 60% of patients continue to have pain relief. Therefore, cordotomy in general is not a long-term treatment for cancer-related pain. However, it is an appropriate treatment for patients with severe debilitating pain related to malignancy. Other articles discuss the use of percutaneous cordotomy for the treatment of noncancer-related pain and the results are less optimal. Lahuerta and colleagues[88] reported the comparison of nonmalignant pain versus malignant pain in 1985, which reflects the general feeling of less optimal results for noncancer pain management; namely, only 20% of patients experienced complete relief of pain (66% with malignant pain) and 40% of patients had no relief at all (compared with 12% in the malignant population).

Despite the eventual loss of efficacy for pain relief in patients with cancer, the short-term results at least for the first year can be quite dramatic. Most of these patients before surgery require significant opioid and other medications without substantial relief of their pain. In large series of follow-up it is obvious that patients are able to come off other pain medications either completely or significantly within the first 6 months of their procedures. Rosomoff and colleagues[79] in their series of 789 patients undergoing 1279 percutaneous cordotomies, reported that 84% of patients at 3 months required no additional analgesic medications for pain control. Half of the patients who still required some pain medications after the procedure still felt that the procedure had decreased their pain and they could return to activities of daily living without significant narcotic requirements. When compared with standard medical management of pain related to malignant disease, percutaneous cordotomy restores significant quality of life in these patients in the first 2 years following the procedure.

Midline Myelotomy

The traditional commissurotomy procedure addresses the need for patients who have bilateral lower extremity, medically refractory pain. In particular, the same general principles apply in patient selection for this procedure as for cordotomies. The advantage for a midline, single lesioning procedure of the anterior commissure is that it addresses bilateral somatic pain with less risk for injury to the motor tracts than 2 separate lesioning procedures of the STT. However, as the following discussion reveals, leg weakness is still a potential complication of this technique. Description of the midline myelotomy (commissurotomy) was first seen in the literature by Armour in 1927.[89] The goal of this procedure is to interrupt the commissural fibers crossing just anterior to the central canal and thereby disrupting the STT bilaterally. Although it is not known how many levels over which to carry a myelotomy needs to occur, in general most reports advocate for coverage extending from T10 inferiorly for several levels to address bilateral lower extremity pain.[34,90–92] An additional advantage to performing a midline myelotomy is the division of the dorsal columns along the midline, which putatively contain visceral pain pathways.[36,37,40] Viswanathan and colleagues[34] recently reviewed their experience with 11 patients who underwent lower thoracic midline myelotomy for the treatment of severe cancer-related pain involving the lower abdomen/pelvis or legs or both. Patients were selected who had bilateral involvement of pain. A good discussion of the technique and outcomes is noted in this article.

An incomplete version of the midline myelotomy was advocated by Gildenberg and Hirshberg in 1984[38] and Nauta and colleagues in 1997[39] purely to address visceral pain. The approach should be rostral enough to encompass the visceral pain pathway of the dorsal columns; and, therefore, lesions are typically planned for the mid to upper thoracic cord (no lower than T8 reported). However, whereas traditional commissurotomy involves a 3-level to 4-level laminectomy, exposing the cord from T10 to L1 typically, a limited midline myelotomy can be done through a 1-level or 2-level laminectomy usually approximately T8 or higher.

Lesioning technique

Patients are positioned prone under general anesthesia and target spinal levels identified, which for most patients range from T10 to L1. After performing a midline laminectomy, a midline durotomy is used to expose the spinal cord. With the operating microscope the point halfway between the dorsal root entry zone is identified in a rostrocaudal direction. The pia along this midline approach is then coagulated with microforceps. And arachnoid knife or similar microblade is then used to first open the pia longitudinally along the midline. This myelotomy is carried anteriorly until the pia from the anterior sulcus is encountered, indicating complete division of the midline.

When neurosurgeons discovered that visceral pain relief was excellent in these patients in addition to the intended bilateral somatic pain reduction. Some, like Mansuy and colleagues,[35] noted this effect despite poor coverage of the anterior commissure. Speculation began to emerge discussing the existence of a dorsal column visceral pain pathway. A limited midline myelotomy that just lesions the dorsal columns and avoids cutting the anterior commissure was then described by Gildenberg and Hirshberg[38] and then further reduced to a small transverse lesion by Nauta and colleagues.[39] The goal is to interrupt the ascending visceral pain pathways postulated by Willis and colleagues[36] and others that mediate nonsomatic pain arising along the midline.

As with other cordotomies, knowledge of the position of the anterior spinal artery is a key to avoiding significant complications. Closure of the dura is performed in routine fashion. Patients are typically placed on a tapering dose of dexamethasone for several days. When successful, patients experience significant reduction in narcotic use within the ensuing days following this procedure.

Complications

Patients who typically are candidates for this procedure are usually in terminal stages of their cancer disease. Hence, high morbidity associated with this surgery is also linked to the poor prognosis of the patient in general. **Table 5** contains the few reports that described outcomes and complications of this rare technique. In general, as expected there will be diminished proprioception in the lower extremities due to division of the dorsal columns, which actually may be difficult to measure in patients with severe bilateral lower extremity pain. Leg weakness on the other hand is a significant complication (27%) likely related to trauma in the micro-environment of the dorsal half of the spinal cord. Dysesthesias resulting in either gait disturbances or, worse, burning sensation in the legs, was not frequently seen (9%) in these few reports, but discussed more commonly in other reviews.

Gildenberg[70] and Meyerson[29] argue for the limited myelotomy involving just the separation of dorsal columns along the midline for treatment of visceral pain only. The results in a limited set of case reports seems to indicate less risk of lower extremity weakness and anterior spinal artery damage. With the option of a percutaneous procedure (percutaneous cordotomy) it can be debated whether the traditional commissurotomy has any advantages other than for neurosurgeons who are not familiar with performing percutaneous cordotomy procedures. However, a limited midline myelotomy appears to have a unique advantage for patients with pure visceral pain associated with malignancies of the abdomen or pelvis.

Prognosis for pain relief

Table 5 lists the outcomes in the few case series reported in the literature for both commissurotomy and limited midline myelotomy. In both types of

---

Table 5
Midline myelotomy results as reported in the literature

Author, Year	No. Patients	Lesion Level	Good Results	Complications	Follow-up Period, mo
Commissurotomy					
Sourek,[108] 1969	25	T10 to conus	Excellent: Majority immediately postoperative	Burning dysesthesia: 12%	36 (n = 3)
Viswanathan et al,[34] 2010	11	T10 to conus (n = 10/11)	Excellent: 45% Good: 27% Poor: 9%	Leg weakness: 27% Urinary retention: 9%	1–41
Limited midline myelotomy (dorsal columns only)					
Gildenberg & Hirshberg,[38] 1984	14	T9–10	Excellent: 75%	None	2–13
Kim & Kwon,[45] 2000	8	C7-T2	Excellent: 25% Good: 38%	Transient paresthesias: 37%	1–4
Nauta et al,[39] 1997	1	T8	Excellent for lower abdomen/pelvis	None	10

Abbreviations: C, cervical; T, thoracic.

procedures, the pain relief was excellent or good in more than half of patients. The difference primarily was, as expected, that commissurotomy was able to provide bilateral lower extremity pain relief as well as visceral pain relief, whereas limited midline myelotomy (in which only the dorsal columns are divided) was effective for visceral pain only. Keeping these results in mind, it appears that with good patient selection, a midline lesioning procedure is an excellent choice for patients with severe midline and/or bilateral lower extremity pain. The patient, in particular, who has abdominal or pelvic organ involvement in addition to bilateral lower extremity pain will do much better with a midline myelotomy versus an anterolateral cordotomy.

SUMMARY

Lesioning of the spinal cord is underused today for patients with severe, medically refractory pain. Lesioning of the spinal cord can have dramatic results in both the treatment of the pain and the need for oral pain medications. This article summarizes the patient selection, surgical technique, and outcomes for the most common spinal cord lesioning methods reported in the literature. Each technique has a unique patient population that benefits from these procedures, and the neurosurgeon who is contemplating offering a lesioning procedure for pain should become familiar with as many of these surgical options as possible. Understanding the spinal cord anatomy of which procedures will address what types of pain is mandatory before considering these procedures. The following points summarize each type of lesioning technique:

DREZ

- Excellent for brachial plexus avulsion pain (54%–91% pain relief), "end-zone" spinal cord injury pain, and inoperable upper thoracic tumors that compress the brachial plexus.
- Lesions are performed with either a radiofrequency electrode or open myelotomy of the dorsal root entry zone.
- Ipsilateral leg weakness can occur in 3% to 14% of patients. Sensory changes appear to be much better tolerated.

Open Cordotomy

- Excellent for unilateral lower extremity pain due to malignancies, such as sarcoma of the hip and legs. Poor results for chronic, nonmalignant pain (such as spinal cord injury–related pain).

- Surgeons need to be comfortable with approach to the anterolateral cord through a posterior durotomy in the thoracic region. Upper open cervical cordotomies have been replaced by percutaneous techniques.
- Injury to the anterior spinal artery and corticospinal tract can result in ipsilateral leg weakness (3%–22%). Urinary retention or incontinence also is reported in a significant portion (11%–33%).
- Mirror pain in 7% to 11% of patients is a unique complication of this procedure.
- May provide a more "complete" or lasting analgesic effect in the lower extremities when compared with percutaneous cordotomies.

Percutaneous Cordotomy

- Excellent for pain related to malignancy in the lower quadrant, including abdominal wall, pelvic bone, and lower extremity (such as carcinomas and sarcomas invading the lower quadrant).
- Poor ability to create significant analgesia in the upper thoracic and upper extremity area above C5.
- Surgeons need to have the appropriate equipment and technique for percutaneous approach to the C1-2 region. This skill has not been taught much in the past 2 decades (since 1990).
- Provides instantaneous relief in most (>90%) patients; however, effects lasting more than a year are rare.
- Ipsilateral leg weakness (1%) and bladder dysfunction (7%–8%) are to be watched for.
- Respiratory complications are unique to this technique, occurring in 3% to 5%, as reported in large series.

Midline Myelotomy

- Patients with visceral pain due to abdominal or pelvic malignancies are ideal candidates for this technique.
- Surgeons should be comfortable with open midline spinal cord approaches. For pure visceral pain treatment, a limited midline myelotomy can be performed with smaller exposure than a commissurotomy aimed at treating both somatic and visceral pain.
- Leg weakness (unilateral or bilateral) occurred in 27% of patients in one report.
- A limited number of cases are reported in the literature. However, the outcomes with respect to visceral pain were good to excellent in more than 50% of patients.

REFERENCES

1. Almeida TF, Roizenblatt S, Tufik S. Afferent pain pathways: a neuroanatomical review. Brain Res 2004;1000(1–2):40–56.
2. Coggeshall RE. Fos, nociception and the dorsal horn. Prog Neurobiol 2005;77(5):299–352.
3. Mertens P, Guenot M, Hermier M, et al. Radiologic anatomy of the spinal dorsal horn at the cervical level (anatomic-MRI correlations). Surg Radiol Anat 2000;22(2):81–8.
4. Romanelli P, Esposito V. The functional anatomy of neuropathic pain. Neurosurg Clin N Am 2004; 15(3):257–68.
5. Willis WD Jr. Dorsal horn neurophysiology of pain. Ann N Y Acad Sci 1988;531:76–89.
6. Elliot KA. Cross-sectional diameters and areas of the human spinal cord. Anat Rec 1945;93:287–93.
7. Xiang JP, Liu XL, Xu YB, et al. Microsurgical anatomy of dorsal root entry zone of brachial plexus. Microsurgery 2008;28(1):17–20.
8. Light AR. Normal anatomy and physiology of the spinal cord dorsal horn. Appl Neurophysiol 1988; 51(2–5):78–88.
9. McCormick PC, Stein BM. Functional anatomy of the spinal cord and related structures. Neurosurg Clin N Am 1990;1(3):469–89.
10. Young PA. The anatomy of the spinal cord pain paths: a review. J Am Paraplegia Soc 1986;9(3–4): 28–38.
11. Zhang H, Xie W, Xie Y. Spinal cord injury triggers sensitization of wide dynamic range dorsal horn neurons in segments rostral to the injury. Brain Res 2005;1055(1–2):103–10.
12. Friedman AH, Nashold BS Jr. DREZ lesions for relief of pain related to spinal cord injury. J Neurosurg 1986;65(4):465–9.
13. Furue H, Katafuchi T, Yoshimura M. Sensory processing and functional reorganization of sensory transmission under pathological conditions in the spinal dorsal horn. Neurosci Res 2004;48(4): 361–8.
14. Nashold BS Jr. Deafferentation pain in man and animals as it relates to the DREZ operation. Can J Neurol Sci 1988;15(1):5–9.
15. Rosenow JM, Henderson JM. Anatomy and physiology of chronic pain. Neurosurg Clin N Am 2003; 14(3):445–62, vii.
16. Romanelli P, Esposito V, Adler J. Ablative procedures for chronic pain. Neurosurg Clin N Am 2004;15(3):335–42.
17. Sampson JH, Cashman RE, Nashold BS Jr, et al. Dorsal root entry zone lesions for intractable pain after trauma to the conus medullaris and cauda equina. J Neurosurg 1995;82(1):28–34.
18. Karatas A, Caglar S, Savas A, et al. Microsurgical anatomy of the dorsal cervical rootlets and dorsal root entry zones. Acta Neurochir (Wien) 2005; 147(2):195–9 [discussion: 199].
19. Nashold BS Jr, Friedman A, Bullitt E. The status of dorsal root entry zone lesions in 1987. Clin Neurosurg 1989;35:422–8.
20. Rath SA, Seitz K, Soliman N, et al. DREZ coagulations for deafferentation pain related to spinal and peripheral nerve lesions: indication and results of 79 consecutive procedures. Stereotact Funct Neurosurg 1997;68(1–4 Pt 1):161–7.
21. Samii M, Moringlane JR. Thermocoagulation of the dorsal root entry zone for the treatment of intractable pain. Neurosurgery 1984;15(6):953–5.
22. Sindou M, Mertens P, Wael M. Microsurgical DREZotomy for pain due to spinal cord and/or cauda equina injuries: long-term results in a series of 44 patients. Pain 2001;92(1–2):159–71.
23. Denkers MR, Biagi HL, Ann O'Brien M, et al. Dorsal root entry zone lesioning used to treat central neuropathic pain in patients with traumatic spinal cord injury: a systematic review. Spine 2002; 27(7):E177–84.
24. Tomycz L, Forbes J, Ladner T, et al. Open thoracic cordotomy as a treatment option for severe, debilitating pain. J Neurol Surg A Cent Eur Neurosurg 2014;75(2):126–32.
25. Atkin N, Jackson KA, Danks RA. Bilateral open thoracic cordotomy for refractory cancer pain: a neglected technique? J Pain Symptom Manage 2010;39(5):924–9.
26. Collins KL, Taren JA, Patil PG. Four-decade maintenance of analgesia with percutaneous cordotomy. Stereotact Funct Neurosurg 2012;90(4): 266–72.
27. Jones B, Finlay I, Ray A, et al. Is there still a role for open cordotomy in cancer pain management? J Pain Symptom Manage 2003;25(2):179–84.
28. Tasker RR. Percutaneous cordotomy. In: Lozano AM, Gildenberg PL, Tasker RR, editors. Textbook of stereotactic and functional neurosurgery. 2nd edition. Berlin: Springer; 2009. p. 2137–48.
29. Meyerson BA. Neurosurgical approaches to pain treatment. Acta Anaesthesiol Scand 2001;45(9): 1108–13.
30. Palma A, Holzer J, Cuadra O, et al. Lateral percutaneous spinothalamic tractotomy. Acta Neurochir (Wien) 1988;93(3–4):100–3.
31. Burchiel K. Surgical management of pain. New York: Thieme; 2002.
32. Nannapaneni R, Behari S, Todd NV, et al. Retracing "Ondine's curse". Neurosurgery 2005;57(2):354–63 [discussion: 354–63].
33. Mullan S, Hosobuchi Y. Respiratory hazards of high cervical percutaneous cordotomy. J Neurosurg 1968;28(4):291–7.
34. Viswanathan A, Burton AW, Rekito A, et al. Commissural myelotomy in the treatment of

intractable visceral pain: technique and outcomes. Stereotact Funct Neurosurg 2010;88(6):374–82.

35. Mansuy L, Lecuire J, Acassat L. Technique de la myélotomie commissurale postérieure. J Chir 1944;60:206–13.

36. Willis WD, Al-Chaer ED, Quast MJ, et al. A visceral pain pathway in the dorsal column of the spinal cord. Proc Natl Acad Sci U S A 1999;96(14):7675–9.

37. Willis WD Jr, Westlund KN. The role of the dorsal column pathway in visceral nociception. Curr Pain Headache Rep 2001;5(1):20–6.

38. Gildenberg PL, Hirshberg RM. Limited myelotomy for the treatment of intractable cancer pain. J Neurol Neurosurg Psychiatr 1984;47(1):94–6.

39. Nauta HJ, Hewitt E, Westlund KN, et al. Surgical interruption of a midline dorsal column visceral pain pathway. Case report and review of the literature. J Neurosurg 1997;86(3):538–42.

40. Gildenberg PL. Myelotomy through the years. Stereotact Funct Neurosurg 2001;77(1–4):169–71.

41. Konrad P, Caputi F, El-Naggar AO. Radiofrequency dorsal root entry zone lesions for pain. In: Lozano AM, Gildenberg PL, Tasker RR, editors. Textbook of stereotactic and functional neurosurgery. 2nd edition. Berlin: Springer; 2009. p. 2251–68.

42. Friedman AH, Bullitt E. Dorsal root entry zone lesions in the treatment of pain following brachial plexus avulsion, spinal cord injury and herpes zoster. Appl Neurophysiol 1988;51(2–5):164–9.

43. Nashold B, Pearlstein R. The DREZ operation. Park Ridge (IL): The American Association of Neurological Surgeons; 1996.

44. Sindou MP, Blondet E, Emery E, et al. Microsurgical lesioning in the dorsal root entry zone for pain due to brachial plexus avulsion: a prospective series of 55 patients. J Neurosurg 2005;102(6):1018–28.

45. Kim YS, Kwon SJ. High thoracic midline dorsal column myelotomy for severe visceral pain due to advanced stomach cancer. Neurosurgery 2000; 46(1):85–90 [discussion: 90–82].

46. Potter K, Saifuddin A. Pictorial review: MRI of chronic spinal cord injury. Br J Radiol 2003; 76(905):347–52.

47. Ochi M, Ikuta Y, Watanabe M, et al. The diagnostic value of MRI in traumatic brachial plexus injury. J Hand Surg Br 1994;19(1):55–9.

48. Bodley R. Imaging in chronic spinal cord injury—indications and benefits. Eur J Radiol 2002;42(2): 135–53.

49. Albert TJ, Vacarro A. Postlaminectomy kyphosis. Spine 1998;23(24):2738–45.

50. Nashold BS Jr, Ostdahl RH. Dorsal root entry zone lesions for pain relief. J Neurosurg 1979;51(1): 59–69.

51. Nashold BS Jr, Bullitt E. Dorsal root entry zone lesions to control central pain in paraplegics. J Neurosurg 1981;55(3):414–9.

52. Rawlings CE 3rd, el-Naggar AO, Nashold BS Jr. The DREZ procedure: an update on technique. Br J Neurosurg 1989;3(6):633–42.

53. Vieira JF, Shieff C, Nashold BS Jr, et al. Impedance measurements of the spinal cord of man and animals. Appl Neurophysiol 1988;51(2–5): 154–63.

54. Makachinas T, Ovelmen-Levitt J, Nashold BS Jr. Intraoperative somatosensory evoked potentials. A localizing technique in the DREZ operation. Appl Neurophysiol 1988;51(2–5):146–53.

55. Tomas R, Haninec P. Dorsal root entry zone (DREZ) localization using direct spinal cord stimulation can improve results of the DREZ thermocoagulation procedure for intractable pain relief. Pain 2005; 116(1–2):159–63.

56. Nashold BS Jr, Ovelmen-Levitt J, Sharpe R, et al. Intraoperative evoked potentials recorded in man directly from dorsal roots and spinal cord. J Neurosurg 1985;62(5):680–93.

57. Oberle J, Antoniadis G, Kast E, et al. Evaluation of traumatic cervical nerve root injuries by intraoperative evoked potentials. Neurosurgery 2002;51(5): 1182–8 [discussion: 1188–90].

58. Konrad PE, Tacker WA. Pyramidal versus extrapyramidal origins of the motor evoked potential. Neurosurgery 1991;29(5):795–6.

59. Husain AM, Elliott SL, Gorecki JP. Neurophysiological monitoring for the nucleus caudalis dorsal root entry zone operation. Neurosurgery 2002;50(4): 822–7 [discussion: 827–8].

60. Nashold BS Jr. Neurosurgical technique of the dorsal root entry zone operation. Appl Neurophysiol 1988;51(2–5):136–45.

61. Iacono RP, Aguirre ML, Nashold BS Jr. Anatomic examination of human dorsal root entry zone lesions. Appl Neurophysiol 1988;51(2–5): 225–9.

62. Yoshida M, Noguchi S, Kuga S, et al. MRI findings of DREZ-otomy lesions. Stereotact Funct Neurosurg 1992;59(1–4):39–44.

63. Raslan AM, McCartney S, Burchiel KJ. Management of chronic severe pain: spinal neuromodulatory and neuroablative approaches. Acta Neurochir Suppl 2007;97(Pt 1):33–41.

64. Prestor B. Microcoagulation of junctional dorsal root entry zone is effective treatment of brachial plexus avulsion pain: long-term follow-up study. Croat Med J 2006;47(2):271–8.

65. Young RF. Clinical experience with radiofrequency and laser DREZ lesions. J Neurosurg 1990;72(5): 715–20.

66. Falci S, Best L, Bayles R, et al. Dorsal root entry zone microcoagulation for spinal cord injury-related central pain: operative intramedullary electrophysiological guidance and clinical outcome. J Neurosurg 2002;97(Suppl 2):193–200.

67. Sindou M. Microsurgical DREZotomy (MDT) for pain, spasticity, and hyperactive bladder: a 20-year experience. Acta Neurochir (Wien) 1995;137(1–2):1–5.

68. Edgar RE, Best LG, Quail PA, et al. Computer-assisted DREZ microcoagulation: posttraumatic spinal deafferentation pain. J Spinal Disord 1993;6(1):48–56.

69. Spiller W, Martin E. The treatment of persistent pain of organic origin in the lower part of the body by division of the anterolateral column of the spinal cord. JAMA 1912;58:1489–90.

70. Gildenberg PL. Ablative spinal cord procedures for cancer pain. In: Lozano AM, Gildenberg PL, Tasker RR, editors. Textbook of stereotactic and functional neurosurgery. 2nd edition. Berlin: Springer; 2009. p. 2159–70.

71. Hodge CJ Jr, Christensen MD. Anterolateral cordotomy. In: Burchiel K, editor. Surgical management of pain. New York: Thieme; 2002. p. 732–44.

72. White JC, Sweet WH, Hawkins R, et al. Anterolateral cordotomy: results, complications and causes of failure. Brain 1950;73(3):346–67.

73. White JC, W.H. S. Anterolateral cordotomy: open versus closed comparison of end results. In: Advances in Pain Research. vol. 3. 1979. p. 911–9.

74. Cowie RA, Hitchcock ER. The late results of anterolateral cordotomy for pain relief. Acta Neurochir (Wien) 1982;64(1–2):39–50.

75. Piscol K. Open spinal surgery for intractable pain. Advances in Neurosurgery 1975;3:157–69.

76. White JC, Sweet WH. Pain and the neurosurgeon: a forty-year experience. Springfield (IL): Charles C. Thomas; 1969.

77. Mansuy L, Sindou M, Fischer G, et al. Spinothalamic cordotomy in cancerous pain. Results of a series of 124 patients operated on by the direct posterior approach. Neurochirurgie 1976;22(5): 437–44 [in French].

78. Gildenberg PL. Percutaneous cervical cordotomy. Appl Neurophysiol 1976;39(2):97–113.

79. Rosomoff HL, Brown CJ, Sheptak P. Percutaneous radiofrequency cervical cordotomy: technique. J Neurosurg 1965;23(6):639–44.

80. Mullan S, Harper PV, Hekmatpanah J, et al. Percutaneous interruption of spinal-pain tracts by means of a strontium90 needle. J Neurosurg 1963; 20:931–9.

81. Kanpolat Y, Ugur HC, Ayten M, et al. Computed tomography-guided percutaneous cordotomy for intractable pain in malignancy. Neurosurgery 2009; 64(Suppl 3):ons187–93 [discussion: ons193–4].

82. Kanpolat Y, Savas A, Ucar T, et al. CT-guided percutaneous selective cordotomy for treatment of intractable pain in patients with malignant pleural mesothelioma. Acta Neurochir (Wien) 2002;144(6): 595–9 [discussion: 599].

83. Tasker RR, Organ LW, Smith KC. Physiological guidelines for the localization of lesions by percutaneous cordotomy. Acta Neurochir (Wien) 1974;(Suppl 21): 111–7.

84. Kanpolat Y. The surgical treatment of chronic pain: destructive therapies in the spinal cord. Neurosurg Clin N Am 2004;15(3):307–17.

85. Kanpolat Y. Percutaneous destructive pain procedures on the upper spinal cord and brain stem in cancer pain: CT-guided techniques, indications and results. Adv Tech Stand Neurosurg 2007;32: 147–73.

86. Krieger AJ, Rosomoff HL. Sleep-induced apnea. 1. A respiratory and autonomic dysfunction syndrome following bilateral percutaneous cervical cordotomy. J Neurosurg 1974;40(2):168–80.

87. Lorenz R, Grumme T, Herrmann HD, et al. Percutaneous cordotomy. Advances in Neurosurgery 1998;3:178–85.

88. Lahuerta J, Lipton S, Wells JC. Percutaneous cervical cordotomy: results and complications in a recent series of 100 patients. Ann R Coll Surg Engl 1985;67(1):41–4.

89. Armour D. Surgery of the spinal cord and its membranes. Lancet 1927;1:691–7.

90. van Roost D, Gybels J. Myelotomies for chronic pain. Acta Neurochir Suppl (Wien) 1989;46:69–72.

91. Atlas of anatomy collection. New York: Thieme Medical Publishers; 2007.

92. Lozano AM, Gildenberg PL, Tasker RR, editors. Textbook of stereotactic and functional neurosurgery. 2nd edition. Berlin: Springer; 2009.

93. Richter HP, Seitz K. Dorsal root entry zone lesions for the control of deafferentation pain: experiences in ten patients. Neurosurgery 1984;15(6):956–9.

94. Thomas DG, Jones SJ. Dorsal root entry zone lesions (Nashold's procedure) in brachial plexus avulsion. Neurosurgery 1984;15(6):966–8.

95. Garcia-March G, Sanchez-Ledesma MJ, Diaz P, et al. Dorsal root entry zone lesion versus spinal cord stimulation in the management of pain from brachial plexus avulsion. Acta Neurochir Suppl (Wien) 1987;39:155–8.

96. Campbell JN, Solomon CT, James CS. The Hopkins experience with lesions of the dorsal horn (Nashold's operation) for pain from avulsion of the brachial plexus. Appl Neurophysiol 1988;51(2–5): 170–4.

97. Ishijima B, Shimoji K, Shimizu H, et al. Lesions of spinal and trigeminal dorsal root entry zone for deafferentation pain. Experience of 35 cases. Appl Neurophysiol 1988;51(2–5):175–87.

98. Saris SC, Iacono RP, Nashold BS Jr. Successful treatment of phantom pain with dorsal root entry zone coagulation. Appl Neurophysiol 1988;51(2–5):188–97.

99. Saris SC, Vieira JF, Nashold BS Jr. Dorsal root entry zone coagulation for intractable sciatica. Appl Neurophysiol 1988;51(2–5):206–11.

100. Kumagai Y, Shimoji K, Honma T, et al. Problems related to dorsal root entry zone lesions. Acta Neurochir (Wien) 1992;115(3–4):71–8.

101. Samii M, Bear-Henney S, Ludemann W, et al. Treatment of refractory pain after brachial plexus avulsion with dorsal root entry zone lesions. Neurosurgery 2001;48(6):1269–75 [discussion: 1275–7].

102. Chen HJ, Tu YK. Long term follow-up results of dorsal root entry zone lesions for intractable pain after brachial plexus avulsion injuries. Acta Neurochir Suppl 2006;99:73–5.

103. Awad AJ, Forbes JA, Jermakowicz W, et al. Experience with 25 years of dorsal root entry zone lesioning at a single institution. Surg Neurol Int 2013;4:64.

104. Konrad PE, Tacker WA Jr. Suprathreshold brain stimulation activates non-corticospinal motor evoked potentials in cats. Brain Res 1990;522(1):14–29.

105. Weigand H, Winkelmuller W. Gehandlung des Deafferentierungsschmerzes durch Hochfrequenzlasion der Hinterwurzeleintrittszone. Dtsch Med Wochenschr 1985;110:216–20.

106. Meglio M, Cioni B. The role of percutaneous cordotomy in the treatment of chronic cancer pain. Acta Neurochir (Wien) 1981;59(1–2):111–21.

107. Rosomoff H. Percutaneous radiofrequency cervical cordotomy for intractable pain. Adv Neurol 1974;4:683–8.

108. Sourek K. Commissural myelotomy. J Neurosurg 1969;31(5):524–7.

Percutaneous Spinal Cord Stimulation for Chronic Pain: Indications and Patient Selection

Sean J. Nagel, MD[a,*], Scott F. Lempka, PhD[a,b],
Andre G. Machado, MD, PhD[a]

KEYWORDS

- Spinal cord stimulation • Failed back surgery syndrome • Complex regional pain syndrome
- Surgical indications • Psychological evaluation • Surgical risk assessment

KEY POINTS

- Percutaneous spinal cord stimulation (pSCS) is an effective treatment of patients with complex regional pain syndrome or failed back surgery syndrome refractory to conventional medical management.
- Although frequently used for other indications, the data supporting the use of pSCS remain limited for other types of chronic, peripheral, neuropathic pain.
- Selecting patients who may benefit from pSCS is based on the cause of the pain, rigorous psychological evaluation, and medical comorbidities, including opioid dependence and risk of perioperative infection.

INTRODUCTION

Percutaneous spinal cord stimulation (pSCS) or dorsal column stimulation is a safe, minimally invasive, reversible treatment of patients with chronic neuropathic pain refractory to conventional medical management (CMM). Electrical stimulation of the dorsal columns was shown to inhibit pain transmission more than 40 years ago by Shealy.[1] Since then, multiple studies have demonstrated superior clinical benefit to other treatments in properly selected patients.[2,3] It is cost-effective over the long-term and complements other therapies in multimodal treatment. However, these devices continue to be used as a treatment of last resort despite known advantages.

INDICATIONS

Spinal cord stimulation (SCS) is currently approved in the United States by the Food and Drug Administration for the treatment of chronic pain of the back or limbs. In Europe, SCS for refractory angina pectoris (RAP) is frequently used in some centers but it is not considered a routine treatment in all countries. Several studies, including eight randomized controlled trials (RCTs) have tested SCS for RAP. However, the studies were small and several had methodological flaws.[4] The Refractory Angina Spinal Cord stimulation and usuAL care (RASCAL), a pilot RCT on the effectiveness and cost-effectiveness of SCS for refractory angina, was recently completed at three centers in the United Kingdom.[4] SCS has also been extensively

Disclosures: Dr. Machado: Consultant: Spinal Modulation, DBI and Functional Neuromodulation; Fellowship Support: Medtronic Possible distribution from Intellectual Property: Enspire, ATI and Cardionomics Scientific Advisory Board: Enspire.
[a] Department of Neurosurgery, Center for Neurological Restoration, Neurological Institute, Cleveland Clinic, 9500 Euclid Avenue, S31, Cleveland, OH 44195, USA; [b] Research Service, Louis Stokes Cleveland Veterans Affairs Medical Center, 10701 East Boulevard, Cleveland, OH 44106-1702, USA
* Corresponding author.
E-mail address: nagels@ccf.org

Neurosurg Clin N Am 25 (2014) 723–733
http://dx.doi.org/10.1016/j.nec.2014.06.005
1042-3680/14/$ – see front matter © 2014 Elsevier Inc. All rights reserved

studied in the treatment of inoperable chronic critical leg ischemia. A 2013 Cochrane review concluded that SCS may be better than conservative treatment alone in both pain relief and amputation risk reduction in select patients.[5] However, the surgical risk of implanting an SCS, coupled with the costs of the implant in patients with expected short life spans (10%–30% mortality in 6 months), continues to favor amputation.[5]

Over the last several years, several international expert panels have convened to establish the indications for pSCS based on a review of the available literature. Though a clear consensus has not been reached on many of the indications, the recommendations for SCS are relatively consistent with some notable exceptions. Almost universally, the panels agree that patients with failed back surgery syndrome (FBSS) or complex regional pain syndrome (CRPS) benefit from pSCS. Those with peripheral neuropathic pain due to illness or injury, including plexopathies, also seem to benefit. However, to date, this has not been evaluated with a properly powered study. Patients with central pain syndromes originating in the brain or spinal cord, including root avulsion, seem to benefit less with SCS except when the posterior columns are only minimally injured in the case of spinal cord injury. A synthesis of these recommendations is compiled into **Table 1**.[6–10] SCS has only been studied in a rigorous RCT on three occasions (see later discussion).

FBSS

In the United States, the most common indication for an SCS implant is FBSS. Patients with FBSS who did not achieve the goals of the spinal operation, specifically the anticipated pain relief, or who developed recurrent pain following surgery and have limited response to nonsurgical therapies may be candidates for SCS. In the United States in 2002, more than 1 million spinal procedures were performed and it estimated that the rate of back surgery is nearly 40% higher in the United States than in any other country.[11] It is difficult to measure the frequency of FBSS in the general population but it is estimated that between 0.02% and 2% of lumbar spinal surgeries have unsuccessful outcomes.[11] Furthermore, the health-related quality of life and economic costs often exceed other chronic pain and medical conditions. Even if only a small portion of these patients were candidates for pSCS, the potential for improvement in health and cost savings could be considerable.

In addition to multiple long-term outcome studies and retrospective case series that support the use of SCS, there were two published RCTs in the last decade that specifically addressed the use of SCS for FBSS. In 2005, North and colleagues[12] published the results from a RCT comparing reoperation to SCS for FBSS in an effort to move SCS ahead of reoperation in the treatment algorithm. Only subjects with radicular pain that exceeded or was equal to the axial back pain were included in the study. Subjects who experienced at least 50% pain relief with the trial were offered a permanent implant with a paddle electrode. Although the sample size was relatively small (24 in the SCS treatment arm and 26 in the reoperation arm), there were statistically significant differences between the two groups. At a mean follow-up of 2.9 years (+/− 1.1 SD), 47% of subjects randomized to SCS versus 12% of subjects randomized to reoperation achieved pain relief of at least 50% (P<.01). Narcotic use remained stable or decreased in subjects randomized to SCS compared with reoperation subjects (P<.025) and 54% of subjects who initially underwent reoperation crossed over compared with only 21% in the SCS group (P = .02). In this study, improvements in work status and activities of daily living were not improved following treatment.

In 2007, Kumar and colleagues[3] reported the outcomes from a RCT that compared SCS to CMM for subjects with FBSS. The Prospective Randomised Controlled Multicentre Trial of the Effectiveness of Spinal Cord Stimulation (PROCESS) tested the hypothesis that SCS plus CMM (SCS+CMM) is more effective than CMM alone. Permanent lead type, percutaneous or paddle, was at the discretion of the surgeon. Unlike the study by North and colleagues,[12] this was not a single institutional experience. The primary endpoint of the study was to calculate the proportion of subjects with at least 50% relief of leg pain at 6 months. One hundred subjects were initially included in the randomization. At 6-month follow-up, 44 subjects in the CMM-alone group were available for follow-up and 50 in the SCS+CMM group. After the 6 months, 28 (64%) of the subjects in the CMM group crossed over and received an implantable system. Twenty-four (48%) of the subjects in the SCS+CMM achieved the primary endpoint versus only four subjects (9%) in the CMM-alone group. Secondary outcomes at 6 months showed statistical significance favoring SCS+CMM versus CMM alone, including improvements in health-related quality of life, superior function, and greater treatment satisfaction. Nine subjects were able to wean off opioids in the SCS+CMM versus only one subject in the CMM group. There was no difference in return to work status between the two groups.

Table 1
Summary of selected recommendations on the indications for SCS

Diagnosis	European Federation of Neurologic Societies (EFNS)[a] (2007)	Practice Parameters for the Use of Spinal Cord Stimulation in the Treatment of Chronic Neuropathic Pain (2007)	British Pain Society (2009)	Austral-Asian Neurostimulation Working Group (2011)	Canadian Pain Society Special Interest Group on Neuropathic Pain (2012)
FBSS	Level B (probably effective) class II evidence: RCT that does not meet class I criteria	A: Well-designed RCTs; well-designed clinical studies; weighing risk vs potential benefit and expert consensus reveals a high likelihood of a favorable outcome	Neuropathic leg pain: good indication (likely to respond); axial pain: intermediate indication	Good indication (likely to respond)	Evidence quality: good; certainty: moderate; strength of recommendation; B
Failed Neck Surgery Syndrome	No evidence	N/A	Neuropathic arm pain: good indication (likely to respond)	Neuropathic arm pain: good indication (likely to respond)	N/A
CRPS I	Level B (probably effective), class II evidence: RCT that does not meet class I criteria	A: Well-designed RCTs; well-designed clinical studies; weighing risk vs potential benefit and expert consensus reveals a high likelihood of a favorable outcome	Good indication (likely to respond)	Intermediate indication (may respond)	Evidence quality: good; certainty: moderate; strength of recommendation; B
CRPS II	D, IV positive case series	A: Well-designed RCTs; well-designed clinical studies; weighing risk vs potential benefit and expert consensus reveals a high likelihood of a favorable outcome	Good indication (likely to respond)	Intermediate indication (may respond)	Evidence quality: good; certainty: moderate; strength of recommendation; B
Peripheral Nerve Injury	D, IV positive case series	Consider as other peripheral neuropathic pain	Good indication (likely to respond)	Intermediate indication (may respond)	Evidence quality: fair; certainty: moderate; strength of recommendation: grade C

(continued on next page)

Table 1
(continued)

Diagnosis	European Federation of Neurologic Societies (EFNS)[a] (2007)	Practice Parameters for the Use of Spinal Cord Stimulation in the Treatment of Chronic Neuropathic Pain (2007)	British Pain Society (2009)	Austral-Asian Neurostimulation Working Group (2011)	Canadian Pain Society Special Interest Group on Neuropathic Pain (2012)
Other Peripheral Neuropathy	D, IV positive case series	B: Well-designed clinical studies; case reports; weighing risk vs potential benefit and expert consensus reveals a good likelihood of a favorable outcome	Intermediate indication (may respond)	Intermediate indication (may respond)	Evidence quality: poor; certainty: low; strength of recommendation: grade I
Postherpetic Neuralgia	D, IV positive case series	B: Well-designed clinical studies; case reports; weighing risk vs potential benefit and expert consensus reveals a good likelihood of a favorable outcome B	Intermediate indication (may respond)	Not indicated (rarely respond)	Evidence quality: poor; certainty: low; strength of recommendation grade I
Intercostal Neuralgia	No evidence	Consider as other peripheral neuropathic pain	Intermediate indication (may respond)	Intermediate indication (may respond)	Evidence quality: poor; certainty: low; strength of recommendation: grade I
Brachial Plexus Injury	D, Class IV: positive case series	B: Well-designed clinical studies; case reports; weighing risk vs potential benefit and expert consensus reveals a good likelihood of a favorable outcome B	Brachial plexopathy: traumatic (partial); postirradiation: good indication (likely to respond)	N/A	Evidence quality: fair; certainty: moderate; strength of recommendation: grade C
Brachial Plexus Root Avulsion	D, IV negative case series for avulsion	N/A	Root avulsion: unresponsive	Avulsion: not indicated (rarely respond)	N/A

Diagnosis					
Amputation Pain	D, IV positive case series	B: Well-designed clinical studies; case reports; weighing risk vs potential benefit and expert consensus reveals a good likelihood of a favorable outcome	Intermediate indication (may respond)	Not indicated (rarely respond)	N/A
Central Pain of Spinal Cord origin	D, IV better success with incomplete lesion	B: Well-designed clinical studies; case reports; weighing risk vs potential benefit and expert consensus reveals a good likelihood of a favorable outcome	Intermediate indication (may respond) unless complete loss of posterior column function (poor response); complete spinal cord transection: unresponsive	Not indicated (rarely respond)	N/A
Central Pain of Brain Origin	D, IV negative case series	N/A	Poor indication (rarely respond)	Not indicated (rarely respond)	N/A
Refractory Angina Pectoris Pain	N/A	N/A	Good indication (likely to respond)	Good indication (likely to respond)	N/A
Peripheral Vascular Disease Pain	N/A	N/A	Good indication (likely to respond)	Intermediate indication (may respond)	N/A
Other	Facial pain: insufficient evidence; diabetic peripheral neuropathy: D, IV positive case series		Perineal or anorectal: poor indication (rarely respond); nonischemic nociceptive pain: unresponsive	Neuropathic pain secondary to peripheral nerve lesion: good indication (likely to respond); nociceptive axial back pain: not indicated (rarely respond)	N/A

a Class IV studies in the EFNS guidelines included uncontrolled studies, case series, case reports, or expert opinion. A Level D grade was not published in the original guidelines by the EFNS. In some instances, the diagnoses were inconsistent from one guideline to the next, requiring minor modifications in organizing the recommendations.
Data from Refs.[6–10]

CRPS

Although less common in the general population, especially compared with FBSS, the treatment of CRPS with SCS is well established and includes one RCT. The trial compared SCS plus physical therapy (PT; SCS+PT) in 36 subjects with PT alone in 18 subjects.[2] At 6 months, pain was reduced by 3.6 cm (in those who received the implant) on the visual analogue scale in the SCS+PT group and it was increased by 0.2 cm (P<.001) in the PT-alone group. The functional status and health-related quality of life did not improve in the SCS+PT group at the 6 month mark. Follow-up was available for subjects implanted in the initial study at 24 months and at 5 years.[13,14] Visual analogue scores, which were significantly better in the SCS+PT group at 2 years (3.0 cm–0 cm; P<.001), showed no difference at 5 years (1.7 cm SCS+PT vs 1.0 cm; P = .25). However, 95% reported they would undergo the treatment again for the same result.

PATIENT SELECTION
Diagnostic Evaluation

Patients referred for pSCS with an established diagnosis of neuropathic pain should be reevaluated at the initial visit. The diagnosis of neuropathic pain is made in the clinic by medical history, the description of pain, and sensory examination. There are many validated pain assessments tools that discern neuropathic from nonneuropathic pain that could be completed before the office visit.[15] Traditionally, it is the causal diagnosis that determines surgical candidacy for pSCS trials and implants. However, the somatosensory phenotype may prove to better predict outcomes than cause alone and allow for individualized therapies.[16] Unrecognized or overlooked conditions are common and should be considered before proceeding with neuromodulation. Patients with surgically remediable compression of the neural elements due to conditions such as degenerative disc disease, ligamentum hypertrophy, and/or foraminal stenosis may be considered for reoperation but could also be considered for SCS as the next alternative. This is a complex decision and takes into account a patient's overall health, surgical candidacy for larger procedures, risk of spinal implantation, and estimated likelihood of benefit from spinal operation versus neuromodulation. Benign tumors, such as schwannomas and neurofibromas, though less likely, may initially have been radiographically undetectable or overlooked at the onset of pain. Standing or dynamic plain radiographs may demonstrate either frank instability or abnormal motion at the facets, across the disc space, or both. Patients with persistent pain after a spinal fusion should be checked for pseudoarthrosis and hardware that is either broken or displaced. A preoperative spinal MRI or radiographic CT myelogram is usually ordered to check the diameter of the spinal canal. Dorsal calcifications or other obstruction may dissuade the surgeon from proceeding or alter the surgical plan (**Fig. 1**). In the future, it may be possible to use functional neuroimaging methods, such as functional MRI, to determine biomarkers of chronic pain that indicate which patients will likely respond well to SCS.[17] Functional neuroimaging may one day provide the tools to tailor the stimulation and medications to each patient (ie, personalized medicine) to maximize therapeutic benefit while minimizing side effects.[18]

Nonsurgical Management

Patients are often referred very late for SCS evaluation, enduring undertreated pain for years or even decades. In the PROCESS study, subjects randomized to the SCS arm, waited on average, 4.7 years (SD 5.1) between the last surgery and implant and a more recent analysis reported a delay of 65.4 months between pain onset and implant.[3,19] The reason for delay is multifactorial but includes patients unwilling to consent to additional surgery and skepticism and/or unfamiliarity with neuromodulation devices on the part of the referring physicians. In some cases, there is a mutual reluctance to end a longstanding physician–patient relationship built around the management of a chronic disease. On average, patients are managed by their primary care physician for approximately 12 months and nearly 40 additional months by a physician who is not an implant specialist.[19] In one study, subjects waited more than 4 months for surgery after referral to an implanting physician so other diagnostic investigations could be completed.[19]

Guidelines for managing neuropathic pain with medical therapy alone are prevalent and include well established class I evidence for many of the pain-alleviating medications, including antidepressants, anticonvulsants (sodium and calcium channel blockers), opioid agonists, cannabinoids, and topical therapies.[20] Most patients with chronic neuropathic pain are trialed initially on oral monotherapy with either a gabapentinoid, tricyclic antidepressant or a serotonin-norepinephrine reuptake inhibitor in addition to complementary therapies such as physical or psychological therapy. The dose should be titrated up if the response is

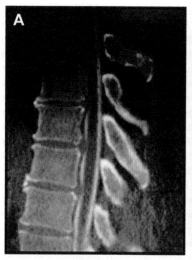
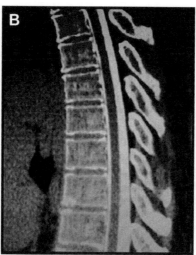
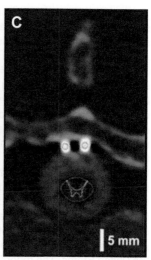

5 mm

Fig. 1. (*A*) CT myelogram of the thoracic spine in a patient with chronic neuropathic pain who underwent evaluation for SCS. There are three contiguous thoracic disc herniations displacing the thecal sac and abutting the spinal cord ventrally. There is a reduced volume of cerebrospinal fluid (CSF) dorsal to the spinal cord. A paddle lead (2 mm thick) would displace considerably more CSF than a percutaneous lead and potentially could cause neurologic symptoms. A percutaneous lead may be a better alternative in this case. (*B*) A normal CT myelogram from a second patient is shown for comparison. (*C*) CT myelogram of a patient with two cylindrical pSCS leads implanted in the epidural space dorsal to the spinal cord. Outlines show the approximate locations of the cylindrical leads as well as the spinal cord.

incomplete or, if there is no relief, the patient should be switched to another class. Combinations of medications should then be tried before considering opioid medications. Failure of opioid medications to control the pain at lower doses should prompt referral for surgical therapy.

Unfortunately, many patients are trialed on one after another of these medications either alone or in combination with an escalating dose of opioids before their pain is deemed refractory. This strategy is both costly and detrimental to outcomes because the likelihood for significant pain relief is reduced with each year of chronic pain.[21,22] Furthermore, it has been shown that those with chronic pain will develop measurable changes in brain function and structure. For example, abnormal hemodynamic activity has been recorded in the insular and anterior cingulate cortex of chronic pain patients compared with normal healthy subjects and gray matter atrophy is accelerated in patients with low back pain.[23,24] Whether these changes are reversible has yet to be determined.

Drug Use or Abuse

The widespread legal and illegal distribution of prescription narcotics over the last two decades has led to an epidemic of overdose deaths in the United States that exceeds 15,000 per year, a rate that has tripled since 1990.[25] The causes are multifactorial and include patient misuse or mixing with unauthorized substances, self-medication to control a comorbid mental health disease, lack of familiarity with opioid conversion, and overestimation of opioid tolerance.[26] In addition, methadone use, in particular, is associated with one-third of opioid-related deaths even though it accounts for only 5% of the prescriptions (this is related to both mixing with unauthorized substances, unapproved dose escalations, and wide variation in conversion guidelines).[26] It is the responsibility of physicians who treat chronic pain to identify at-risk patients, counsel those on chronic opioids about the risks, and make a concerted effort to reduce the chance of death in their patient population. In fact, this is frequently the first hurdle that a patient should clear when seen in clinic for evaluation. Signs of drug abuse include dose escalation without a practitioner's approval, lost or stolen prescriptions, requests for frequent refills, loss of opioid medications, and obtaining opioids from multiple prescribers or other sources.

Drug abuse or aberrant drug-related behaviors that may lead to abuse need to be considered before proceeding with neurostimulation therapy. In one evidence-based review of subjects exposed to chronic opioid analgesic therapy with nonmalignant pain, 3.27% developed abuse or addiction and additional 11.5% showed aberrant drug-related behaviors.[27] Urine toxicology screening of chronic pain patients receiving prescriptions for narcotics found that 20.4% of patients had either no opioid in their urine or a nonprescribed opioid.[27] However, there are several predictive screening questions that can be used to minimize the chance of inadvertently operating on a drug abuser or someone with tendencies. These include the disclosure of any previous or current history of alcohol or illicit drug use, a family history for alcohol or illicit drug use, prior treatment in a drug rehabilitation facility, use of multiple drugs, use of needles, and use of tobacco. It is important to discuss who the prescribing physician is and what the anticipated plan will be postoperatively. Prescription drug monitoring programs are now available in several states in the United States. The reporting systems are often the only evidence that a patient may have drug use or abuse problems. The details and usefulness of these systems vary from state to state.

Psychological Testing

Failure to control pain and improve quality of life following a technically successful surgical implant is not uncommon.[28] Furthermore, many patients may experience a loss of efficacy despite adequate coverage when pSCS is used long-term. Some failures may be preventable through appropriate psychological evaluation and treatment.[14] Although, many chronic pain patients in the United States undergo psychological consultation as a condition of approval for a neuromodulation device, the initial visit is an opportunity to explore inconsistencies in the patient's history, physical examination, pain rating, and imaging, as well as nonorganic signs of a major underlying psychiatric disorder. In fact, up to 50% of patients with chronic pain may have an underlying or undiagnosed personality disorder.[29] In particular, patients grouped into cluster B, especially those with antisocial personality disorders or borderline personality disorders, are difficult to manage.[30] Patients with a psychological need to be cared for by others, such as those with dependent personality disorders, are likely to have false-positive trials and to pose greater management risk. Along those same lines, those who depend on the medical system may not be prepared for the improvement they may find with neurostimulation therapy.[30] Doleys[30,31] has written extensively on the patient psychological factors that are more or less likely to influence patient outcomes following SCS. Patients with specific, well-localized pain with a clear-cut cause who are psychologically intact are most likely to achieve a good outcome. On the other hand, patients who place too much emphasis on the implant and who disregard the influence of psychosocial factors are more likely to have a negative outcome. Unlike almost any other surgical procedures, physician perceptions about pain can also influence treatment outcomes, especially when they acknowledge that chronic pain is a multifactorial disease process and treatment is long-term.[30] Physicians should not focus solely on the subjective relief of pain intensity. Rather, it is useful to discuss improvements in function or quality of life. Realistic expectations about pain relief are discussed along with an outline of the steps needed to achieve long-term benefits. It is important that the patients are ready and willing to undergo lifestyle modifications. This often comes in the form of tobacco cessation, eagerness to return to work, willingness to lose weight and exercise, commitment to wean off of medications (especially opioids), and willingness to continue with physical therapy exercises.

The psychological evaluation should consist of a clinical interview (with a significant other if available) and validated tests. As of now, there is no universally accepted psychological test that is used to screen potential SCS candidates.[28] The Minnesota Multiphasic Personality Inventory (MMPI) was the most commonly used assessment test in a systematic literature review conducted between the years 1967 and 2009.[32] Six studies identified in this article, reported that depression was associated with poorer outcome after SCS but SCS did, in some instances, improve premorbid depression.[33] Other premorbid psychological conditions, such as mania, hysteria, and hypochondriasis, were inconclusive as predictors. In another review, presurgical somatization, depression, anxiety, and poor coping, along with older age and longer pain duration, predicted poor outcomes.[32]

Medical Comorbidities

In general, pSCS is a well-tolerated, minimally invasive operation that does not require general anesthesia. Therefore, it lends itself to the management of chronic pain even in patients with an American Society of Anesthesiologists (ASA) class III or, in some cases, class IV who have comorbidities that would preclude more invasive operations requiring general anesthesia. Even so, the risk of a minimally invasive operation will still exceed the risks of nearly all nonsurgical treatments. Consequently, the physician should proceed with caution in a high-risk patient because, in one study, the risk of mortality in a large sample of subjects undergoing elective surgery was 7.3% in the ASA 4 group.[34] Patients with very poor nutrition or hypalbuminemia may be at increased risk for wound breakdown over the hardware sites. In morbidly obese patients or those with sleep apnea or chronic obstructive pulmonary disease, extended time in the prone position may increase the risk of airway compromise mandating judicious use of sedation. Active treatment with an antiplatelet or anticoagulant medication that cannot be stopped is an absolute contraindication, as are untreated bleeding disorders. In patients who carry a high risk of stroke or thrombosis when not therapeutically anticoagulated, opting for a permanent implant without a trial may be the safest option to minimize the total time off anticoagulants. Patients with implanted pacemakers or defibrillators are able to have an SCS device implanted and vice versa.[35] However, the manufacturers of both devices should be queried before proceeding. Bipolar stimulation settings should minimize the chance of an inadvertent shock being delivered or interfere with pacing. In general, patients who do not have the cognitive capacity to use or understand the device, or who are unwilling or unable to return for intermittent follow-up and programming, are not suitable candidates for neuromodulation therapy.

Minimizing the Risk of Infection

A postoperative infection of the surgical site that involves a nonbiological implantable device, specifically an SCS system, will usually necessitate hardware removal and lengthy antibiotic treatment. Unfortunately, this process not only poses a serious risk to the patient but also reverses the clinical benefit and, in so doing, erodes the cost savings of the operation.[36,37] Fortunately, postoperative infection can be minimized through careful patient selection and through the use of proven perioperative prophylaxis. The estimated risk of postoperative infection following SCS varies between studies with a recent review of SCS complications citing a range of 2.5% to 14% in the published literature with a mean of approximately 5%.[37] This is in line with the infection rate of 4.5% (32 patients) reported by single center with a large experience that included 707 cases of SCS, a rate that doubled in its diabetic patients.[38]

Patients should be screened for a history of poor wound healing, malnutrition, malignancy, immunosuppression (especially secondary to chronic steroid use), evidence of active infections, history of prior hardware-related infections, and diabetes. Although not all of these factors are modifiable, extra attention to wound care or an infectious disease consultation may be helpful in certain situations. In addition to routine presurgical testing, screening, and decolonizing for asymptomatic nasal carriage of *Staphylococcus aureus* with mupirocin has been shown to reduce the incidence of surgical infection.[39] Preoperative hospitalization also increases the infection risk up to four times and, in general, SCS should not be undertaken in a patient admitted to the hospital for another reason (and likely after a recent hospitalization).[40] Preoperative bathing with chlorhexidine has not been shown to reduce surgical site infection.[41] Preoperative urinalysis and treatment of bacteriuria in patients undergoing implant of a foreign body has limited support in the literature but is frequently recommended.[42] Given the overall low costs and low risks associated with these preventative options, inclusion in the preoperative protocol for physicians who implant neuromodulation devices should be a consideration.

The risk of infection is significantly increased in those who are actively smoking. Even 4 weeks of abstinence from smoking reduces the risk of infection.[43] Because this is a modifiable risk factor with other obvious health benefits, some practitioners elect not to trial or implant patients who are actively smoking because this may be an indirect surrogate for a commitment to adopting the healthy lifestyle that predicts a long-term clinical success.

SUMMARY

Although pSCS is a well-described treatment of FBSS and refractory neuropathic pain, it remains underused in these patient populations. Early referral for pSCS therapy should be considered in patients who require long-term opioid medication to achieve pain control, especially in light of the number of deaths from prescription painkillers. Diagnostic workup can reveal anatomic findings that may underlie the pain condition. In these cases, it is important to carefully judge and discuss with the patient the advantages and disadvantages of each treatment modality. Psychological factors contribute significantly to the patient's pain, their ability to cope, and the likelihood of long-term clinical success and should not be overlooked. In general, ordinarily high-risk surgical candidates may still be considered for pSCS because it does not require general anesthesia. Every effort should be made to minimize the risk of infection, which often requires explant of the device if it does occur. Improvements in the devices have enabled an ever-expanding array of programming combinations, longer battery life, and improved patient satisfaction.

REFERENCES

1. Shealy CN, Mortimer JT, Reswick JB. Electrical inhibition of pain by stimulation of the dorsal columns: preliminary clinical report. Anesth Analg 1967; 46(4):489–91.

2. Kemler MA, Barendse GA, van Kleef M, et al. Spinal cord stimulation in patients with chronic reflex sympathetic dystrophy. N Engl J Med 2000;343(9): 618–24.

3. Kumar K, Taylor RS, Jacques L, et al. Spinal cord stimulation versus conventional medical management for neuropathic pain: a multicentre randomised controlled trial in patients with failed back surgery syndrome. Pain 2007;132(1–2):179–88.

4. Eldabe SF, Raphael JF, Thomson SF, et al. The effectiveness and cost-effectiveness of spinal cord stimulation for refractory angina (RASCAL study): study protocol for a pilot randomized controlled trial. Trials 2013;14(57):1–9.

5. Ubbink DT, Vermeulen H. Spinal cord stimulation for non-reconstructable chronic critical leg ischaemia. Cochrane Database Syst Rev 2013;(2):CD004001.

6. Mailis A, Taenzer P. Evidence-based guideline for neuropathic pain interventional treatments: spinal cord stimulation, intravenous infusions, epidural injections and nerve blocks. Pain Res Manag 2012; 17(3):150.

7. Cruccu G, Aziz TZ, Garcia-Larrea L, et al. EFNS guidelines on neurostimulation therapy for neuropathic pain. Eur J Neurol 2007;14(9):952–70.

8. North R, Shipley J. Practice parameters for the use of spinal cord stimulation in the treatment of chronic neuropathic pain. Pain Med 2007;8:S200–75.

9. The British Pain Society. Spinal cord stimulation for the management of pain: recommendations for best clinical practice. London: The British Pain Society; 2009.

10. Atkinson L, Sundaraj SR, Brooker C, et al. Recommendations for patient selection in spinal cord stimulation. J Clin Neurosci 2011;18(10):1295–302.

11. Taylor RS, Taylor RJ. The economic impact of failed back surgery syndrome. British Journal of Pain 2012;6(4):174–81.

12. North RB, Kidd DH, Farrokhi F, et al. Spinal cord stimulation versus repeated lumbosacral spine surgery for chronic pain: a randomized, controlled trial. Neurosurgery 2005;56(1):98–107.

13. Kemler MA, De Vet HC, Barendse GA, et al. The effect of spinal cord stimulation in patients with chronic reflex sympathetic dystrophy: two years' follow-up of the randomized controlled trial. Ann Neurol 2004;55(1):13–8.

14. Kemler MA, de Vet HC, Barendse GA, et al. Effect of spinal cord stimulation for chronic complex regional pain syndrome type I: five-year final follow-up of patients in a randomized controlled trial. J Neurosurg 2008;108(2):292–8.

15. Cruccu GF, Truini A. Tools for assessing neuropathic pain. PLoS Med 2009;6(4):e1000045.

16. Arning KF, Baron R. Evaluation of symptom heterogeneity in neuropathic pain using assessments of sensory functions. Neurotherapeutics 2009;6:738–48.

17. Moens M, Sunaert S, Mariën P, et al. Spinal cord stimulation modulates cerebral function: an fMRI study. Neuroradiology 2012;54(12):1399–407.

18. Davis KD, Moayedi M. Central mechanisms of pain revealed through functional and structural MRI. J Neuroimmune Pharmacol 2013;8(3):518–34.

19. Kumar K, Rizvi S, Nguyen R, et al. Impact of wait times on spinal cord stimulation therapy outcomes. Pain Pract 2013 Oct 25. [Epub ahead of print].

20. Baron R, Binder A, Wasner G. Neuropathic pain: diagnosis, pathophysiological mechanisms, and treatment. Lancet Neurol 2010;9(8):807–19.

21. Kumar KF, Hunter GF, Demeria D. Spinal cord stimulation in treatment of chronic benign pain: challenges in treatment planning and present status, a 22-year experience. Neurosurgery 2006;58(3):481–96.

22. Kumar K, Wilson JR. Factors affecting spinal cord stimulation outcome in chronic benign pain with suggestions to improve success rate. In: Sakas D, Simpson B, Krames E, editors. Operative neuromodulation. Vienna (Austria): Springer-Verlag; 2007. p. 91–9.

23. Malinen S, Vartiainen N, Hlushchuk Y, et al. Aberrant temporal and spatial brain activity during rest in patients with chronic pain. Proc Natl Acad Sci U S A 2010;107(14):6493–7.

24. Apkarian AV, Sosa Y, Sonty S, et al. Chronic back pain is associated with decreased prefrontal and thalamic gray matter density. J Neurosci 2004; 24(46):10410–5.

25. CDC. Available at: Http://Www.cdc.gov/vitalsigns/PainkillerOverdoses/index.html. Accessed December, 2013.

26. Webster LR, Cochella S, Dasgupta N, et al. An analysis of the root causes for opioid-related overdose deaths in the United States. Pain Med 2011;12:S26–35.

27. Fishbain DA, Cole B, Lewis J, et al. What percentage of chronic nonmalignant pain patients exposed to chronic opioid analgesic therapy develop abuse/addiction and/or aberrant drug-related behaviors? A structured evidence-based review. Pain Med 2008;9(4):444–59.

28. Beltrutti D, Lamberto A, Barolat G, et al. The psychological assessment of candidates for spinal cord stimulation for chronic pain management. Pain Pract 2004;4(3):204–21.

29. Gatchel RJ. Comorbidity of chronic pain and mental health disorders: the biopsychosocial perspective. Am Psychol 2004;59(8):795–805.

30. Doleys DM. Psychological issues and evaluation for patients undergoing implantable technology. In: Krames ES, Peckham PH, Rezai AR, editors. Neuromodulation. London: Elsevier; 2009. p. 69–77.

31. Doleys DM. Psychological factors in spinal cord stimulation therapy: brief review and discussion. Neurosurg Focus 2006;21(6):1–6.

32. Celestin J, Edwards RR, Jamison RN. Pretreatment psychosocial variables as predictors of outcomes following lumbar surgery and spinal cord stimulation: a systematic review and literature synthesis. Pain Med 2009;10(4):639–53.

33. Sparkes E, Raphael JH, Duarte RV, et al. A systematic literature review of psychological characteristics as determinants of outcome for spinal cord stimulation therapy. Pain 2010;150(2):284–9.

34. Prause GF, Ratzenhofer-Comenda BF, Pierer GF, et al. Can ASA grade or Goldman's cardiac risk index predict peri-operative mortality? A study of 16,227 patients. Anaesthesia 1997;52(3):203–6.

35. Kosharskyy B, Rozen D. Feasibility of spinal cord stimulation in a patient with a cardiac pacemaker. Pain Physician 2006;9:249–52.

36. Manca A, Kumar K, Taylor RS, et al. Quality of life, resource consumption and costs of spinal cord stimulation versus conventional medical management in neuropathic pain patients with failed back surgery syndrome (PROCESS trial). Eur J Pain 2008;12(8): 1047–58.

37. Bendersky D, Yampolsky C. Is spinal cord stimulation safe? A review of its complications. World Neurosurg 2013. pii:S1878-8750(13)00758-4.

38. Mekhail NA, Mathews M, Nageeb F, et al. Retrospective review of 707 cases of spinal cord stimulation: indications and complications. Pain Pract 2011; 11(2):148–53.

39. Bode LG, Kluytmans JA, Wertheim HF, et al. Preventing surgical-site infections in nasal carriers of staphylococcus aureus. N Engl J Med 2010; 362(1):9–17.

40. Anderson DJ. Surgical site infections. Infect Dis Clin North Am 2011;25(1):135–53.

41. Webster J, Osborne S. Preoperative bathing or showering with skin antiseptics to prevent surgical site infection. Cochrane Database Syst Rev 2012;(9): CD004985.

42. Feely M, Collins C, Daniels P, et al. Preoperative testing before noncardiac surgery: guidelines and recommendations. Am Fam Physician 2013;87(6): 414–8.

43. Sorensen LT, Karlsmark TF, Gottrup F. Abstinence from smoking reduces incisional wound infection: a randomized controlled trial. Ann Surg 2003;238: 1–5.

Intrathecal Pain Pumps
Indications, Patient Selection, Techniques, and Outcomes

Robert Bolash, MD[a], Nagy Mekhail, MD, PhD[b],*

KEYWORDS

- Intrathecal pain pumps • Intrathecal drug delivery • Chronic pain • Intractable spasticity

KEY POINTS

- Intrathecal drug delivery allows continual administration of analgesics directly to their site of action within the cerebrospinal fluid (CSF), providing pain relief to patients who are intolerant or refractory to other routes of administration.
- Success with intrathecal therapy requires careful patient selection, an understanding of the pain mechanisms, and reasonable patient expectations.
- A trial of intrathecal drug therapy often precedes implant of the intrathecal drug delivery system. The trialing period enables both patient and physician to assess efficacy and immediate side effects of the intrathecal analgesia.
- Sustained improvement in both pain score and functional measures have been demonstrated when intrathecal drug delivery is used for both neuropathic and nociceptive pain.

INTRODUCTION

Intrathecal drug delivery systems represent an important therapeutic strategy for a subset of refractory chronic pain patients. Only morphine and the N-type calcium channel blocker ziconotide are Food and Drug Administration (FDA) approved for intrathecal administration, although a much wider variety of agents are currently in use for both nociceptive or neuropathic pain conditions.[1]

The continuous administration of analgesics via the intrathecal route results in higher subarachnoid drug concentrations and can achieve improved pain scores while mitigating many of the side effects seen with systemic administration of these same medications. Quality-of-life measures and overall health care utilization costs are decreased in select patients when intrathecal drug delivery is compared with conventional medical management alone, underscoring the importance of this route of delivery in an increasingly cost-conscious health care arena.[2–11]

INDICATIONS

Although intrathecal drug delivery systems have been widely used for treating intractable pain due to various malignancies, the delivery of neuraxial opiates for chronic nonmalignant pain states continues to gain favor in parallel with a growing body of evidence supporting their use.[12] By delivering opiates in close proximity to their site of action on the dorsal horn of the spinal cord, analgesia is achieved at doses much lower than when these same medications are administered systemically. Additionally, adverse effects are often mitigated and concerns about opiate diversion and analgesic compliance are attenuated when medications are administered via an

[a] Department of Pain Management, Cleveland Clinic, 9500 Euclid Avenue/C25, Cleveland, OH 44195, USA;
[b] Evidence Based Pain Medicine Research, Department of Pain Management, Cleveland Clinic, 9500 Euclid Avenue/C25, Cleveland, OH 44195, USA
* Corresponding author.
E-mail address: mekhain@ccf.org

Neurosurg Clin N Am 25 (2014) 735–742
http://dx.doi.org/10.1016/j.nec.2014.06.006

implanted drug delivery system. Newer intrathecal delivery systems are capable of providing patient-controlled analgesia on demand via a personal therapy manager.[13]

Although opiates have multiple established routes of delivery, the recent discovery of the non-opiate analgesic ziconotide necessitates direct administration into the CSF and has efficacy exclusively via the intrathecal route. As ziconotide use increases so will the number of patients with intrathecal drug delivery systems. Although outside of the scope of this discussion, intrathecal drug delivery systems are also widely used in the treatment of spasticity in both pediatric and adult populations.[14,15]

Consideration of the administration of intrathecal analgesics is typically reserved for those patients who fail, or are unable to tolerate, conservative treatment modalities, including opiate and nonopiate pharmacotherapy, as well as nonpharmacological adjuncts, such as interventional procedures or physical modalities. A pain diagnosis should be well established, classifying the pain as either nociceptive or neuropathic, and serve to guide the selection of intrathecal agents. Additionally, the pain should be chronic and present throughout most of the day, necessitating round-the-clock analgesic dosing. The source of the pain should not be easily correctable via an alternative intervention or any alternative surgical treatment should be deemed to pose a greater risk than treatment of the condition with intrathecal analgesics.

The development of intolerable side effects precluding the use of oral opiates represents a subset of patients who may achieve analgesic benefit from these same agents when administered directly into the CSF. This includes patients who achieve substantial pain relief from oral opiates but develop intolerable sedation, constipation, and other adverse effects. On administration of these same agents into the intrathecal space, many patients achieve analgesia while avoiding the adverse cognitive and gastrointestinal side effects (**Box 1**).

PATIENT SELECTION

Judicious patient selection is perhaps the most important strategy for achieving lasting success with continuous intrathecal drug therapy and involves multidisciplinary decision making with the input of interventionalists, mental health professionals, patients and their caregivers. Several stepwise algorithms to identify candidates for consideration of intrathecal drug delivery have been suggested, all with a focus on evaluating

> **Box 1**
> **Indications for consideration of intrathecal drug delivery**
>
> - An established pain diagnosis has been made classifying the symptoms as neuropathic, nociceptive, or mixed.
> - The pain complaint should be chronic or both chronic and progressive in nature owing to either a malignant or nonmalignant cause.
> - Pain should be present throughout nearly the entire day.
> - Patients have failed to achieve analgesia with conservative nonpharmacologic modalities
> - Patients who are refractory or intolerant to orally administered analgesics
> - Corrective treatment addressing the pain generator is not warranted.
> - Surgical contraindications to implanting prosthetic hardware and accessing the intrathecal space are absent (eg, bacteremia or anticoagulation).

and optimizing the multiple comorbidities on which chronic pain has an impact.[12,16]

First, pain practitioners identify patients, establish a pain diagnosis, and determine that more conservative options have been exhausted. Second, intrathecal drug delivery is presented to patients and expectations, comprehension, and support networks are assessed. Because administration of analgesics via the intrathecal route offers pain control, rather than pain elimination, realistic expectations should be set by practitioners and anticipated outcomes quantified among patients. Third, patients are evaluated and treated for psychological comorbidities that may be barriers to success with the therapy. The psychological evaluation is particularly important when considering the use of ziconotide because worsening mood disorders, cognitive impairment, and suicidal ideation have been observed with its use.[1,17,18] Although not demonstrated prospectively, preexisting psychopathology is thought to predispose patients to new adverse psychiatric events after initiation of ziconotide therapy, and many physicians consider psychosis a contraindication to the use of ziconotide.[1]

The multidisciplinary team should focus on how best to optimize patient success with intrathecal therapy rather than accepting intrathecal analgesia as a strategy of last resort. Patient dissatisfaction with intrathecal therapy remains a significant reason for premature revision or removal of intrathecal drug delivery systems, with only 51% of patients reporting satisfaction with the therapy 12 months after implant.[19] These dissatisfied patients represent a significant cost to the health care system. At the authors' institution, 11% of all patients who have undergone a successful trial undergo a surgical explant of the permanent drug delivery system due to dissatisfaction with the long-term therapy.[36]

TECHNIQUES

Perhaps somewhat unique to implantable therapies in interventional pain management is the opportunity for patient and physician to ascertain some measure of patient success and satisfaction with the therapy prior to implanting prosthetic hardware. Similar to a short-term temporary trial of spinal cord stimulation, the decision to proceed with implant of an intrathecal drug delivery system is often proceeded by a brief trial wherein medication is administered through a temporary intrathecal catheter. Throughout this trial period, pain relief is quantified, side effects are noted, and patient outcomes are assessed. Contingent on a favorable trial, an intrathecal drug delivery system consisting of a medication reservoir, pump, and intrathecal catheter is surgically implanted.

Trialing

The decision to implant an intrathecal pump for many pain diagnoses is often contingent on patients' success with a trial of intrathecal analgesic therapy. The trial serves multiple purposes, including the ability to assess a change in pain score or improvement in function. Conversely, a trial can assess a decrease in opiate-related adverse effects or a decrease in reliance on oral analgesics.[20] Also, the trial may provide additional data for the psychological assessment by providing insight into the patients mental status, enabling quantification of the consistency of response to the trial medication, and observing a snapshot of patient expectations.[16]

There are no prospective data demonstrating that a single trialing method is superior to another, and practitioners can accomplish an intrathecal trial via either continuous or intermittent epidural or intrathecal administration.[16,21] Despite a consensus committee recommendation outlining a trialing technique algorithm (**Fig. 1**), the choice is often individualized based on practitioner preference, infrastructure for patient care throughout the trial period, and an estimate of the duration needed to assess response to the medication.[16]

An epidural trial avoids the need for dural puncture and the potential for a resultant postdural puncture headache but requires that a 10-fold increase in opiate dose is administered. Additionally, an epidural trial excludes any contribution that the fluid dynamics of the CSF may have on the trial medication. Whereas a positive epidural opiate trial yields favorable information, a negative epidural trial does not exclude the possibility of potential success with intrathecal administration.[20]

An intrathecal trial can be accomplished via a single bolus, multiple bolus, or continuous infusion technique via a catheter inserted into the intrathecal space. The infusion permits administration of the intrathecal medication continuously, a technique that most similarly mimics the pharmacokinetics of delivery with an implanted pump, and avoids fluctuating drug levels seen with repeated intermittent bolus.[20]

The endpoint of an intrathecal trial is often defined in both research protocols and clinical practice as a greater than or equal to 50% decrease in pain.[6,16,22–24] Many investigators also prefer to see improved functionality and decreased reliance on oral opiate analgesic as clear endpoints of a successful trial. A trial may be deemed a failure if measurable pain relief is not achievable, adverse effects of the trial medication outweigh the observed benefits, patient satisfaction is low, or psychological barriers become apparent throughout the trial period.

Selecting Pharmacotherapy

Although morphine and ziconotide are currently the only FDA-approved pain medications for intrathecal use, a variety of monotherapies or combination agents, including hydromorphone, fentanyl, sufentanil, bupivacaine, clonidine, and baclofen, are in use. Nonapproved agents are recommended throughout established consensus statement algorithms, even as first-line therapies for the treatment of both neuropathic and nociceptive pain.[1] In light of its off-label use, a study to validate the safety and efficacy of intrathecal hydromorphone is currently in a phase 3 FDA clinical trial. Baclofen also carries an FDA approval for intrathecal use but is primarily used for spasticity and appears only late in the treatment algorithm for neuropathic pain.

Intrathecal trials are often performed with a single agent, such as morphine or ziconotide. A consensus committee has proposed 2 algorithms for the selection of agents for long-term intrathecal therapy. The choice of agents and stepwise decision recommendations differ based on the cause of the pain as either neuropathic (**Table 1**) or nociceptive (**Table 2**). Monotherapy is typically recommended at the initial stages of the algorithm, whereas combination agents with synergistic

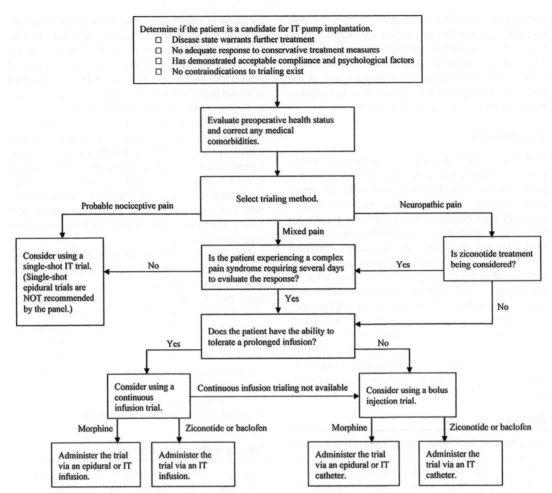

Fig. 1. Trialing technique algorithm. IT, intrathecal. (*From* Deer TR, Prager J, Levy R, et al. Polyanalgesic Consensus Conference 2012: recommendations on trialing for intrathecal (intraspinal) drug delivery: report of an interdisciplinary expert panel. Neuromodulation 2012;15(5):420–35; with permission.)

mechanisms of actions are used in the later steps.[1,25,26]

Type of Device

Intrathecal drug delivery requires implant of an infusion pump consisting of (1) a medication reservoir, (2) a mechanical pump, and (3) a catheter implanted into the intrathecal space. Both nonprogrammable and programmable pumps are available in the marketplace, as are a variety of catheter systems.

A nonprogrammable, fixed-rate pump delivers a continuous volume of medication into the intrathecal space by maintaining a consistent flow at a fixed daily rate. Although these systems are lower in cost, any change in dose necessitates a change of the concentration of medication in the reservoir.

A programmable pump can deliver variable doses by modulating the medication flow rate. Two programmable pump systems are presently available: the SynchroMed II (Medtronic, Minneapolis, Minnesota) and Prometra (Flowonix, Mt. Olive, New Jersey). Complex changes in dose can be preset by a physician, and an option to deliver a bolus dose can be administered on demand by patients using an external wireless transponder with the SynchroMed II system. Various reservoir sizes are available and selection is often contingent on patient habitus and the anticipated refill interval.

Surgical Implant

The intrathecal drug reservoir is typically placed in the abdominal wall with a tunneled subcutaneous catheter placed into the thecal sac. In preparation for surgical implant, the anterior abdominal

Table 1
Polyanalgesic algorithm for intrathecal therapies in neuropathic pain

Line 1	Morphine	Ziconotide		Morphine + bupivacaine
Line 2	Hydromorphone	Hydromorphone + bupivacaine or hydromorphone + clonidine		Morphine + clonidine
Line 3	Clonidine	Ziconotide + opioid	Fentanyl	Fentanyl + bupivacaine or Fentanyl + clonidine
Line 4	Opioid + clonidine + bupivacaine		Bupivacaine + clonidine	
Line 5	Baclofen			

Line 1: morphine and ziconotide are approved by the FDA for intrathecal (IT) therapy and are recommended as first-line therapy for neuropathic pain. The combination of morphine and bupivacaine is recommended for neuropathic pain on the basis of clinical use and apparent safety. Line 2: hydromorphone, alone or in combination with bupivacaine or clonidine, is recommended. Alternatively, the combination of morphine and clonidine may be used. Line 3: third-line recommendations for neuropathic pain include clonidine, ziconotide plus an opioid, and fentanyl alone or in combination with bupivacaine or clonidine. Line 4: the combination of bupivacaine and clonidine (with or without an opioid drug) is recommended. Line 5: baclofen is recommended on the basis of safety, although reports of efficacy are limited.

From Deer TR, Prager J, Levy R, et al. Polyanalgesic Consensus Conference 2012: recommendations for the management of pain by intrathecal (intraspinal) drug delivery: report of an interdisciplinary expert panel. Neuromodulation 2012;15(5):436–64; with permission.

reservoir site is marked at the midpoint between the costal margin and the iliac crest. This presurgical marking is typically done with the participation of the patient to ensure comfort with the location above the beltline because skin tissue can shift substantially intraoperatively.

The patient is positioned in the operating room in the lateral decubitus position with the side of the reservoir site up. The procedure begins by directing a Tuohy needle toward the thecal sac and advancing it in a paramedian plane until the dura is punctured. The stylette is removed and CSF flow is noted through the needle. A catheter is then threaded into the subarachnoid space. Leaving the Tuohy needle in place, an incision is made caudal to the needle insertion site through the skin and subcutaneous tissues with deep dissection proceeding until the supraspinous

Table 2
Polyanalgesic algorithm for intrathecal therapies in nociceptive pain

Line 1	Morphine	Hydromorphone	Ziconotide	Fentanyl
Line 2	Morphine + bupivacaine	Ziconotide + opioid	Hydromorphone + bupivacaine	Fentanyl + bupivacaine
Line 3	Opioid (morphine, hydromorphone, or fentanyl) + clonidine			Sufentanil
Line 4	Opioid + clonidine + bupivacaine		Sufentanil + bupivacaine or clonidine	
Line 5	Sufentanil + bupivacaine + clonidine			

Line 1: morphine and ziconotide are approved by the FDA for intrathecal (IT) therapy and are recommended as first-line therapy for nociceptive pain. Hydromorphone is recommended based on widespread clinical use and apparent safety. Fentanyl has been upgraded to first-line use by the consensus conference. Line 2: bupivacaine in combination with morphine, hydromorphone, or fentanyl is recommended. Alternatively, the combination of ziconotide and an opioid drug can be used. Line 3: recommendations include clonidine plus an opioid (ie, morphine, hydromorphone, or fentanyl) or sufentanil monotherapy. Line 4: the triple combination of an opioid, clonidine, and bupivacaine is recommended. An alternate recommendation is sufentanil in combination with either bupivacaine or clonidine. Line 5: the triple combination of sufentanil, bupivacaine, and clonidine is suggested.

From Deer TR, Prager J, Levy R, et al. Polyanalgesic Consensus Conference 2012: recommendations for the management of pain by intrathecal (intraspinal) drug delivery: report of an interdisciplinary expert panel. Neuromodulation 2012;15(5):436–64; with permission.

ligament is encountered. A nonabsorbable suture is anchored to the supraspinous ligament and the Tuohy needle is withdrawn leaving the catheter in place. The catheter is then anchored to the supraspinous ligament. Free CSF flow through the catheter system is confirmed after it is secured.

The reservoir pocket is then created by incising along the previously marked site on the anterior abdominal wall. A 1-inch deep subcutaneous pocket is expanded using blunt dissection caudal to the incision. The pump reservoir is inserted and anchored to the deep layer of the pocket to prevent rotation or flipping.

Finally, the intrathecal catheter and pump are connected by tunneling the dorsally secured catheter to the ventrally placed pump reservoir. Any redundant catheter is placed deep to the intrathecal pump to prevent strain when the patient bends or rotates. The incisions are closed in sequential fashion and the device is primed and programmed to begin drug delivery.

OUTCOMES

There is an expanding body of literature demonstrating the efficacy of intrathecal drug therapy for both neuropathic and nociceptive pain states due to malignant and nonmalignant etiologies.[12,27] Although more widely accepted as an option for end-of-life pain, the use of intrathecal analgesics for nonmalignant pain states continues to grow as the body of supporting evidence noting improved function expands. Ziconotide is gaining more widespread acceptance, owing in part to the absence of the need for continued dose escalation once a therapeutic level is determined.[28]

Cancer-Related Pain

End-of-life pain states represent a subgroup of patients in which intrathecal drug delivery has widespread acceptance and a demonstrated success. In a multicenter trial, 119 patients with either cancer-related pain or intolerable side effects with chronic opiate therapy were implanted with an intrathecal drug delivery system with the option to deliver a patient-controlled bolus: 90% of patients demonstrated a greater than or equal to 50% reduction in pain score 1 month after commencing intrathecal therapy, and the marked reduction was sustained throughout the 4-month study endpoint.[24]

The efficacy of intrathecal drug delivery has demonstrated benefits in conjunction with simultaneous medical management in patients with refractory cancer pain. Although clinical success with intrathecal therapy was defined by a less

rigorous greater than or equal to 20% decrease in pain score in this trial, patients in the intrathecal drug delivery group achieved success more often than those managed with conventional medical management alone. Additionally, measures of fatigue and alertness were improved in those treated with an intrathecal drug delivery, resulting in improved quality of life.[9]

Ziconotide has also demonstrated efficacy in the management of end-of-life pain due to both neoplastic and AIDS-related pain states. In a double-blind placebo-controlled trial, patients were administered ziconotide or placebo during a titration and maintenance period with a crossover arm for nonresponders. Mean pain scores decreased 53.1% in the treatment arm, with 52.9% of patients reporting moderate to complete pain relief throughout the study period.[29]

Nonmalignant Chronic Pain

Success with chronic intrathecal opiate therapy was assessed in a cohort of 57 patients over a 3-year period after implant of an intrathecal pump for primarily nonmalignant (96%) causes. Visual analog pain scores were decreased between implant and first pump refill, and pain scores remained low throughout the 3-year observation period. Oral opiate intake was decreased on placement of the intrathecal pump from a mean daily morphine equivalent dose of 183.9 mg/d at baseline to 43.5 mg/d at 1-year follow-up.[30,31]

Vertebral compression fractures were managed with intrathecal morphine in a cohort of 24 Italian patients who were refractory to oral and transdermal opiate delivery routes. Mean pain scores decreased from 8.7 to 1.9, whereas measures of quality of life, ambulation, and perceived health status improved after initiating intrathecal morphine therapy. Although the mean dose of intrathecal morphine escalated in the cohort at 1-year follow-up, all the patients were able to eliminate the need for any supplemental oral analgesics.[32]

Ziconotide has demonstrated a similar efficacy in nonmalignant pain states. In a randomized, double-blind, placebo-controlled trial, 169 patients with nonmalignant pain received ziconotide via continuous infusion throughout a 6-day hospital stay. A 31.2% improvement in pain scores was seen in the treatment arm compared with 6% in the placebo-treated group.[33]

Given the increasing trend toward measuring success with interventional pain therapy in terms of function and psychological outcomes rather than simply a reduction in patient-reported pain scores, 30 patients with nonmalignant chronic pain conditions were assessed prospectively over 24 months after implant of an intrathecal drug delivery system. The evaluative, affective, and sensory components of the McGill Pain Questionnaire improved throughout the study period, with 92% of patients returning to the workplace and 82% of retired patients requiring less assistance at home after beginning intrathecal therapy.[34]

Several investigators addressed the factors affecting opioid dose escalation in large cohorts of chronic nonmalignant pain patients managed with intrathecal therapy. Age has been inconsistently shown to predict the need for rapid dose escalation, with tolerance developing more slowly in the elderly in one study.[27,35] Preoperative factors, including gender, comorbid conditions, and duration and dose of oral therapy, as well as diagnosis were screened to predict subsets of patients who would require rapid intrathecal opiate dose escalation. The only subgroup found significantly associated with the need for rapid dose escalation was those with neuropathic pain.[35] In another cohort, the addition of bupivacaine to the intrathecal opiate was shown to mitigate the need for rapid dose escalation compared with therapy with opiate alone.[19]

SUMMARY

Success with intrathecal drug delivery hinges on multiple factors, including a thorough understanding of the pain condition, careful patient selection, meaningful trialing, and concordance between patient expectations and outcomes. With advances in the longevity and decreases in the cost of intrathecal drug delivery hardware, coupled with a growing body of evidence demonstrating meaningful functional outcomes, intrathecal drug delivery will continue to play a growing role in the treatment of chronic pain syndromes.

REFERENCES

1. Deer TR, Prager J, Levy R, et al. Polyanalgesic Consensus Conference 2012: recommendations for the management of pain by intrathecal (intraspinal) drug delivery: report of an interdisciplinary expert panel. Neuromodulation 2012;15(5):436–64.
2. Biggs SA, Duarte RV, Raphael JH, et al. Influence of a latent period in QALY analysis: pilot study of intrathecal drug delivery systems for chronic nonmalignant pain. Br J Neurosurg 2011;25(3):401–6.
3. de Lissovoy G, Brown RE, Halpern M, et al. Cost-effectiveness of long-term intrathecal morphine therapy for pain associated with failed back surgery syndrome. Clin Ther 1997;19(1):96–112.
4. Deer TR, Caraway DL, Kim CK, et al. Clinical experience with intrathecal bupivacaine in combination with opioid for the treatment of chronic pain related to failed back surgery syndrome and metastatic cancer pain of the spine. Spine J 2002;2(4):274–8.
5. Guillemette S, Witzke S, Leier J, et al. Medical cost impact of intrathecal drug delivery for noncancer pain. Pain Med 2013;14(4):504–15.
6. Kumar K, Hunter G, Demeria DD. Treatment of chronic pain by using intrathecal drug therapy compared with conventional pain therapies: a cost-effectiveness analysis. J Neurosurg 2002;97(4):803–10.
7. Mueller-Schwefe G, Hassenbusch SJ, Reig E. Cost effectiveness of intrathecal therapy for pain. Neuromodulation 1999;2(2):77–87.
8. Roberts LJ, Finch PM, Goucke CR, et al. Outcome of intrathecal opioids in chronic non-cancer pain. Eur J Pain 2001;5(4):353–61.
9. Smith TJ, Staats PS, Deer T, et al, Implantable Drug Delivery Systems Study Group. Randomized clinical trial of an implantable drug delivery system compared with comprehensive medical management for refractory cancer pain: impact on pain, drug-related toxicity, and survival. J Clin Oncol 2002;20(19):4040–9.
10. Thimineur MA, Kravitz E, Vodapally MS. Intrathecal opioid treatment for chronic non-malignant pain: a 3-year prospective study. Pain 2004;109(3):242–9.
11. Winkelmüller M, Winkelmüller W. Long-term effects of continuous intrathecal opioid treatment in chronic pain of nonmalignant etiology. J Neurosurg 1996; 85(3):458–67.
12. Ver Donck A, Vranken JH, Puylaert M, et al. Intrathecal drug administration in chronic pain syndromes. Pain Pract 2014;14(5):461–76.
13. Medtronic (2007, February) retrieved from: medtronic personal therapy manager for synchromed ii physician implant manual. Available at: http://professional.med tronic.com/wcm/groups/mdtcom_sg/@mdt/@neuro/documents/documents/idd-ptm8835-manl.pdf. Accessed July 21, 2014.
14. Dan B, Motta F, Vles JS, et al. Consensus on the appropriate use of intrathecal baclofen (ITB) therapy in paediatric spasticity. Eur J Paediatr Neurol 2010; 14(1):19–28.
15. McIntyre A, Mays R, Mehta S, et al. Examining the effectiveness of intrathecal baclofen on spasticity in individuals with chronic spinal cord injury: a systematic review. J Spinal Cord Med 2014; 37(1):11–8.
16. Deer TR, Prager J, Levy R, et al. Polyanalgesic Consensus Conference–2012: recommendations on trialing for intrathecal (intraspinal) drug delivery: report of an interdisciplinary expert panel. Neuromodulation 2012;15(5):420–35.
17. Maier C, Gockel HH, Gruhn K, et al. Increased risk of suicide under intrathecal ziconotide treatment? - a warning. Pain 2011;152(1):235–7.
18. Thompson JC, Dunbar E, Laye RR. Treatment challenges and complications with ziconotide

monotherapy in established pump patients. Pain Physician 2006;9(2):147–52.

19. Veizi IE, Hayek SM, Narouze S, et al. Combination of intrathecal opioids with bupivacaine attenuates opioid dose escalation in chronic noncancer pain patients. Pain Med 2011;12(10):1481–9.

20. Przybyl JS, Follett KA, Caraway D. Intrathecal drug delivery: general considerations. Semin Pain Med 2003;1(4):228–33.

21. Grider JS, Harned ME, Etscheidt MA. Patient selection and outcomes using a low-dose intrathecal opioid trialing method for chronic nonmalignant pain. Pain Physician 2011;14(4):343–51.

22. Anderson VC, Burchiel KJ, Cooke B. A prospective, randomized trial of intrathecal injection vs. epidural infusion in the selection of patients for continuous intrathecal opioid therapy. Neuromodulation 2003; 6(3):142–52.

23. Kumar K, Kelly M, Pirlot T. Continuous intrathecal morphine treatment for chronic pain of nonmalignant etiology: long-term benefits and efficacy. Surg Neurol 2001;55(2):79–86.

24. Rauck RL, Cherry D, Boyer MF, et al. Long-term intrathecal opioid therapy with a patient-activated, implanted delivery system for the treatment of refractory cancer pain. J Pain 2003;4(8):441–7.

25. Pope JE, Deer TR. Ziconotide: a clinical update and pharmacologic review. Expert Opin Pharmacother 2013;14(7):957–66.

26. Wallace MS, Rauck RL, Deer T. Ziconotide combination intrathecal therapy: rationale and evidence. Clin J Pain 2010;26(7):635–44.

27. Hayek SM, Deer TR, Pope JE, et al. Intrathecal therapy for cancer and non-cancer pain. Pain Physician 2011;14(3):219–48.

28. Ellis DJ, Dissanayake S, McGuire D, et al, Elan Study 95-002 Group. Continuous intrathecal infusion of ziconotide for treatment of chronic malignant and nonmalignant pain over 12 months: a prospective, open-label study. Neuromodulation 2008; 11(1):40–9.

29. Staats PS, Yearwood T, Charapata SG, et al. Intrathecal ziconotide in the treatment of refractory pain in patients with cancer or AIDS: a randomized controlled trial. JAMA 2004;291(1):63–70.

30. Atli A, Theodore BR, Turk DC, et al. Intrathecal opioid therapy for chronic nonmalignant pain: a retrospective cohort study with 3-year follow-up. Pain Med 2010;11(7):1010–6.

31. Belverud S, Mogilner A, Schulder M. Intrathecal pumps. Neurotherapeutics 2008;5(1):114–22.

32. Saltari MR, Shaladi A, Piva B, et al. The management of pain from collapse of osteoporotic vertebrae with continuous intrathecal morphine infusion. Neuromodulation 2007;10(2):167–76.

33. Wallace MS, Charapata SG, Fisher R, et al, Ziconotide Nonmalignant Pain Study 96-002 Group. Intrathecal ziconotide in the treatment of chronic nonmalignant pain: a randomized, double-blind, placebo-controlled clinical trial. Neuromodulation 2006;9(2):75–86.

34. Duse G, Davià G, White PF. Improvement in psychosocial outcomes in chronic pain patients receiving intrathecal morphine infusions. Anesth Analg 2009; 109(6):1981–6.

35. Mekhail N, Mahboobi R, Farajzadeh Deroee A, et al. Factors that might impact intrathecal drug delievery (IDD) dose escalation: a longitudinal study. Pain Pract 2014;14(4):301–8.

36. Bolash RB, Udeh B, Saweris Y, et al. Longevity and Cost of Implantable Intrathecal Drug Delivery Systems for Chronic Pain Management: A Retrospective Analysis of 365 Patients. Neuromodulation "in press".

Microvascular Decompression for Trigeminal Neuralgia

Burak Sade, MD[a],*, Joung H. Lee, MD[b]

KEYWORDS

- Microvascular decompression • Management • Trigeminal neuralgia • Surgical • Treatment

KEY POINTS

- Microvascular decompression (MVD) has proven to be a safe and effective option for patients with medically intractable trigeminal neuralgia (TN).
- MVD provides a high rate of early pain relief, with relatively low recurrence and complication rates in experienced hands, as compared with other surgical modalities such as the percutaneous techniques and stereotactic radiosurgery.
- MVD should be considered as the first line of surgical treatment in patients with TN, including carefully selected candidates in the elderly population (provided that there are no significant medical comorbidities associated), and in whom the pathophysiology of the pain is most likely to be the neurovascular compression and no other alternative mechanisms (ie, multiple sclerosis, herpetic neuralgia) are likely.

INTRODUCTION

Trigeminal neuralgia (TN) is one of the many types of facial pain syndromes,[1] which is thought to occur as a result of the ignition of hyperexcitable axons at the trigeminal root and neuronal somata at the trigeminal ganglion.[1,2] Compression of the root entry zone (REZ) of the nerve by the neighboring offending artery, which was initially proposed by Jannetta,[3] and for which the microvascular decompression (MVD) procedure was introduced thereafter, has been shown to contribute to the demyelination process within the trigeminal nerve, a main finding in patients with TN.[2]

In contemporary neurosurgery, the first line of management for patients suffering from this debilitating problem is medical treatment (ie, Carbamazepine, gabapentin). In cases of failed medical therapy or drug intolerance, or simply when patients do not prefer to take these medications for a long period of time, other treatment options, including MVD, should be considered[4]:

- MVD
- Percutaneous techniques:
  - Glycerol rhizotomy
  - Balloon compression
  - Radiofrequency rhizotomy
- Gamma Knife radiosurgery (GKRS)

SURGICAL TECHNIQUE
Patient Selection

Establishing the diagnosis accurately
One cannot overemphasize the significance of establishing accurate clinical diagnosis of TN in ensuring a favorable postoperative outcome for MVD. The patient's description of the pain, and

Disclosures: None.
[a] Department of Neurosurgery, Beyin ve Sinir Cerrahisi ABD, Dokuz Eylul Universitesi Hastanesi, Balcova, Izmir 35340, Turkey; [b] The Hycy and Howard Neuroscience Institute, Providence St. Joseph Medical Center, 501 S. Buena Vista Street, Burbank, CA 91505, USA
* Corresponding author.
E-mail address: burak.sade@deu.edu.tr

neurosurgery.theclinics.com

the neurologic examination, should leave no doubt that what is being dealt with is TN before referring to any radiologic study or intervention. Miller and colleagues[5] reported that patients presenting with type 1 TN pain (50% episodic pain), according to the classification of Burchiel,[1] had significantly higher chance of having a favorable outcome following MVD for TN than patients with type II pain (84% vs 64%). In this context, one also has to keep in mind the possibility of multiple sclerosis–induced neuralgia and postherpetic neuralgia before proceeding with MVD.

Age as a factor in the decision-making process

Age has been an important factor for neurosurgeons in choosing the appropriate treatment option for patients with TN, and traditionally, there has been a tendency to offer percutaneous procedures or GKRS rather than MVD to patients with advanced age. However, recent studies have shown no significant differences in complications or short-term and long-term outcome of MVD in elderly patients than in younger ones.[6,7] One study concluded that although complications show a tendency to increase with advanced age, age itself does not act as a risk factor in isolation.[8]

Significance of radiographic findings

The significance of demonstrating a close anatomic relationship or contact between the vessels and the trigeminal nerve preoperatively has been debated in the literature, because this finding has also been reported quite commonly in patients without TN.[9,10] However, when preoperative assessment of the neurovascular relationships of the region is desired, 3D constructive interference in steady state magnetic resonance (MR) (**Fig. 1**), which is a heavily T2-weighted sequence with very high resolution of the cerebrospinal fluid (CSF) tissue contrast and high-resolution 3D time-of-flight MR angiography[9] may provide adequate information to the surgeon in most cases.

The other important detail when reviewing preoperative radiological studies would be the tentorial alignment and angle. The authors' group has shown previously that a steeper tentorial angle

would result in a decreased distance between the trigeminal nerve and the acoustico-facial nerve complex, limiting the operative field between these cranial nerves.[11]

Surgical Approach and Patient Positioning

In the authors' practice, they use the "simplified retrosigmoid approach" for MVD procedures.[12] Following induction of general anesthesia, the patient is placed in the supine position with the head rotated to the contralateral side and slightly flexed, and it is verified that the jugular vein is free of compression (**Fig. 2**A). The ipsilateral shoulder may be elevated and supported by a shoulder roll.

Procedure

Incision

A 4 to 5 cm curvilinear skin incision is placed using the asterion as the main landmark (see **Fig. 2**B). Approximately one-third of the incision remains above, and two-thirds are below the asterion.

Craniectomy and dural opening

A triangular craniectomy is performed using a cutting drill and Kerrison rongeurs so that the upper lateral corner of the triangle sits at the junction of the transverse and sigmoid sinuses (see **Fig. 2**C). During this stage, one needs to be prepared for the possibility of brisk bleeding from the emissary veins or sinuses themselves. In individuals with generously aerated mastoid bones, one can enter wide air cells, which could potentially result in CSF rhinorrhea. Therefore, when encountered, these should be appropriately plugged and sealed.

A Y-shaped dural opening is performed creating 2 triangular flaps based on the sinuses. Following this, the cerebellum is retracted gently and the lateral cerebellomedullary cistern is entered to drain CSF (see **Fig. 2**D); this should be done with care so as to minimize cerebellar trauma, which can potentially result in serious swelling.

Intradural dissection and retraction

The microscope is tilted upwards. It cannot be overemphasized that the cerebellar retraction remains

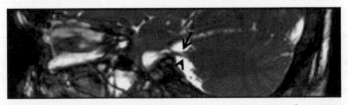

Fig. 1. Preoperative 3D constructive interference in steady state sequence MR of a patient with right-sided TN demonstrating a contact between the trigeminal nerve and a superior cerebellar artery loop on the right. *Arrow,* superior cerebellar artery; *arrowhead,* trigeminal nerve.

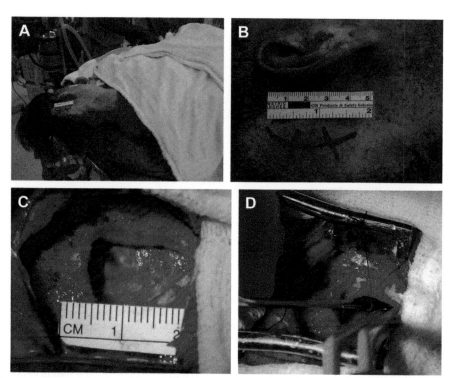

Fig. 2. (*A*) Positioning for MVD procedure. (*B*) Marking of the incision with the asterion as the main landmark. (*C*) Craniectomy bordering the transverse and sigmoid sinuses. (*D*) Intradural stage of the procedure after the posterior fossa is decompressed.

very mild and gentle throughout the surgery. In fact, with adequate CSF drainage and arachnoidal opening, the cerebellum falls out of the operative field without necessitating any significant retraction for the most part of the procedure. Also, one has to keep in mind that excessive retraction of the petrosal surface of the cerebellum can result in injury to the cochlear nerve. Therefore, a more petrotentorial retraction would not only yield a better access to the trigeminal nerve but also lower the risk of this potential complication.

Intraoperative neuromonitoring
Routine use of intraoperative monitoring of the facial and cochlear nerves has been described and advocated by some groups in the literature. However, in the authors' practice, they do not feel the need to do so on a routine basis, as the core of the surgery takes place relatively far from the acoustico-facial nerve complex and, with appropriate retraction, the risk of nerve damage is reduced.

Petrosal veins
The issue of whether to preserve or sacrifice the superior petrosal vein/complex (SPV) is probably one of the most controversial aspects of MVD (**Fig. 3**). SPV drains the anterior aspect of the brain stem and cerebellum and empties into the superior

petrosal sinus. Its most common tributaries are the vein of the cerebellopontine fissure, vein of the middle cerebellar peduncle, transverse pontine vein, pontotrigeminal vein, and the veins draining the lateral surface of the cerebellum.[13]

At times, it may be necessary to sacrifice this vein (complex) to improve exposure of the REZ of the trigeminal nerve, but it is often possible to work around without sacrificing it (**Fig. 4**A). There have been reports in the literature along with anecdotal experience of many surgeons, suggesting that its sacrifice may result in venous infarction of the cerebellum.[13] However, considering how many times

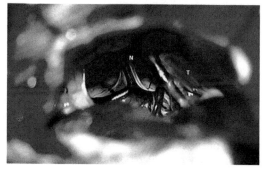

Fig. 3. A SPV complex partially obstructing the view of the trigeminal nerve. N, trigeminal nerve; T, tentorium.

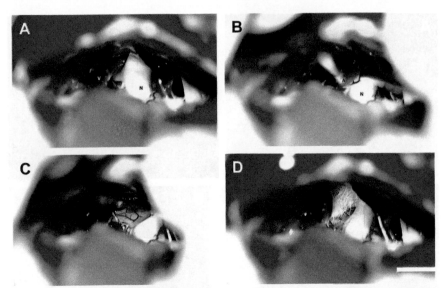

Fig. 4. (*A*) Dissection at the dorsal aspect of the trigeminal nerve in between 2 petrosal veins. Note the absence of any offending vessels in the dorsal aspect. (*B*) A superior cerebellar artery loop compressing the nerve ventrally. (*C*) View after the artery has been dissected away. (*D*) After the Teflon sponge has been placed. A, superior cerebellar artery; N, trigeminal nerve; V, superior petrosal vein.

this is done and how rare this complication is, variations of anatomy and collaterals in a given patient are likely to play an important role here. When this complication is encountered, excessive cerebellar retraction is more likely to be the culprit. The authors' practice has been to try to preserve the vein or veins whenever possible, and especially if it is of a significant caliber. However, in cases where it is not possible to achieve a satisfactory exposure, its sacrifice may be justified.

Identifying the vascular conflict and decompression of the nerve

In up to 75% of the cases, the offending vessel is the superior cerebellar artery.[4,14,15] Pure venous compression is seen in approximately 12% and small arteries in 15%. Multivessel compression consisting of an artery and a vein is reported in as many as 56% of the patients.[14]

At this stage of the procedure, once the trigeminal nerve is exposed by generous arachnoid dissection, it is very important to visualize the REZ because a readily visible vascular contact against the more peripheral aspect of the cisternal segment of the nerve may detract the surgeon's attention from a more relevant offending vessel at the REZ. Similarly, ventral aspect of the nerve should always be explored whether or not one identifies a contacting vessel dorsal to the nerve (see **Fig. 4**B; **Fig. 5**). Once the true offender or offenderd are identified, pieces of Teflon sponge are then positioned in between the nerve and the vessels, thereby eliminating the compression. Here, it would be important to make

sure that the whole surface that is in contact is decompressed (see **Fig. 4**C, D).

In cases where no arterial culprit can be identified despite a meticulous exploration and a nearby vein appears to be in contact with the REZ, the vein may be considered as the offending vessel and cushioned away from the nerve or sectioned, provided that the vein is not of a significant caliber. However, in such cases, the outcome may be somewhat less satisfactory.

Absence of vascular conflict

In about 15% of the patients undergoing MVD, despite satisfactory exploration, no offending vessel can be identified.[16] In these cases, controlled traumatization of the nerve using the bipolar forceps (without coagulation), thereby causing some degree

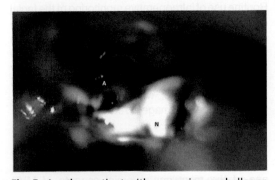

Fig. 5. Another patient with a superior cerebellar artery loop compressing the nerve ventrally. A, superior cerebellar artery; N, trigeminal nerve.

of neuropraxia, has been shown to be effective, albeit, with a shorter-lasting effect. It is important to remember though that manipulation of the trigeminal nerve may result in significant bradycardia, which often resolves once the manipulation is discontinued.

Closure

Following the decompression and hemostasis, the intradural compartment is rigorously irrigated to clean any residual blood clot or debris. In the authors' practice, they reapproximate the dural leaves using 3 to 4 sutures without pursuing any water tightness. This reapproximation is followed by tailoring a gel-foam sandwich consisting of 2 layers of gel foam with a layer of gel film in between. At this stage, it is very important to make sure that the mastoid air cells are appropriately sealed if encountered at the time of opening. Following this, the craniectomy defect is covered by a burr-hole cover, and the subsequent layers of skin are closed in the usual manner.

Complications

The most significant complications and their most likely causes following MVD for TN are as follows:

- Cerebellar swelling/hematoma: excessive cerebellar retraction (more common) or petrous vein sacrifice (rarely)
- Arterial/venous infarct of the cerebellum and/or the brain stem: inadvertent vascular sacrifice/injury
- Hearing loss: excessive cerebellar retraction
- CSF rhinorrhea: inadequate sealing of opened mastoid air cells
- CSF leak from the wound: inadequate closure of the wound, or poor wound healing.

Recovery

In the authors' practice, they apply a tight head-wrap in the operating room and keep it on for the first 48 hours, after which they keep the incision exposed to open air. Prophylactic antibiotics are continued for 24 hours postoperatively. Patients are mobilized the next morning after surgery and are usually discharged within 2 days after surgery, unless they have severe dizziness, which is relatively rare following MVD for TN.

CLINICAL OUTCOME
Long-term Outcome

The MVD procedure has proven to be an effective and durable treatment option for patients with TN. Initial pain relief can be as high as 98%.[4] The largest review of series, performed by Barker and colleagues,[14] showed that 70% of the patients were free of pain and medications at 10 years. In the same report, the annual rate of recurrence was reported as less than 1%. The most significant factors that play a role for a favorable outcome are as follows[5,14,17]:

- Type 1 TN, namely, more than 50% of the pain being in the episodic form
- Identification of an obvious offending vessel on imaging studies preoperatively
- Identification of an offending artery intraoperatively.

Postradiosurgery MVD

The feasibility of MVD following a failed GKRS treatment as a salvage procedure is a matter of extensive debate in the neurosurgical community. Most opinions expressed on the subject are based on anecdotal experience and there are scant data in the literature. For instance, Sekula and colleagues[18] reported that, contrary to general belief, thickened arachnoid was seen in only 3%, and adhesions between the trigeminal nerve and the vessels were seen in 21% of the patients. However, this was significant enough to abort the procedure in 4%. Approximately 60% of the patients reported good to excellent outcome following surgery, which may be seen as reasonable for a salvage procedure, but one has to keep in mind the high rate (32%) of new-onset numbness or dysesthesias in the postoperative period.

Comparison with Other Surgical Modalities

An extensive review by Tatli and colleagues[19] looked at the outcomes of various surgical modalities in the literature that had a minimum 5 years of follow-up. Their findings suggested that

- MVD provided the highest rate of long-term patient satisfaction and lowest rate of pain recurrence
- Among the percutaneous techniques, compared with MVD:
  - Glycerol rhizotomy had a low initial pain relief and a high pain recurrence rate
  - Balloon compression had a high rate of facial hypoesthesia, and a higher rate of postoperative trigeminal motor dysfunction
  - Radiofrequency rhizotomy provided a high rate of initial pain relief, but showed a high rate of long-term failure and also higher rate of serious complications, such as corneal hypoesthesia, keratitis, and anesthesia dolorosa.

- GKRS showed a low initial pain relief and a lower pain-free rate in the follow-up period compared with MVD.

Interestingly, the retrospective cohort study of Wang and colleagues,[20] which looked at the trends in the surgical treatment modalities for patients admitted to US hospitals between 1988 and 2008 with a diagnosis of TN, found that the preference of MVD over other modalities increased by 194% from 1988 to 2008, whereas percutaneous procedures decreased by 92%. Following its introduction in the early 1990s, the use of GKRS peaked in 2004 and declined since then.

SUMMARY

In the authors' experience, and in the data available in the literature, MVD has proven to be a safe and effective option for patients with medically intractable TN. It provides a high rate of early pain relief, with relatively low recurrence and complication rates in experienced hands, as compared with other surgical modalities such as the percutaneous techniques and stereotactic radiosurgery. As a matter of fact, as phrased by Sindou, it is an anatomic-based operation; therefore, it is actually a conservative method as compared with the destructive procedures.[21]

In conclusion, it is the authors' opinion that MVD should be considered the first line of surgical treatment in patients with TN, including carefully selected candidates in the elderly population (provided that there are no significant medical comorbidities associated), and in whom the pathophysiology of the pain is most likely to be the neurovascular compression and no other alternative mechanisms (ie, multiple sclerosis, herpetic neuralgia) are likely.

REFERENCES

1. Burchiel KJ. A new classification for facial pain. Neurosurgery 2003;53:1164–7.
2. Devor M, Govrin-Lippmann R, Rappaport ZH. Mechanism of trigeminal neuralgia: an ultrastructural analysis of trigeminal root specimens obtained during microvascular decompression surgery. J Neurosurg 2002; 96:532–43.
3. Jannetta PJ. Arterial compression of the trigeminal nerve at the pons in patients with trigeminal neuralgia. J Neurosurg 1967;26(Suppl):159–62.
4. Sade B, Lee JH. Tic douloureux. In: Nader R, Sabbagh AJ, editors. Neurosurgery case review. New York: Thieme; 2010. p. 76–8.
5. Miller JP, Magill ST, Acar F, et al. Predictors of long-term success after microvascular decompression for trigeminal neuralgia. J Neurosurg 2009;110:620–6.
6. Günther T, Gerganov VM, Stieglitz L, et al. Microvascular decompression for trigeminal neuralgia in the elderly: long-term treatment outcome and comparison with younger patients. Neurosurgery 2009;65: 477–82.
7. Sekula RF, Frederickson AM, Jannetta PJ, et al. Microvascular decompression for elderly patients with trigeminal neuralgia: a prospective study and systemic review with meta-analysis. J Neurosurg 2011;114:172–9.
8. Rughani AI, Dumont TM, Lin CT, et al. Safety of microvascular decompression for trigeminal neuralgia in the elderly. J Neurosurg 2011;115:202–9.
9. Garcia M, Naraghi R, Zumbrunn T, et al. High resolution 3D-constructive interference in steady-state MR imaging and 3D time-of-flight MR angiography in neurovascular compression: a comparison between 3T and 1.5T. AJNR Am J Neuroradiol 2012; 33:1251–6.
10. Peker S, Dincer A, Pamir MN. Vascular compression of the trigeminal nerve is a frequent finding in asymptomatic individuals: 3T MR imaging of 200 trigeminal nerves using 3D CISS sequences. Acta Neurochir 2009;151:1081–8.
11. Sade B, Lee JH. Significance of the tentorial alignment in approaching the trigeminal nerve and the ventral petrous region through the suboccipital retrosigmoid technique. J Neurosurg 2007;107: 932–6.
12. Yamashima T, Lee JH, Tobias S, et al. Surgical procedure "simplified retrosigmoid approach" for C-P angle lesions. J Clin Neurosci 2004;11:168–71.
13. Masuoka J, Matsushima T, Hikita T, et al. Cerebellar swelling after sacrifice of the superior petrosal vein during microvascular decompression for trigeminal neuralgia. J Clin Neurosci 2009;16:1342–4.
14. Barker FG, Jannetta PJ, Bissonette DJ, et al. The long-term outcome of microvascular decompression for trigeminal neuralgia. N Engl J Med 1996;334: 1077–83.
15. Thomas KL, Vilensky JA. The anatomy of vascular compression in trigeminal neuralgia. Clin Anat 2014;27:89–93.
16. Reveulta-Gutierrez R, Martinez-Anda J, Coll JB, et al. Efficacy and safety of root compression of trigeminal nerve for trigeminal neuralgia without evidence of vascular compression. World Neurosurg 2013;80:385–9.
17. Zhang H, Lei D, You C, et al. The long-term outcome predictors of pure microvascular decompression for primary trigeminal neuralgia. World Neurosurg 2013; 79:756–62.
18. Sekula RF, Frederickson AM, Jannetta PJ, et al. Microvascular decompression after failed gamma knife surgery for trigeminal neuralgia: a safe and effective rescue therapy? J Neurosurg 2010; 113(1):45–52.

19. Tatli M, Satici O, Kanpolat Y, et al. Various surgical modalities for trigeminal neuralgia: literature study of respective long-term outcomes. Acta Neurochir 2008;150:243–55.

20. Wang DD, Ouyang D, Englot DJ, et al. Trends in surgical treatment for trigeminal neuralgia in the United States of America from 1988 to 2008. J Clin Neurosci 2013;20:1538–45.

21. Sindou M. Trigeminal neuralgia: a plea for microvascular decompression as the first surgical option. Anatomy should prevail. Acta Neurochir 2010;152:361–4.

Percutaneous Treatments for Trigeminal Neuralgia

Symeon Missios, MD[a], Alireza M. Mohammadi, MD[a], Gene H. Barnett, MD, MBA[a,b],*

KEYWORDS

- Trigeminal neuralgia • Balloon compression • Glycerol rhizotomy
- Radiofrequency thermocoagulation

KEY POINTS

- Minimally invasive percutaneous techniques used in the treatment of trigeminal neuralgia include balloon compression, glycerol rhizotomy, and radiofrequency thermocoagulation.
- All 3 percutaneous techniques offer a high rate of initial pain relief. However, long-term pain relief and recurrence rates vary widely among studies.
- Permanent complications are rare for each procedure. Complications may include facial hyperalgesia or dysethesias, masseter weakness, corneal analgesia, and, rarely, cranial nerve deficits.
- In certain circumstances, like multiple sclerosis-related trigeminal neuralgia or elderly patients who are not candidates for intracranial surgery, such minimally invasive procedures could be considered as a preferred treatment option.

INTRODUCTION

Trigeminal neuralgia (TN) is a neurologic condition affecting 3 to 27 persons per 100,000 population. It is defined by paroxysmal electric shocklike painful attacks in 1 or more trigeminal nerve branches, with an estimated 15,000 new cases diagnosed per year in the United States.[1–4] Treatment of TN is quite diverse, ranging from pharmacologic, radiosurgery, and other minimally invasive percutaneous techniques to major intracranial nerve exploration and decompression. Percutaneous treatment modalities for TN consist of balloon compression (BC), glycerol rhizotomy (GR), and radiofrequency thermocoagulation (RT). All 3 of these treatments are generally safe, efficient, and effective, and rely on the principle of inducing pain relief by directed injury to the trigeminal nerve.[5]

Since the inception of these techniques a few decades ago, there have been numerous publications. However, a clear consensus has not been reached regarding their specific indications and degree of efficacy. In some centers, percutaneous techniques are used as a first line of procedural treatment,[6–8] whereas in others they are reserved for patients in whom microvascular decompression (MVD) is unsuitable or in refractory cases previously treated with another modality.[9] They are valuable in providing pain relief and treatment to the elderly and to patients with multiple medical comorbidities who would not be candidates for MVD.[9] Although similar in terms of their surgical approach and overall effectiveness, differences do exist in the type of injury inflicted (mechanical, chemical, or thermal) and the type of anesthesia that can be used. GR and RT can be performed without the use of general anesthesia, allowing direct feedback to be obtained from the patient. Despite their favorable complication profile and good outcomes, the recurrence rate of TN after use of these procedures can be significant.[10] There have been attempts to identify positive and negative predictors affecting long-term treatment success. The presence of atypical

[a] Department of Neurosurgery, Neurological Institute, The Rose Ella Burkhardt Brain Tumor and Neuro-Oncology Center, Cleveland Clinic, 9500 Euclid Avenue, S73, Cleveland, OH 44195, USA; [b] Cleveland Clinic Lerner College of Medicine of Case Western Reserve University, 9500 Euclid Avenue, NA21, Cleveland, OH 44195
* Corresponding author. The Rose Ella Burkhardt Brain Tumor and Neuro-Oncology Center, Department of Neurosurgery, Neurological Institute, Cleveland Clinic, 9500 Euclid Avenue, S73, Cleveland, OH 44195.
E-mail address: barnetg@ccf.org

Neurosurg Clin N Am 25 (2014) 751–762
http://dx.doi.org/10.1016/j.nec.2014.06.008
1042-3680/14/$ – see front matter © 2014 Elsevier Inc. All rights reserved

facial pain symptoms is a negative predictor of long-term success of all percutaneous treatment modalities[5,11,12] and there have been attempts to standardize a classification system for TN based on the characteristics of the facial pain.[13] TN is a common pain syndrome in patients with multiple sclerosis, found in 2% of patients with multiple sclerosis,[14] and can be disabling. The presence of multiple sclerosis also serves as a negative predictor, rendering any type of surgical interventions less effective and leading to increased recurrence rates.[15,16]

The aim of this article is to describe the percutaneous treatments available for TN and outline their characteristics, technique, indications, and efficacy.

BC

Percutaneous BC of the trigeminal ganglion was first introduced by Mullan and Lichtor in 1983.[17] The procedure evolved from prior work performed by Shelden, Pudenz, Taarnhoj, and their colleagues in the 1950s, who described that it was actually compression and not decompression of the trigeminal nerve that may offer pain relief.[18,19] The procedure involves the percutaneous insertion of a Fogarty balloon catheter through foramen ovale into Meckel's cave and subsequent inflation of the balloon and induction of mechanical injury to the Gasserian ganglion. Anatomic cadaver studies confirmed the extent of mechanical injury induced by this procedure[20] and rabbit models revealed that BC created a preferential injury to the myelinated axons from the trigeminal sensory root and extensive transganglionic degeneration of the trigeminal cranial nerve brain stem complex,[21] thus interfering with pain transmission and sparing light touch sensation and the corneal reflex.

Procedure

We typically perform the procedure with the patient under general anesthesia using a short-acting anesthetic in a biplanar angiography suite or operating room. The patient is placed on the operating table in the supine position with the neck gently extended at 15°. The foramen ovale is identified and positioned so that it is between the ramus of the mandible and the maxilla on the submental vertex view, and the overlying skin is marked as the entry point. The patient's cheek is prepped and draped in the usual fashion and the skin is punctured by a 20-gauge spinal needle, which is advanced to the region of the foramen ovale under fluoroscopic guidance (**Fig. 1**). Lateral views are used to determine the depth of the needle and submental vertex views are valuable to

establish the trajectory for the needle. A skin puncture is made immediately above the first puncture site and a 14-gauge introducer needle is advanced along the 20-gauge needle, again using biplanar fluoroscopy, and also puncturing the foramen. The 20-gauge needle is removed and a 4-French Fogarty balloon catheter is passed through the 14-gauge needle and inflated with 0.75 mL of iodinated contrast. Compression is maintained for 60 seconds (90 seconds for TN related to multiple sclerosis). For recurrent BC procedures, the balloon inflation time is extended by an additional 30 seconds for each previous BC procedure (eg, 90 and 120 seconds of compression for second and third BC procedures, respectively)[15]; at times, the volume of inflation is increased as well.

Despite the simplicity and long experience with this procedure, there is no consensus among neurosurgeons on the value of several parameters involved with percutaneous BC.[9] Regarding the shape of the inflated balloon within Meckel's cave, a dumbbell shape has been described to be optimal, but a precise definition does not exist.[9,17] Balloon volumes ranging between 0.35 and 1 mL have been used in the past and compression times have varied from 60 to 75 seconds[6,14,22,23] to longer than 3 minutes.[8,24,25] The intraluminal balloon pressure has also been considered and higher pressures have been associated with increased rates of postoperative dysesthesias and masseter weakness, whereas lower pressures have been associated with increased rates of recurrence.[5,26,27] Kouzounias and colleagues[9] in 2010 reported on the factors that influence the outcome of percutaneous BC. Balloon shape was among the strongest predictors with a pear-shaped or dumbbell-shaped balloon having a positive impact on outcome, whereas a persistent elliptical balloon was typically associated with an unsuccessful procedure. In the same study, compression duration of longer than 60 seconds did not affect outcome. In the author's experience (GHB), presence of a small 'nipple' at the posterior superior portion of the balloon indicates herniation of the balloon into the ambient cistern and is predictive of V1 branch compression. This is to be avoided when triggers are only in V2 and or V3 distribution so as to limit the risk of corneal anesthesia.

Discussion

There is a large experience with the use of percutaneous BC for TN and several reported large series exist in the literature.[7,8,23–26,28–33] Rates of initial pain relief are high ranging from 91% to 100%[25,26]; however, long-term pain relief rates

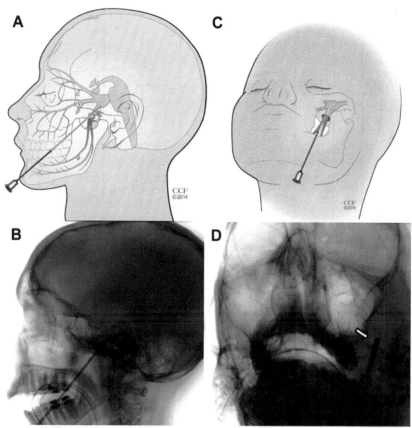

Fig. 1. Lateral and oblique (*A, C*) schematic and corresponding fluoroscopic (*B, D*) views of a percutaneous approach to the foramen ovale. The trajectory involves an entry point positioned 2.5 cm lateral to the corner of the mouth and aimed toward the ipsilateral foramen ovale (marked by *arrow* in *D*) under fluoroscopic guidance. (*Courtesy of* The Cleveland Clinic, Cleveland, Ohio.)

range from 68% to 91%, with an average follow-up of 1 to 10.7 years.[7,8,23,24,26,30–33] Recurrence rates range from 10% to 14% at 2 years,[23,26] 15% to 19%[23,29] at 3 years, and 19.2% to 32.5% at 5 years (**Table 1**).[8,23,24]

Complications of the procedure include development of significant dysesthesias in a trigeminal distribution and rates vary from 0% to 15%.[7,8,23–26,28–33] Disruption of the corneal reflex and subsequent corneal analgesia is rare and was not observed in all studies with 100 or more patients, except one where the rate was 3%.[24] Trigeminal motor weakness typically involves the masseter and has been reported at rates of 0% to 33%, but typically resolves within 12 months. Cranial nerve palsies are less common and have been reported at rates of 0% to 1.9%. Last, postoperative morbidity including infection and meningitis can occur at a rate of 0% to 5% depending on the study examined.[7,8,23–26,28–33]

There are very few comparisons of the efficacy and complications of the different percutaneous techniques in the literature and the results are

varied at times conflicting. No randomized comparisons exist and most studies are retrospective reviews. Lopez and colleagues[10] in 2004 in a review of the different procedures described higher rates of pain relief, but also higher rates of complications with RT compared with BC. Kouzounias and colleagues[34] in 2010 compared BC with GR and reported similar efficacy between the 2 procedures, but lower rates of complications with GR.

In our institution, BC is used mostly for elderly patients who are not a candidate for MVD or those patients with multiple sclerosis-related TN. In our recent report comparing BC, GR, and other surgical and radiosurgical modalities on treatment of multiple sclerosis-related TN, which included 82 patients who underwent BC, BC had the highest rate of initial pain relief (95%) and median pain-free interval (28 months), when performed as an initial procedure. The rates decreased to 71% initial pain relief and 17-month median pain-free interval when performed as a repeat procedure. Temporary

Table 1
Summary of series regarding the use of percutaneous BC for trigeminal neuralgia

Author (year)	No. of Patients (n)	Patients Previously Treated (n)	Follow-up (y)	Initial Pain Relief <3 m (%)	Long-term Pain Relief, >1 y (%)	Early Recurrence <2 y (%)	Late Recurrence >2 y (%)	Dysesthesias (%)	Anesthesia Dolorosa (%)	Trigeminal Motor Weakness (%)	Corneal Anesthesia (%)	Cranial Nerve Deficits (%)	Herpes Reactivation (%)	Meningitis (%)	Other Postoperative Morbidity/Mortality (%)
Fraioli et al,[31] 1989	159	13	3.5	89.9	90.2	NR	9.8	7.6	0.6	6.9	0	0	0	0	0
Frank and Fabrizi,[32] 1989	212	NR	<3	NR	75	NR	25	NR	0	9	0	0.9	0	0	0
Lichtor and Mullan,[33] 1990	100	37	1–10	100	80	4	20	4	0	NR	0	1	0	0	0
Lobato et. al,[26] 1990	144	62	0.5–4.5	100	91.3	6.2	9.7	19	0	12	0	0	NR	NR	0
Abdennebi et al,[28] 1995	150	NR	4	94.6	69.3	9.3	30	10.7	0.6	6.7	2.7	1.5	0	0	0
Brown and Gouda,[30] 1997	141	NR	2	92	74	NR	26	6	0	16	0	0	0	0	5
Abdennebi et. al,[24] 1997	200	NR	4.25	94.5	67.5	14	32.5	7.5	1.5	5	2.5	1.5	0	0	0.5
Correa and Teixera,[7] 1998	158	72	3	89.8	91.7	10.1	8.2	15	0	33	0	1.9	3.8	1.3	0
Skirving and Dan,[8] 2001	496	20	10.7	>99	80.8	9.8	19.2	3.8	0	3.4	0	1.6	NR	0	0
Liu et al,[25] 2007	276	22	1.5	91.3	NR	5.2	NR	4.0	0	50	0.4	1.1	NR	NR	0
Chen et al,[23] 2011	130	57	8.9	93.8	70.5	14	29.5	20.7	0	6.2	2.3	1.5	33.1	0	0
Baabor et al,[29] 2011	206	66	>3	93	85	7	15	44	0	NR	1.7	0.5	0	0	0

numbness was reported in 53% of initial procedures and 29% of repeat.[15]

GR

The discovery of the beneficial effects of glycerol in patients with TN was accidental. In an attempt to develop a method of lesioning the Gasserian ganglion using the Leksell gamma knife in Stockholm in the late 1970s, patients were injected with tantalum powder, a radiopaque metal dust intended to be used as a marker, and glycerol as the vehicle.[35] It was discovered that the injection alone produced pain relief, and in 1981 Hakanson developed the technique of percutaneous glycerol rhizolysis and published the first series of 75 patients.[36] Glycerol injection induces changes in osmolarity and subsequent demyelination and axonal damage.[37] Animal studies using a rat neuroma model revealed evidence that glycerol exerts its major effect on the large-diameter fibers.[38] Glycerol injection in patients abolished the components of the trigeminal root potential corresponding to the A-delta and C-fibers, minutes after the injection.[39]

Procedure

The procedure is usually performed under light intravenous anesthesia (usually propofol) or general anesthesia with the patient in a semisitting position. A 20-gauge is advanced toward the foramen ovale using the external Härtel guidelines and the assistance of fluoroscopy in a similar fashion as in the BC procedure. When the needle passes the foramen ovale, the stylet is removed and spontaneous flow of the cerebrospinal fluid (CSF) is confirmed. If there is no CSF flow, the needle is advanced slightly. CSF flow does not guarantee proper placement because, if the needle is too lateral or deep, it can enter the subtemporal subarachnoid space. Cisternography is performed by injected contrast medium (iohexol) through the needle with a 1-mm syringe. After visualization of the cistern, 0.5 mL of anhydrous sterile glycerol is injected intracisternally. The needle is then removed and the patient is transferred to a postprocedure room, kept seated upright with the head flexed for 2 hours to prevent leakage of fluid into the posterior fossa, and then discharged later the same day.

Discussion

Several large series of patients with TN treated with percutaneous GR have been reported representing variations in the technique and length of follow-up. Cisternography has not been routinely used in every study. A total of 22 series were reviewed encompassing more than 6000 patients (range, 30–3370) published between 1983 and 2011.[11,37,40–58] Very high rates of initial pain relief were noticed after the injection, ranging from 73% to 99.6%. The duration of follow-up varies widely among the studies, ranging from 6 months to 11 years. Given the wide variability of follow-up times, recurrence rates are difficult to estimate. The average risk of early recurrence, within the first 2 years after treatment ranges from 2% to 45% with an average of 20% and the risk of late recurrence (>2 years after treatment) ranges from 10% to 72% with an average of approximately 50% (**Table 2**).[11,37,40–58]

Percutaneous glycerol rhizolysis is an overall safe procedure with a low risk of significant morbidity. The most common postoperative finding is a disturbance of facial sensation that typically lasts for a few hours to 1 or 2 weeks.[59] Complications include facial hypesthesia lasting longer than 2 weeks and the rates range from 0% to 30%.[11,37,40–58] The wide variability is a result of the variation in technique among the different studies. The incidence of painful facial dysesthesia and allodynia typically ranges between 0% and 4% with few studies reporting rates as high as 11% and 26%.[38,47,53–55] Serious infectious complications are rare after percutaneous GR. Reactivation of latent herpes simplex virus has been described at a rate ranging from 3% to 77% and cases of aseptic meningitis have a frequency of 0%–7%.[11,37,40–59] The etiology of aseptic meningitis after percutaneous GR remains unclear; however, the frequency of cases has decreased since the replacement of contrast medium from the previously used metrizamide to iohexol, which is used currently. Similarly, the rates of other cranial neuropathies and bacterial meningitis are low and both range between 0% and 2% with inadvertent and unrecognized entry into the oral cavity being the most common etiology for bacterial meningitis after percutaneous GR.

There have been few studies trying to identify positive predictive factors of pain relief after percutaneous GR. A prospective analysis of factors related to pain relief was published in 2005 by Bruce Pollock[52] and reports that predictive factors for success included patients without any constant facial pain, patients with immediate facial pain during glycerol injection, and patients with new trigeminal deficits after percutaneous GR. Repeat GR remains safe and effective. Bender and colleagues[60] and Harries and colleagues[61] described their experience with 100 or more patients with repeat GR and reported similar rates of initial and long-term pain relief to the initial GR

Table 2
Summary of series regarding the use of percutaneous GR for trigeminal neuralgia

Author (year)	No. of Patients (n)	Patients Previously Treated (n)	Follow-up (y)	Initial Pain Relief <3 m (%)	Long-term Pain Relief >1 y (%)	Early Recurrence <2 y (%)	Late Recurrence >2 y (%)	Dysesthesias (%)	Anesthesia Dolorosa (%)	Trigeminal Motor Weakness (%)	Corneal Anesthesia (%)	Cranial Nerve Deficits (%)	Herpes Reactivation (%)	Meningitis (%)	Other Postoperative Morbidity/ Mortality (%)
Arias,[40] 1986	100	0	3	95	84	4	16	10	0	0	2	0	10	0	2
Beck et al,[41] 1986	58	22	1.5	NR	72	21	NR	2	0	0	2	2	9	0	4
Dieckmann et al,[44] 1987	252	NR	2–5	89	63	11	37	2	0	NR	NR	NR	77	1	0
Saini,[53] 1987	469	266	1–6	77	17	41	83	23	5.5	3.4	5	0	3.2	0	0
Burchiel,[43] 1988	60	NR	1	80	53	20	47	10	0	0	7	0	5	1.7	0
Young,[58] 1988	162	28	0.5–5.6	90	86	13	18.5	3.1	0	0	3.1	0	37.6	0.6	1.8
Ischia et al,[49] 1990	112	24	3.5	92	71	11	20.5	3	0	0	0.9	0	0	0	0
North et al,[11] 1990	85	33	0.5–4.5	85	40	40	60	2.3	0	0	2.3	1.1	0	0	4.7
Fujimaki et al,[47] 1990	135	36	3–5	96	26	35	70	29	1.5	NR	NR	NR	NR	NR	NR
Slettebo et al,[54] 1993	60	39	4.5	93	50	20	45	10	0	NR	NR	NR	NR	NR	2
Bergenheim and Hariz,[42] 1995	99	53	1	97	76	24	NR	7	1	NR	5	0	0	0	0
Erdem and Alkan,[45] 2001	157	NR	4	98	62	10	38	8.9	NR	NR	NR	NR	NR	NR	NR
Jagia et al,[50] 2004	115	NR	0.5–3	82	71	18	29	40	0	NR	2.8	0	3.6	0.7	0
Kondziolka and Lunsford,[37] 2005	1174	NR	2–11	90	77	10	23	NR	NR	NR	NR	NR	NR	NR	0.1
Henson et al,[48] 2005	79	15	2.5	80	47	20	53	34	0	2.5	0	1.2	NR	3.8	0
Pollock,[52] 2005	98	50	2.4	75	50	39	50	8	0	0	7	NR	12	0	2
Xu-Hui et al,[57] 2011	3370	624	13.1	99.5	65	21	35	4	NR	0.06	1.8	0.39	NR	0.03	0.2

procedure without changes in the durability of procedure or increase in morbidity and especially no cases of anesthesia dolorosa.

In our institution, we use GR for the same indications as for BC, as described. In our experience of GR for multiple sclerosis-related TN patients, which included 89 patients, patients undergoing GR as an initial procedure had 74% initial pain relief and a median pain-free interval of 28 months, and the repeat procedures had an initial pain relief rate of 70% and a median pain-free interval of 12 months. Temporary numbness was seen in 10% of initial and 18% of repeat procedures.[15]

RT

Electrocoagulation of peripheral branches of the trigeminal nerve and later of the Gasserian ganglion were performed as early as 1913 by Rethi.[62] The technique was further developed by Kirschner between 1931 and 1933, who developed a special head frame to guide the electrode insertion through the foramen ovale and reported 250 cases in 1936 and 113 cases in 1942.[63–65] The technique had a high rate of complications, however, and a substantial advance was made in 1969 when Sweet introduced a less painful and safer technique that included electrophysiologic stimulation, controlled lesion production, and short-acting anesthesia.[63,66,67] Another major innovation occurred in 1978 when Tew and colleagues introduced the use of image guided fluoroscopy and in 1982 when van Loveren, Tew, and Keller introduced the Tew curved-tip electrode (Radionics, Burlington, MA, USA).[68,69]

One of the potential mechanisms of pain relief using this technique is the differential thermocoagulation of trigeminal rootlets which proposes that the action potentials of nociceptive fibers (A-δ and C) are blocked at lower temperatures than those that transmit tactile sensation.[66,70] Histologic animal studies, however, indicated that the induced injury affected all sizes of nerve fibers, regardless of their myelination status[71]; therefore, the success of the procedure may rely on reducing the overall sensory input to the trigeminal root.

Procedure

The procedure is performed under light intravenous anesthesia (usually propofol). The patient is placed on the operating table in the supine position with the neck gently extended at 15°. A 20-gauge needle is advanced toward the foramen ovale in a similar fashion as in the BC procedure. When the needle passes the foramen ovale, the stylet is removed and replaced by the electrode. Once the electrode is in proper position, the patient is awakened and stimulation mapping takes place to identify optimal locations for lesioning by inducing paresthesias in the same pattern as the TN. Typically 0.1 to 0.4 V at 50 pulses per second are required to reproduce symptoms, but up to 1 V may be required in patients who have had prior treatments. Lesions are then performed at a temperature of 60°C to 80°C for 30 to 120 seconds. The duration of lesioning depends on the voltage threshold of response during stimulation. After the lesioning, with the patient fully awake, sensory testing of the patient's face is conducted to assess both pinprick sensation as well as light touch. Additional lesions may be performed. After hypalgesia has been achieved, the motor function of the trigeminal nerve is also tested.

Discussion

Several large published series exist, totaling greater than 7000 patients with follow-up ranging from 1 to 14 years.[12,31,32,66,72–84] The rates of initial pain relief have been reported as high as 97% to 100%.[66,75,83] Rates of long-term pain relief range from 25% to 95%,[12,31,32,66,72–84] but defining long-term recurrence rates becomes difficult because of the variable durations of follow-up for each study. Kanpolat and colleagues[75] in 2001 reported on their experience with 1600 patients and described 52.3% of pain relief at 10-year follow-up and 41% pain relief at 20-year follow-up. In the same study, pain relief rates were better for patients having undergone multiple procedures and 94.2% and 100% patients reported pain relief at 10 years and 20 years, respectively. Taha and colleagues[82] in 1995 described a 25% recurrence rate after 14 years in a group of 154 patients and the rate of recurrence correlated with the degree of sensory deficits elicited during the procedure: The more mild the hypalgesia noted, the higher the recurrence rate. In the same study, 15% of patients recurred within 5 years, 7% within 5 to 10 years and 3% within 10 to 15 years (**Table 3**).

Complications include persistent sensory deficit and paresthesias as a result of the lesioning and the rates range from 0.9% to 9% among the large patient series.[12,31,32,66,72–84] Tew and colleagues[83] reported on their experience with 1200 patients and noted a decrease in their rate of postoperative dysesthesias from 27% to 11% for minor and 5% to 2% for major symptoms, with the use of a curved electrode. Similarly, the rates of anesthesia dolorosa decreased from 1.6% to 0.2%. Other strategies to decrease the risks of postoperative dysesthesias involved frequent sensory testing during treatment and an awake and actively

Table 3
Summary of series regarding the use of percutaneous RT for trigeminal neuralgia

Author (year)	No. of Patients (n)	Patients Previously Treated (n)	Follow-up (y)	Initial Pain Relief, <3 m (%)	Long-term Pain Relief, >1 y (%)	Early Recurrence <2 y (%)	Late Recurrence >2 y, (%)	Dysesthesias (%)	Anesthesia Dolorosa (%)	Trigeminal Motor Weakness (%)	Corneal Anesthesia (%)	Cranial Nerve Deficits (%)	Herpes Reactivation (%)	Meningitis (%)	Other Postoperative Morbidity/Mortality (%)
Nugent,[72] 1982	643	NR	4.7	NR	77	NR	23	5	1	25	8	NR	NR	NR	NR
Fraioli et al,[31] 1989	533	35	6.5	99.2	90	NR	10	15	1.5	3	3	0.2	0	0	0
Frank and Fabrizi,[32] 1989	700	NR	>3	NR	75	NR	25	0.6	0.6	8	1	0.2	0	0	0
Miserocchi et al,[77] 1989	111	NR	1-7	NR	80	NR	20	6	0	NR	2	0	0	0	0
Broggi et al,[73] 1990	1000	NR	9.3	94.8	80	13	18	5.2	1.5	10.5	20	0.5	0	0	0
Ischia et al,[49] 1990	162	0	3.7	95	67	26	33	3	2	3	3.7	0.5	0	0	3.7
Taha et al,[82] 1995	154	NR	15	99	75	7	25	3	0	14	5	0	0	0	0
Oturai et al,[79] 1996	185	NR	8	85	51	30	49	5	0	NR	15	0	NR	NR	NR
Spendel et al,[80] 1997	182	NR	0.5-10	95	87	NR	12.5	1	0	NR	NR	NR	NR	NR	0
Zakrzewska,[12] 1999	48	0	0.5-4.5	95	60	20	40	10	0	12	12	NR	NR	NR	0
Mathews and Scrivani,[76] 2000	258	NR	3	NR	75	NR	25	8	0	28	2	0	NR	0	0
Kanpolat et al,[75] 2001	1600	440	1-25	98	75	8	25	1.8	0.8	4	5.7	0.8	0	0	0.9
Tronnier et al,[84] 2001	206	94	14	85	25	50	75	1	0	NR	0	0.8	NR	NR	0.8
Son et al,[66] 2011	38	0	3	100	70	18	30	20	0	16	0	0	0	0	0

participating patient. Corneal anesthesia has been reported ranging from 0% to 17%.[12,31,32,66,72–84] Trigeminal motor paresis has been reported ranging from 3%[31,74] to as high as 65%[81] and in most cases the deficit is partial and transient. Reactivation of herpes simplex virus has been reported in 3% of patients[83] and the rate of cranial nerve palsies have ranged between 0% and 1%.[12,31,32,66,72–84] Severe morbidity is rare, but there have been reports of intracranial hemorrhage and brain stem injury after percutaneous RT,[85–87] as well as rare cases of CSF rhinorrhea.[88]

In an attempt to decrease the rate of complications associated with percutaneous RT, there have been efforts to improve targeting accuracy via the use of intraoperative computed tomography neuronavigation and frameless stereotactic cannulation of the foramen ovale with good success.[89–91] Xu and colleagues[92] described their experience with 54 patients and reported increased rates of long-term pain relief (85% vs 54% at 12 months and 62% vs 35% at 36 months) in the patients undergoing percutaneous RT with navigation compared with standard procedure. In a later study by Yang and colleagues[93] of 79 patients in 2010, there was no difference in pain relief outcomes between the navigation and control groups, and navigation was only successful in decreasing median time for needle placement (14 vs 40 min).

Although at one time the procedure of choice for percutaneous treatment of TN, we seldom use this treatment currently and rely on BC and GR. In our limited experience with multiple sclerosis-related TN patients undergoing RT (15 patients), they exhibited 86% and 75% immediate pain relief rates for initial and repeat procedures, respectively; however, short median times to recurrence were noted at 5 months for initial treatment and 9 months for repeat procedures.[15]

SUMMARY

Percutaneous treatments of TN are associated with excellent short-term pain relief rates and low morbidity and mortality. Procedures can be easily repeated in cases of recurrence and they offer a valuable treatment option for patients with greater perioperative risk. There are no randomized, controlled, clinical studies directly comparing the safety and efficacy of percutaneous procedures or with other treatment modalities like MVD or radiosurgery. However, at least in certain circumstances like multiple sclerosis-related TN, which is known to have a high recurrence rate regardless of the type of treatment modality, or elderly patients who are not candidates for a major intracranial surgery, such minimally invasive procedures could be considered as preferred treatment options.

REFERENCES

1. Cruccu G, Bonamico LH, Zakrzewska JM. Cranial neuralgias. Handb Clin Neurol 2010;97:663–78.
2. Hall GC, Carroll D, Parry D, et al. Epidemiology and treatment of neuropathic pain: the UK primary care perspective. Pain 2006;122(1–2): 156–62.
3. Katusic S, Beard CM, Bergstralh E, et al. Incidence and clinical features of trigeminal neuralgia, Rochester, Minnesota, 1945-1984. Ann Neurol 1990;27(1):89–95.
4. Rozen TD. Trigeminal neuralgia and glossopharyngeal neuralgia. Neurol Clin 2004;22(1):185–206.
5. Cheng JS, Lim DA, Chang EF, et al. A review of percutaneous treatments for trigeminal neuralgia. Neurosurgery 2013. [Epub ahead of print].
6. Broggi G, Ferroli P, Franzini A. Treatment strategy for trigeminal neuralgia: a thirty years experience. Neurol Sci 2008;29(Suppl 1):S79–82.
7. Correa CF, Teixeira MJ. Balloon compression of the Gasserian ganglion for the treatment of trigeminal neuralgia. Stereotact Funct Neurosurg 1998;71(2): 83–9.
8. Skirving DJ, Dan NG. A 20-year review of percutaneous balloon compression of the trigeminal ganglion. J Neurosurg 2001;94(6):913–7.
9. Kouzounias K, Schechtmann G, Lind G, et al. Factors that influence outcome of percutaneous balloon compression in the treatment of trigeminal neuralgia. Neurosurgery 2010;67(4):925–34 [discussion: 934].
10. Lopez BC, Hamlyn PJ, Zakrzewska JM. Systematic review of ablative neurosurgical techniques for the treatment of trigeminal neuralgia. Neurosurgery 2004;54(4):973–82 [discussion: 982–3].
11. North RB, Kidd DH, Piantadosi S, et al. Percutaneous retrogasserian glycerol rhizotomy. Predictors of success and failure in treatment of trigeminal neuralgia. J Neurosurg 1990;72(6):851–6.
12. Zakrzewska JM, Jassim S, Bulman JS. A prospective, longitudinal study on patients with trigeminal neuralgia who underwent radiofrequency thermocoagulation of the Gasserian ganglion. Pain 1999;79(1):51–8.
13. Burchiel KJ. A new classification for facial pain. Neurosurgery 2003;53(5):1164–6 [discussion: 1166–7].
14. Hooge JP, Redekop WK. Trigeminal neuralgia in multiple sclerosis. Neurology 1995;45(7):1294–6.
15. Mohammad-Mohammadi A, Recinos PF, Lee JH, et al. Surgical outcomes of trigeminal neuralgia in patients with multiple sclerosis. Neurosurgery 2013;73(6):941–50.

16. Bender MT, Pradilla G, Batra S, et al. Glycerol rhizotomy and radiofrequency thermocoagulation for trigeminal neuralgia in multiple sclerosis. J Neurosurg 2013;118(2):329–36.

17. Mullan S, Lichtor T. Percutaneous microcompression of the trigeminal ganglion for trigeminal neuralgia. J Neurosurg 1983;59(6):1007–12.

18. Taarnhoj P. Decompression of the trigeminal root and the posterior part of the ganglion as treatment in trigeminal neuralgia; preliminary communication. J Neurosurg 1952;9(3):288–90.

19. Shelden CH, Pudenz RH, Freshwater DB, et al. Compression rather than decompression for trigeminal neuralgia. J Neurosurg 1955;12(2):123–6.

20. Urculo E, Martinez L, Arrazola M, et al. Macroscopic effects of percutaneous trigeminal ganglion compression (Mullan's technique): an anatomic study. Neurosurgery 1995;36(4):776–9.

21. Brown JA, Hoeflinger B, Long PB, et al. Axon and ganglion cell injury in rabbits after percutaneous trigeminal balloon compression. Neurosurgery 1996; 38(5):993–1003 [discussion: 1003–4].

22. Broggi G. Percutaneous retrogasserian balloon compression for trigeminal neuralgia. World Neurosurg 2013;79(2):269–70.

23. Chen JF, Tu PH, Lee ST. Long-term follow-up of patients treated with percutaneous balloon compression for trigeminal neuralgia in Taiwan. World Neurosurg 2011;76(6):586–91.

24. Abdennebi B, Mahfouf L, Nedjahi T. Long-term results of percutaneous compression of the gasserian ganglion in trigeminal neuralgia (series of 200 patients). Stereotact Funct Neurosurg 1997;68(1–4 Pt 1):190–5.

25. Liu HB, Ma Y, Zou JJ, et al. Percutaneous microballoon compression for trigeminal neuralgia. Chin Med J (Engl) 2007;120(3):228–30.

26. Lobato RD, Rivas JJ, Sarabia R, et al. Percutaneous microcompression of the gasserian ganglion for trigeminal neuralgia. J Neurosurg 1990;72(4): 546–53.

27. Zanusso M, Curri D, Landi A, et al. Pressure monitoring inside Meckel's cave during percutaneous microcompression of gasserian ganglion. Stereotact Funct Neurosurg 1991;56(1):37–43.

28. Abdennebi B, Bouatta F, Chitti M, et al. Percutaneous balloon compression of the Gasserian ganglion in trigeminal neuralgia. Long-term results in 150 cases. Acta Neurochir (Wien) 1995;136(1–2):72–4.

29. Baabor MG, Perez-Limonte L. Percutaneous balloon compression of the gasserian ganglion for the treatment of trigeminal neuralgia: personal experience of 206 patients. Acta Neurochir Suppl 2011;108:251–4.

30. Brown JA, Gouda JJ. Percutaneous balloon compression of the trigeminal nerve. Neurosurg Clin N Am 1997;8(1):53–62.

31. Fraioli B, Esposito V, Guidetti B, et al. Treatment of trigeminal neuralgia by thermocoagulation, glycerolization, and percutaneous compression of the gasserian ganglion and/or retrogasserian rootlets: long-term results and therapeutic protocol. Neurosurgery 1989;24(2):239–45.

32. Frank F, Fabrizi AP. Percutaneous surgical treatment of trigeminal neuralgia. Acta Neurochir (Wien) 1989;97(3–4):128–30.

33. Lichtor T, Mullan JF. A 10-year follow-up review of percutaneous microcompression of the trigeminal ganglion. J Neurosurg 1990;72(1):49–54.

34. Kouzounias K, Lind G, Schechtmann G, et al. Comparison of percutaneous balloon compression and glycerol rhizotomy for the treatment of trigeminal neuralgia. J Neurosurg 2010;113(3):486–92.

35. Leksell L. Trigeminal neuralgia. Some neurophysiologic aspects and a new method of therapy. Lakartidningen 1971;68(45):5145–8 [in Swedish].

36. Hakanson S. Trigeminal neuralgia treated by the injection of glycerol into the trigeminal cistern. Neurosurgery 1981;9(6):638–46.

37. Kondziolka D, Lunsford LD. Percutaneous retrogasserian glycerol rhizotomy for trigeminal neuralgia: technique and expectations. Neurosurg Focus 2005;18(5):E7.

38. Burchiel KJ, Russell LC. Glycerol neurolysis: neurophysiological effects of topical glycerol application on rat saphenous nerve. J Neurosurg 1985;63(5): 784–8.

39. Sweet WH, Poletti CE, Macon JB. Treatment of trigeminal neuralgia and other facial pains by retrogasserian injection of glycerol. Neurosurgery 1981;9(6):647–53.

40. Arias MJ. Percutaneous retrogasserian glycerol rhizotomy for trigeminal neuralgia. A prospective study of 100 cases. J Neurosurg 1986;65(1):32–6.

41. Beck DW, Olson JJ, Urig EJ. Percutaneous retrogasserian glycerol rhizotomy for treatment of trigeminal neuralgia. J Neurosurg 1986;65(1): 28–31.

42. Bergenheim AT, Hariz MI. Influence of previous treatment on outcome after glycerol rhizotomy for trigeminal neuralgia. Neurosurgery 1995;36(2): 303–9 [discussion: 309–10].

43. Burchiel KJ. Percutaneous retrogasserian glycerol rhizolysis in the management of trigeminal neuralgia. J Neurosurg 1988;69(3):361–6.

44. Dieckmann G, Bockermann V, Heyer C, et al. Five-and-a-half years' experience with percutaneous retrogasserian glycerol rhizotomy in treatment of trigeminal neuralgia. Appl Neurophysiol 1987; 50(1–6):401–13.

45. Erdem E, Alkan A. Peripheral glycerol injections in the treatment of idiopathic trigeminal neuralgia: retrospective analysis of 157 cases. J Oral Maxillofac Surg 2001;59(10):1176–80.

46. Febles C, Werner-Wasik M, Rosenwasser RH. A comparison of treatment outcomes with gamma knife radiosurgery versus glycerol rhizotomy in the management of trigeminal neuralgia. Int J Radiat Oncol Biol Phys 2003;57(Suppl 2):53.

47. Fujimaki T, Fukushima T, Miyazaki S. Percutaneous retrogasserian glycerol injection in the management of trigeminal neuralgia: long-term follow-up results. J Neurosurg 1990;73(2):212–6.

48. Henson CF, Goldman HW, Rosenwasser RH, et al. Glycerol rhizotomy versus gamma knife radiosurgery for the treatment of trigeminal neuralgia: an analysis of patients treated at one institution. Int J Radiat Oncol Biol Phys 2005;63(1):82–90.

49. Ischia S, Luzzani A, Polati E. Retrogasserian glycerol injection: a retrospective study of 112 patients. Clin J Pain 1990;6(4):291–6.

50. Jagia M, Bithal PK, Dash HH, et al. Effect of cerebrospinal fluid return on success rate of percutaneous retrogasserian glycerol rhizotomy. Reg Anesth Pain Med 2004;29(6):592–5.

51. Lunsford L. Trigeminal neuralgia: treatment by glycerol rhizotomy, vol. 3. New York: McGraw-Hill; 1985.

52. Pollock BE. Percutaneous retrogasserian glycerol rhizotomy for patients with idiopathic trigeminal neuralgia: a prospective analysis of factors related to pain relief. J Neurosurg 2005;102(2):223–8.

53. Saini SS. Reterogasserian anhydrous glycerol injection therapy in trigeminal neuralgia: observations in 552 patients. J Neurol Neurosurg Psychiatry 1987;50(11):1536–8.

54. Slettebo H, Hirschberg H, Lindegaard KF. Long-term results after percutaneous retrogasserian glycerol rhizotomy in patients with trigeminal neuralgia. Acta Neurochir (Wien) 1993;122(3–4):231–5.

55. Steiger HJ. Prognostic factors in the treatment of trigeminal neuralgia. Analysis of a differential therapeutic approach. Acta Neurochir (Wien) 1991; 113(1–2):11–7.

56. Waltz TA, Dalessio DJ, Copeland B, et al. Percutaneous injection of glycerol for the treatment of trigeminal neuralgia. Clin J Pain 1989;5(2):195–8.

57. Xu-Hui W, Chun Z, Guang-Jian S, et al. Long-term outcomes of percutaneous retrogasserian glycerol rhizotomy in 3370 patients with trigeminal neuralgia. Turk Neurosurg 2011;21(1):48–52.

58. Young RF. Glycerol rhizolysis for treatment of trigeminal neuralgia. J Neurosurg 1988;69(1): 39–45.

59. Linderoth B, Lind G. Retrogasserian glycerol rhizolysis in trigeminal neuralgia. In: Quinones-Hinojosa A, editor. Schmidek and Sweet: operative neurosurgical techniques, vol. 2, 6th edition. New York: Saunders; 2012. p. 1393–408.

60. Bender M, Pradilla G, Batra S, et al. Effectiveness of repeat glycerol rhizotomy in treating recurrent trigeminal neuralgia. Neurosurgery 2012;70(5): 1125–33 [discussion: 1133–4].

61. Harries AM, Mitchell RD. Percutaneous glycerol rhizotomy for trigeminal neuralgia: safety and efficacy of repeat procedures. Br J Neurosurg 2011;25(2): 268–72.

62. Rethi A. Die elektrolytische Behandlung der Trigeminusneuralgen. Munch Med Wochenschr 1913; 60:295–6.

63. Wilkins R. Trigeminal neuralgia: historical overview with emphasis on surgical treatment. New York: Thieme; 2002.

64. Kirschner M. Zur Behandlung der Trigeminusneuralgie: Erfahrungen an 250 Fallen. Arch Klin Chir 1936;186:325–34.

65. Kirschner M. Die Behandlung der Trigeminusneuralgie (Nach Erfahrungen an 113 Kranken). Munch Med Wochenschr 1942;89:235–9.

66. Son BC, Kim HS, Kim IS, et al. Percutaneous radiofrequency thermocoagulation under fluoroscopic image-guidance for idiopathic trigeminal neuralgia. J Korean Neurosurg Soc 2011;50(5):446–52.

67. Sweet WH, Wepsic JG. Controlled thermocoagulation of trigeminal ganglion and rootlets for differential destruction of pain fibers. 1. Trigeminal neuralgia. J Neurosurg 1974;40(2):143–56.

68. Tew JM Jr, Keller JT, Williams DS. Application of stereotactic principles to the treatment of trigeminal neuralgia. Appl Neurophysiol 1978;41(1–4):146–56.

69. van Loveren H, Tew JM Jr, Keller JT, et al. A 10-year experience in the treatment of trigeminal neuralgia. Comparison of percutaneous stereotaxic rhizotomy and posterior fossa exploration. J Neurosurg 1982; 57(6):757–64.

70. Letcher FS, Goldring S. The effect of radiofrequency current and heat on peripheral nerve action potential in the cat. J Neurosurg 1968;29(1):42–7.

71. Smith HP, McWhorter JM, Challa VR. Radiofrequency neurolysis in a clinical model. Neuropathological correlation. J Neurosurg 1981;55(2):246–53.

72. Nugent GR. Technique and results of 800 percutaneous radiofrequency thermocoagulations for trigeminal neuralgia. Appl Neurophysiol 1982; 45(4–5):504–7.

73. Broggi G, Franzini A, Lasio G, et al. Long-term results of percutaneous retrogasserian thermorhizotomy for "essential" trigeminal neuralgia: considerations in 1000 consecutive patients. Neurosurgery 1990; 26(5):783–6 [discussion: 786–7].

74. Ischia S, Luzzani A, Polati E, et al. Percutaneous controlled thermocoagulation in the treatment of trigeminal neuralgia. Clin J Pain 1990;6(2):96–104.

75. Kanpolat Y, Savas A, Bekar A, et al. Percutaneous controlled radiofrequency trigeminal rhizotomy for the treatment of idiopathic trigeminal neuralgia: 25-year experience with 1,600 patients. Neurosurgery 2001;48(3):524–32 [discussion: 532–4].

76. Mathews ES, Scrivani SJ. Percutaneous stereotactic radiofrequency thermal rhizotomy for the treatment of trigeminal neuralgia. Mt Sinai J Med 2000;67(4):288–99.

77. Miserocchi G, Cabrini G, Motti ED, et al. Percutaneous selective thermorhizotomy in the treatment of "essential" trigeminal neuralgia. The importance of lesion selectivity. J Neurosurg Sci 1989;33(2):179–83.

78. Nugent R. Surgical treatment: radiofrequency gangliolysis and rhizotomy. Stoneham (MA): Butterworth-Heinemann; 1991.

79. Oturai AB, Jensen K, Eriksen J, et al. Neurosurgery for trigeminal neuralgia: comparison of alcohol block, neurectomy, and radiofrequency coagulation. Clin J Pain 1996;12(4):311–5.

80. Spendel MC, Deinsberger R, Lanner G. Operative treatment of trigeminal neuralgia. Stereotact Funct Neurosurg 1997;68(1–4 Pt 1):187–9.

81. Sweet WH. Treatment of trigeminal neuralgia by percutaneous rhizotomy. Philadelphia: WB Saunders; 1990.

82. Taha JM, Tew JM Jr, Buncher CR. A prospective 15-year follow up of 154 consecutive patients with trigeminal neuralgia treated by percutaneous stereotactic radiofrequency thermal rhizotomy. J Neurosurg 1995;83(6):989–93.

83. Tew J Jr, Morgan C, Grande A. Percutaneous stereotactic rhizotomy in the treatment of intractable facial pain, vol. 2. Philadelphia: Saunders; 2012.

84. Tronnier VM, Rasche D, Hamer J, et al. Treatment of idiopathic trigeminal neuralgia: comparison of long-term outcome after radiofrequency rhizotomy and microvascular decompression. Neurosurgery 2001;48(6):1261–7 [discussion: 1267–8].

85. Berk C, Honey CR. Brain stem injury after radiofrequency trigeminal rhizotomy. Acta Neurochir (Wien) 2004;146(6):635–6 [discussion: 636].

86. Rath GP, Dash HH, Bithal PK, et al. Intracranial hemorrhage after percutaneous radiofrequency trigeminal rhizotomy. Pain Pract 2009;9(1):82–4.

87. Savas A, Sayin M. Subarachnoid bleeding into the superior cerebellopontine cistern after radiofrequency trigeminal rhizotomy: case report. Acta Neurochir (Wien) 2010;152(3):561–2.

88. Ugur HC, Savas A, Elhan A, et al. Unanticipated complication of percutaneous radiofrequency trigeminal rhizotomy: rhinorrhea: report of three cases and a cadaver study. Neurosurgery 2004; 54(6):1522–4 [discussion: 1524–6].

89. Bale RJ, Laimer I, Martin A, et al. Frameless stereotactic cannulation of the foramen ovale for ablative treatment of trigeminal neuralgia. Neurosurgery 2006;59(4 Suppl 2):ONS394–401 [discussion: ONS402].

90. Lin MH, Lee MH, Wang TC, et al. Foramen ovale cannulation guided by intra-operative computed tomography with integrated neuronavigation for the treatment of trigeminal neuralgia. Acta Neurochir (Wien) 2011;153(8):1593–9.

91. Gusmao S, Oliveira M, Tazinaffo U, et al. Percutaneous trigeminal nerve radiofrequency rhizotomy guided by computerized tomography fluoroscopy. Technical note. J Neurosurg 2003;99(4): 785–6.

92. Xu SJ, Zhang WH, Chen T, et al. Neuronavigator-guided percutaneous radiofrequency thermocoagulation in the treatment of intractable trigeminal neuralgia. Chin Med J (Engl) 2006;119(18): 1528–35.

93. Yang JT, Lin M, Lee MH, et al. Percutaneous trigeminal nerve radiofrequency rhizotomy guided by computerized tomography with three-dimensional image reconstruction. Chang Gung Med J 2010; 33(6):679–83.

Surgical Options for Complex Craniofacial Pain

Mayur Sharma, MD, Andrew Shaw, MD,
Milind Deogaonkar, MD*

KEYWORDS

- Craniofacial pain • Neuropathic pain • Surgical treatment • Peripheral field/nerve stimulation
- Spinal cord stimulation • Ganglion neuromodulation • Motor cortex stimulation
- Deep brain stimulation

KEY POINTS

- Surgical treatment of complex craniofacial pain syndromes has been shown to achieve significant pain relief (>50%) in medically refractory pain syndromes.
- Appropriate patient selection, risks, and benefits associated with each of these therapies, presence of comorbidities, sensory deficits accompanying the area of pain, and insight into the programming parameters are the key points that need to be considered before selecting these surgical options for complex craniofacial pain syndromes.
- Given the reversibility and minimal invasiveness of peripheral nerve/field stimulation, this modality is being explored at a rapid pace and is preferred by both patients and surgeons.
- Motor cortex stimulation and deep brain stimulation can be considered for patients who fail other less invasive neurostimulation therapy for complex craniofacial pain syndromes.
- There is paucity of reliable data in the literature on the efficacy of these therapies for complex craniofacial pain syndromes and prospective randomized controlled studies are warranted to establish their therapeutic value.
- Peripheral nerve/field stimulation therapy, ganglion stimulation, motor cortex stimulation, and deep brain stimulation therapy are still investigational and off-label therapies for complex craniofacial syndromes.

INTRODUCTION

Craniofacial pain is a common condition that affects approximately 10% to 25% of the adult population worldwide with a significant impact on their quality of life.[1–3] The International Headache Society (2004) classified craniofacial pain into 14 different categories, which provides a useful template in establishing a uniform clinical diagnosis.[4] Women are more frequently affected with craniofacial pain, in the ratio of 2:1.[1] The common causes of face pain include trigeminal neuralgia (tic douloureux or Fothergill disease), trigeminal neuropathic pain, and persistent idiopathic facial pain (PIFP, or atypical face pain). A population-based study reported the lifetime prevalence of trigeminal neuralgia and PIFP to be 0.3% and 0.03% respectively.[5] Of these, trigeminal neuropathic pain and PIFP are complex pain syndromes that are often difficult to manage with medications alone.

Department of Neurosurgery, Center of Neuromodulation, Wexner Medical Center, The Ohio State University, 480 Medical Center Drive, Columbus, OH 43210, USA
* Corresponding author.
E-mail address: milind.deogaonkar@osumc.edu

Neurosurg Clin N Am 25 (2014) 763–775
http://dx.doi.org/10.1016/j.nec.2014.07.001
1042-3680/14/$ – see front matter © 2014 Elsevier Inc. All rights reserved.

According to the International Association for the study of pain, neuropathic pain is defined as "pain initiated or caused by a primary lesion or dysfunction in the nervous system."[6,7] Neuropathic pain can be further classified as peripheral or central (depending on the site of the disorder) and acute or chronic (lasting >3 months).[6,7] Trigeminal neuropathic facial pain (TNP) is defined as a constant burning, cramping, pricking, deep aching, or electric shock–like facial pain along the distribution of trigeminal nerve branches.[6,8] TNP is often associated with sensory dysfunctions such as paresthesia or dysesthesia, which can manifest as cold, pricking, tingling, or itching sensations along the distribution of pain.[6] The most severe form of facial pain, with complete numbness in the distribution of pain, is referred to as anesthesia dolorosa. TNP can result from surgery, traumatic injury, and herpetic infection (shingles) of the areas innervated by the branches of trigeminal nerve, including the sinuses, teeth, face, or skull.[9,10] TNP develops in a delayed fashion typically many days to months following the initial insult.[11] In addition, iatrogenic injury to the trigeminal nerve by nerve ablation, rhizotomy, or ganglion ablation to treat trigeminal neuralgia can initiate trigeminal deafferentation or neuropathic pain.

PIFP (atypical face pain) is defined as "Persistent facial pain that does not have the characteristics of the cranial neuralgias and cannot be attributed to other disorders" (International Headache society, 2004).[4] This entity was first described by neurosurgeons Frazier and Russell, in 1924.[12] This condition is often described as severe persistent unilateral facial pain that is deep or poorly localized and usually burning or crushing in nature. Furthermore, there is a normal work-up without an associated sensory loss or other neurologic deficits.[2,4] There may be a history of surgical or traumatic injury to the face, teeth, or gums before the onset; however, there is no demonstrable local cause that can endorse the persistence of this facial pain. PIFP is usually not confined within the anatomic distribution of the branches of trigeminal nerve and is often a diagnosis of exclusion.[2,13] This condition affects approximately 1 in 100,000 adults, with no clear gender predilection, although the clinical presentation is more common in women.[2]

PATHOPHYSIOLOGY OF COMPLEX FACE PAIN

Multiple mechanisms have been postulated in the pathophysiology of neuropathic face pain, which accounts for a wide variety of clinical presentations in patients with similar diseases.[6] Therefore, patients with different pain generators and clinical presentations differ in their responses to treatment and overall outcome. As such, patients with posttraumatic TNP may have a different mechanism of pain onset compared with those with a spontaneous origin of TNP.[11,14] Surgical or traumatic injury to the trigeminal nerve results in impaired functioning of both small unmyelinated and large myelinated nerve fibers with subsequent demyelination of the trigeminal nerve.[2,14] The phenomenon of abnormal temporal summation of pain signals and reduced temperature thresholds with hot/cold hyperalgesias in patients with TNP can be attributed to hyperexcitability of central neurons and hypersensitization of peripheral C fibers/free nerve endings respectively.[2,11,14] This process initiates as a result of interaction between chemicals (histamine, substance P, calcitonin gene–related peptide, glutamate, prostaglandins, bradykinins) released following tissue injury and peripheral nociceptors/free nerve endings, which subsequently can result in alteration in central pain pathways (central hypersensitization) over a period of time. Gender differences have been implicated in the interaction of chemical mediators with peripheral nociceptors and peripheral pain pathways, which may account for the higher incidence of chronic pain conditions in women.[15] The pathophysiology of postherpetic trigeminal neuropathic pain (PHN) involves dysfunction of both peripheral and central pain pathways in varying proportions in different patients.[16,17] This phenomenon can be attributed to the differences in clinical findings between patients with facial and truncal PHN and those with acute and chronic PHN.[17]

The pathophysiology of PIFP is also not completely understood. PIFP was initially thought to be a component of a somatoform disorder because most patients had associated psychiatric disorders.[2,9] However, various neuropathic mechanisms have recently been implicated in the pathogenesis of this disorder.[2] The specific pathophysiologic mechanisms underlying the onset of neuropathic pain have not yet been elucidated, but with ongoing research it might be possible to identify precise mechanisms and thus target therapy accordingly.

PAIN PATHWAYS AND NODES OF INTERVENTION

The pathways related to pain transmission are complex and include both sensory and affective components. The somatic sensations from the skin of the face, forehead, scalp up to the vertex, and mucous membranes of the nasal cavity and paranasal sinuses are carried by branches of the trigeminal nerve. The sensory cell bodies of these first-order neurons lie in the trigeminal or gasserian ganglion in the posterior aspect of the floor of the middle cranial fossa. The sensory fibers of the ganglion are carried in the spinal trigeminal tract to synapse on the second-order neurons within the main sensory nucleus, mesencephalic nucleus, or spinal trigeminal nucleus in the pons. The spinal nucleus of the trigeminal primarily receives afferents related to tactile, nociceptive, and thermal sensations. The subnucleus interpolaris and subnucleus caudalis of the spinal trigeminal nuclei are associated with touch/dental pain and nociception/thermal sensations respectively.[2] The first-order neurons synapse diffusely on second-order neurons across different segments from medulla to cervical cord level. These second-order neurons then cross the midline and ascend in the trigeminothalamic tract to synapse diffusely on the third-order neurons within the ventral posterior lateral (VPL)/ventral posterior medial and ventral posterior inferior nuclei of the thalamus. These third-order neurons then project to the primary and secondary somatosensory cortices for the perception and characterization of the nociceptive stimulus. The thalamic relay station perceives pain as a dull aching sensation and the precise nature of nociceptive stimulus is defined at the cortical level. This pathway constitutes the lateral pain pathways. The medial pain pathways involve the projection of trigeminothalamic tract to the medial thalamic nuclei, limbic system, anterior cingulate cortex, and reticular formation to modulate the affective or emotional aspect of nociceptive stimuli.[18]

Various nodes of surgical intervention in patients with complex face pain include (1) peripheral neuromodulation (peripheral nerve stimulation [PNS] or ganglion stimulation), (2) spinal cord stimulation, (3) deep brain stimulation, and (4) motor cortex stimulation. The selection of a particular treatment modality needs to be individualized based on (1) risk/benefit ratio, (2) presence of sensory loss, and (3) associated comorbidities.

SURGICAL MANAGEMENT OF COMPLEX FACE PAIN

Because of the inadequate understanding of the basic pathophysiology underlying complex face pain, the management of this condition is often difficult and unsatisfactory. Complex face pain is often refractory to conventional medical management. Tolerance, dependence, and side effects of medications used to treat this condition provide an impetus to steer toward surgical options. Various surgical modalities are discussed later.

Peripheral Neuromodulation

Peripheral trigeminal nerve/field stimulation (PNS/peripheral field/nerve stimulation)

This treatment modality for neuropathic pain was first introduced by Wall and Sweet[19] in 1967. Of 8 patients with intense cutaneous pain, 4 experienced pain relief for more than half an hour following stimulation of infraorbital, mandibular, and other nerves.[19,20] However, it was not until the reintroduction of this modality by Weiner and Reed[21] in 1999 that this therapy gained wider clinical acceptance. In their study of 13 patients with occipital neuralgia, 12 patients experienced greater than 50% pain relief at a mean follow-up of 1.5 to 6 years.[21] Since then, there has been a growing interest and literature in the use of this modality for complex craniofacial pain and other regional pain syndromes.[10,11,20,22–29]

Clinical assessment, indications, and prerequisite for peripheral field/nerve stimulation PNS The results of peripheral field/nerve stimulation (PFNS)/PNS therapy depend on appropriate patient selection. It is crucial to differentiate patients with TNP/PIFP and those with classic trigeminal neuralgia. The prerequisites for this therapy are the following:

1. Patients with severe, chronic, refractory neuropathic pain (posttraumatic, postherpetic, occipital neuralgia, occipital headaches, or cervicogenic pain) that is affecting the patient's quality of life. In addition, nonsurgical options such as pharmacotherapy, physical therapy, transcutaneous nerve stimulation, trigger point injections, nerve blocks, Botox, or acupuncture should be exhausted before consideration of this therapy.[20,30]
2. There should be some preservation of sensation in the distribution of pain, because functioning vibrotactile receptors are mandatory for this therapy to be successful.[20,30] In addition, placing an electrode directly below a patch of allodynia for field stimulation can sometimes aggravate the pain. In these situations bracketing the pain can be useful.[30]
3. The pain should be either in the distribution of a single nerve or should be able to be covered by the length of available electrode(s) for PNS and PFNS, respectively, to be successful.[30]
4. Patients should be devoid of underlying psychiatric disorders (depression, anxiety, personality disorders, somatization, drug dependence) or for gains secondary to their chronic pain disorder, which can be identified by neuropsychological assessment.[10,11,20,30]
5. Similar to spinal cord stimulator placement, a successful PNS/PFNS stimulation trial is

mandatory before permanent placement of PNS/PFNS.[31,32] An externalized trial involves percutaneous placement of the electrodes in the distribution of pain with the externalized leads connected to an external pulse generator for a period of 5 to 12 days. Patients are asked to perform activities to maximize their pain and are taught to self-adjust the programming parameters so as to maximize the pain relief. The duration of the trial is variable between implanters and can be based on response and need for reprogramming. Improvement of greater than 50% of pain relief on a visual analog scale (VAS) is generally considered a successful trial.[10,11,20,30]

6. Nerve blocks and transcutaneous electrical nerve stimulation (TENS) therapy does not accurately predict the likelihood of success of PNS/PFNS therapy and should never be considered as a surrogate trial for PNS/PFNS. Nevertheless, success with nerve blocks/TENS therapy might guide the placement of electrodes.[10,20,30,33]

Contraindications of PFNS/PNS

1. Patients on anticoagulation therapy or bleeding disorders[10,30]
2. Ongoing psychiatric issues or major cognitive impairment
3. Inadequate family support
4. Patients on immunosuppression therapy or active infection
5. Ongoing medicolegal issues or litigation related to chronic pain
6. Patients requiring serial magnetic resonance imaging (MRI) that cannot be substituted with other imaging modalities.

Surgical technique Following written informed consent, the patient is brought to the operating room and placed in a supine position with the head turned to the side opposite to their pain.[10,11,20,30] Trial placement of electrodes is performed under monitored anesthesia with liberal use of local anesthetic. This technique allows the implanter to verify appropriate coverage with the implanted electrodes. In addition, lidocaine is the local anesthetic of choice because systemic side effects are less severe in the event of an arterial injection. Permanent placement is performed under general anesthesia using routine sterile techniques. The electrodes are typically placed in a lateral to medial direction in the epifascial plane under fluoroscopic guidance using standard anatomic landmarks. Occipital neuralgias are an exception, because electrodes can be placed in medial to lateral direction.[34] Four or 8 contact cylindrical leads (Quad, Octad, Quad Plus, or Quad

Compact; Medtronic, Inc, Minneapolis, MN) are placed either close to the nerve or in the region of pain, which is demarcated before surgery. We preferentially use an ON-Q tunneler (I-Flow, Lake Forest, CA) for the placement of cylindrical leads by virtue of its flexibility and atraumatic tip. In PNS, a paddle electrode can be used as an overlay or in a sandwich technique by placing paddle leads on each side of a peripheral nerve after adequate surgical exposure.[35] In addition, ultrasonography guidance can be used to aid the placement of the electrode into the correct plane or to identify the nerve.[36] The electrodes are placed at the level of C2 or directed toward the ipsilateral mastoid to cross the course of occipital nerves for occipital pain. For trigeminal neuropathic pain, the incision is made behind the hairline in a supra-auricular or temporal region and electrodes are implanted along the affected divisions of the trigeminal nerve. The supraorbital electrode should be placed well above the eyebrow and infraorbital electrode below the orbit to the base of the nose. For cluster headache, occipital stimulation alone or a combination of supraorbital and infraorbital stimulation can be useful. In addition, a combination of occipital, supraorbital, or infraorbital stimulation can be used for headaches depending on the area and distribution of pain. The electrodes are secured to the skin after creating a strain-relief loop using a nonabsorbable suture such as silk or Dacron during the trial. Following a successful trial, the trial electrodes are removed and new permanent electrodes are placed, mirroring the exact location of the trial. During permanent implantation, the strain-relief loops of electrodes are similarly secured to the fascia after creating a subcutaneous pocket using nonabsorbable sutures and leads are tunneled beneath the skin of the neck to the generator pocket that is created in the infraclavicular region (**Figs. 1** and **2**).

Programming parameters We prefer to use a low rate (20–50 Hz), low pulse width (60–250 milliseconds, occasionally 450 milliseconds), and low amplitude (1.5–2 V) for initial PFNS programming. A simple bipolar configuration limits the number of cathodes and is effective in reducing the energy used and thus prolonging the battery life. A guarded cathode has not been shown to be useful in PFNS therapy.

Review of literature Most of the published literature on PNS/PFNS has reported significant improvement (>50% on VAS) in localized chronic pain intensity. The supraorbital nerve is the most common nerve stimulated (24 cases) followed by the infraorbital nerve (14 cases), occipital nerve (5 cases), and mandibular nerve (2 cases). More

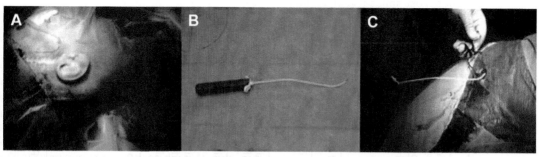

Fig. 1. (*A*) The position of the patient during placement of supraorbital PFNS for postsurgical complex craniofacial pain. (*B*) An ON-Q tunneler bended according to the forehead curvature for optimal placement of supraorbital PFNS. (*C*) A 2-cm to 2.5-cm supra-auricular incision for the introduction of an ON-Q tunneler. ([*B*] I-Flow, Lake Forest, CA.)

than 70% of patients experienced greater than 50% relief in chronic pain intensity in these studies, with follow-up ranging between 3 months and 4 years. Wound breakdown and hardware-related issues were the primary complications seen in these case series (**Table 1**).[11,20,28,37–42]

Sphenopalatine ganglion stimulation for headache and facial pain

Radiofrequency thermocoagulation of the sphenopalatine ganglion (SPG) has been found to be effective in patients with cluster headaches and those with Sluder neuralgia.[43,44] Electric stimulation of sphenopalatine ganglion has recently been shown to be effective in relieving both acute cluster headache pain and the associated autonomic symptoms.[45] This technique involves placement of a needle at the ipsilateral SPG in the pterygopalatine fossa using a percutaneous infrazygomatic approach under fluoroscopic guidance. Of 5 patients with 18 acute attacks of cluster headache over a period of 3 months, short-term (up to

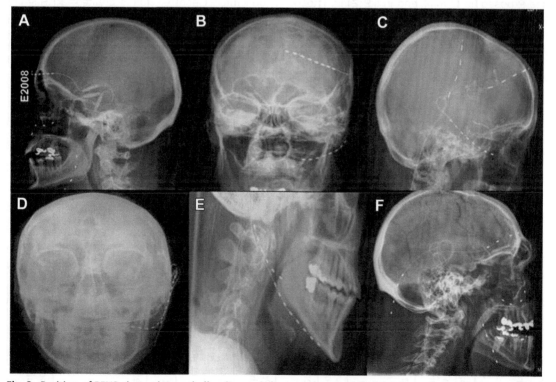

Fig. 2. Position of PFNS electrodes on skull radiograph for complex craniofacial pain syndromes (*A*); supraorbital, infraorbital, and mandibular electrodes (*B*); supraorbital and infraorbital electrodes (*C*); supraorbital and infraorbital electrodes, and along the vertex in the area of pain (*D*); infraorbital electrode (*E*); preauricular and mandibular nerve electrodes (*F*); supraorbital, infraorbital, mandibular, and occipital nerve.

Table 1
Summary of the case series in the literature assessing the efficacy of PFNS for complex craniofacial pain syndromes

Author, Year	Patients (N)	Causes	Area of PFNS Implantation	Results	Follow-up
Dunteman,[38] 2002	2	Postherpetic (2)	Supraorbital (2)	Effectively treated	2 y
Johnson & Burchiel,[11] 2004	10	Postherpetic (4) Posttraumatic (5) Atypical face pain (1)	Supraorbital (8) Infraorbital (2)	50% pain relief in 70% of patients Medication use declined in 70% of patients Two failures (50%) in postherpetic group	26.6 ± 4.7 mo
Slavin et al,[20] 2006	30	Craniofacial pain	Occipital (21) Supraorbital (7) Infraorbital (6) In 19 patients more than 1 nerve was stimulated	73% of patients had >50% pain relief	35 mo
Asensio-Samper et al,[37] 2008	1	Posttraumatic	Supraorbital	VAS 9–10 out of 10 to 2 out of 10 following PFNS	4 y
Reverberi et al,[28] 2009	1	Trigeminal neuropathic pain	Supraorbital and infraorbital	>50% reduction in pain intensity	5 mo
Surjya Prasad Upadhyay et al,[41] 2010	1	Postherpetic	Supraorbital	>50% reduction in pain intensity with improvement in quality of life	8 wk
Yakovlev & Resch,[42] 2010	1	Atypical face pain	Mandibular nerve	>50% reduction in pain intensity	12 mo
Lenchig et al,[39] 2012	1	Posttraumatic	Supraorbital and infraorbital	>50% reduction in pain intensity with improvement in quality of life	3 mo
Stidd et al,[40] 2012	3	Posttraumatic (2) Postherpetic (1)	Supraorbital and infraorbital (2) Supraorbital (1)	>50% reduction in pain intensity	6–27 mo
Feletti et al,[10] 2013	6	Posttraumatic (2) Postsurgical (1) Postherpetic (1) PIFP (2)	Supraorbital (1) Infraorbital (2) Occipital nerve (1) Supraorbital nerve + infraorbital nerve + occipital nerve (1) Occipital nerve + infraorbital nerve + mandibular nerve (1)	VAS from 10 out of 10 to 2.7 out of 10	17 mo
Our experience (unpublished data)	80	Craniofacial pain	Supraorbital + infraorbital + mandibular + occipital nerve	80% of patients had >50% improvement	60 mo

1 hour) electric stimulation of the SPG completely aborted the pain in 11 attacks, partially aborted the pain in 3 attacks, and there was minimal/no relief in 4 attacks.[45] Following the beneficial effect of this therapy in patients with cluster headache, this modality has gained interest in treating patients with migranous headache.[46] The mechanism of action of this therapy involves interruption of the postganglionic parasympathetic outflow and regulating the sensory inputs and processing in the nucleus caudalis of trigeminal.[46] However, the literature on SPG neuromodulation for headaches and face pain is mostly from small series of patients and needs to be validated by randomized clinical trials and long-term studies.

Cervical Spinal Cord Stimulation for Craniofacial Pain

Thoracic spinal cord stimulation is a well-established treatment modality for patients with failed back syndrome and complex regional pain syndromes.[47–49] There are few studies evaluating the role of high cervical spinal cord stimulator for treating head or face pain.[50–52] The procedure is usually performed in a similar manner to a standard thoracic spinal cord stimulator in 2 stages (trial followed by permanent implantation) with somatosensory evoked potential monitoring. The quadripolar paddle leads are implanted in a retrograde manner following a C1 hemilaminotomy. With fluoroscopic guidance the proximal contacts are directed at the cervicomedullary junction.[52] A study reported the success of this therapy in relieving left-side trigeminal neuralgia pain in a patient with advanced multiple sclerosis.[51] Another study evaluating the efficacy of cervical spinal cord stimulator in 41 patients with intractable upper limb and face pain concluded that patients with face pain did not respond to this therapy.[50] A recent retrospective study on the efficacy of cervicomedullary spinal cord stimulator in patients with TNP, PHN, trigeminal deafferentation pain (TDP), occipital neuralgia, and poststroke face pain concluded that cervicomedullary junction stimulator is a favorable option for patients with TDP, TNP, and PHN, whereas those with occipital neuralgic pain rarely responded to this therapy.[52] Of 35 patients in this study, 71.4% (25 patients) had a successful trial followed by permanent implantation. This therapy provided greater than 50% relief in pain intensity in 70% of patients with TDP (n = 7), 80% with TNP (n = 4), 100% both with PHN (n = 2) and poststroke pain (n = 1), and only 28.6% of patients (n = 2) with occipital neuralgia.[52] The drawback of this nonrandomized study was its retrospective nature and small sample size. Therefore randomized controlled studies are required to validate this therapy for complex craniofacial pain syndromes.

Trigeminal Nucleus Caudalis Dorsal Root Entry Zone Ablative Procedures for Complex Craniofacial Pain

Nucleus caudalis dorsal root entry zone (DREZ) ablation has been shown to be effective in relieving refractory trigeminal neuropathic pain, atypical headache, complex craniofacial pain, anesthesia dolorosa, postherpetic neuralgia, refractory pain associated with multiple sclerosis, brain stem infarction, and terminal cancers.[53–55] This technique was first described in a patient with anesthesia dolorosa by Urban and Nashold[29] in 1982. The subnucleus caudalis of the spinal trigeminal nucleus is primarily associated with receiving and integrating nociceptive/thermal sensations, therefore lesioning at this node might interrupt the pain pathways and spontaneous pain generation in patients with deafferentation pain syndromes.[54] Trigeminal tractotomy and nucleotomy (TR-NC) involves lesioning the descending spinal trigeminal tracts in the medulla along with the nucleus caudalis, whereas nucleus caudalis DREZ involves lesioning the whole substantia gelatinosa at the nucleus caudalis.[56] Nucleus caudalis DREZ ablation is usually performed using an open surgical approach, whereas trigeminal TR-NC is performed percutaneously under image guidance.[53–57] Kanpolat and colleagues[57] reported significant pain relief in 19 of 21 patients with atypical face pain following computed tomography–guided TR-NC surgery. In another study, this group reported that 16 of 17 patients with atypical face pain responded to TR-NC therapy and 1 patient with failed therapy subsequently responded to a trigeminal DREZ procedure.[56] Bullard and Nashold[53] evaluated the efficacy of caudalis DREZ surgery for complex craniofacial pain and reported that 96%, 76%, 68%, and 67% of patients experienced good to excellent pain relief immediately, at 1 month, 3 months, and 1 year after surgery, respectively. Another study reported complete and permanent pain relief in 2 of 6 patients with intractable facial pain, 3 patients had significant improvement, and pain recurred in 2 patients several weeks to months after the procedure.[55] Ipsilateral arm/leg ataxia is the most common complication encountered in up to 90% of patients who underwent caudalis DREZ before 1989; however, following the introduction of a 90° bend in the electrodes, which allowed better placement of lesions, this complication has decreased to 33% to 39%.[54,58] This complication can be attributed to injury to spinocerebellar, cuneocerebellar, fasciculus cuneatus, or corticospinal tracts during placement of lesioning electrodes and generally resolves within 10 days following surgery with current technical advances.[54] Overall, nucleus caudalis DREZ lesioning can be associated with significant life-threatening surgical complications during exposure and manipulation of the brainstem. Some studies have advocated TR-NC as a first-step procedure followed by DREZ lesioning for intractable face pain, given the minimal invasiveness, low complication rate, and high efficacy associated with TR-NC.[56,57]

Motor Cortex Stimulation for Complex Craniofacial Pain

Motor cortex stimulation (MCS) has been used for a variety of chronic medically refractory pain syndromes such as facial neuropathic pain, atypical face pain, poststroke central pain, thalamic pain, brachial plexus avulsion pain, phantom limb pain, postherpetic neuralgia, Wallenberg syndrome pain, complex regional pain syndrome, multiple sclerosis pain, spinal cord injury, or pain secondary to posttraumatic brain injury.[59–62] MCS for refractory TNP was first reported in 1993 with 60% to 90% relief in pain intensity at 8 to 28 months.[63] Since then numerous studies have evaluated the efficacy of this modality for complex craniofacial pain, and MCS is now considered one of the last resorts in the management of these medically refractory conditions.[59] Most of these studies are retrospective case series or small prospective randomized trials, and there is a paucity of literature on the efficacy of MCS for chronic neuropathic face pain in large multicenter randomized controlled trials.[59,64] Monsalve[59] evaluated the efficacy of MCS for facial chronic neuropathic pain in a systematic review and reported that, of 126 relevant studies (MCS for chronic pain) and 118 patients, 100 (84.7%) patients underwent permanent implantation and 84% of these had good pain relief. Raslan and colleagues[65] reported that 8 of 11 patients underwent successful permanent implantation of MCS for trigeminal neuropathic pain in their retrospective case series. Of these 8 patients, 5 (62.5%) continued to experience significant pain relief at a mean follow-up of 33 months, and the other 3 patients failed MCS at 6 months follow-up.[65] Another review reported response rates of 72.6% and 45.3% with invasive and noninvasive brain stimulation respectively for chronic pain.[64] In a prospective randomized controlled trial evaluating the efficacy of MCS in 7 patients (total of 16 patients) with chronic craniofacial pain syndromes, 6 of the 7 patients reported significant pain relief.[66]

In our experience of 26 patients with trigeminal neuropathic and poststroke pain who underwent epidural MCS, 50% of them achieved greater than 50% alleviation in the intensity of pain. Overall MCS efficacy was good or satisfactory in 60% of patients with chronic painful conditions.[66] Another prospective double-blinded crossover trial comparing the efficacy of MCS between On and Off states in patients with chronic neuropathic conditions reported that MCS in the On state has significant benefits in terms of both pain relief and improvement in quality of life with no loss of efficacy over time.[67] Velasco and colleagues[68] in a double-blind study reported 100% pain relief in 2 patients with thalamic pain (V2/V3 distribution) and postherpetic neuralgia (V1 distributions) with MCS. We prefer programming parameters of 40-Hz frequency (25–55 Hz), 60–180-millisecond pulse width, 1.5-V to 4-V amplitude (according to the seizure threshold), and bipolar stimulation with cathodes over the motor cortex and anodes over the sensory cortex. Chronic stimulation is usually done in a cycling mode with 3 hours in the On state and 3 hours Off state and should not produce paresthesia. Pain relief is generally achieved several minutes following the onset of stimulation. The common complications associated with MCS include seizures, wound infections, hemorrhage, brain edema, and neurologic deficits.[59] Overall, MCS is a safe and effective treatment of chronic refractory neuropathic pain syndromes that have failed other modalities of treatment. However, large prospective randomized controlled trials are required to validate this modality as a primary therapy for patients with complex craniofacial pain syndromes (**Fig. 3**).

Deep Brain Stimulation for Complex Craniofacial Pain

Deep brain stimulation (DBS) can be a last resort for a variety of neuropathic and chronic pain syndromes that are refractory to medical therapy or other neurmodulatory techniques. DBS has gained significant popularity with improving efficacy, safety, and applications beyond movement disorders. There is great interest in the role of DBS for chronic pain conditions that are refractory to other conventional therapies. DBS can be used for refractory pain syndromes such as neuropathic pain, deafferentation pain, brachial plexus avulsion pain, chronic low back pain, failed back surgery syndrome, and cluster headaches.[61,69–71] DBS therapy for chronic pain dates back to 1954 when stimulation of the septal region was shown to achieve significant pain relief in patients with psychiatric disorders.[69] Since

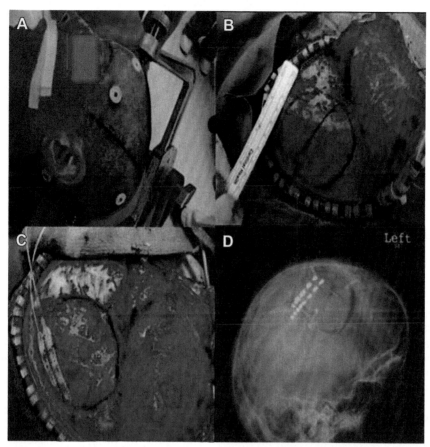

Fig. 3. (*A*, *B*) The position of the patient and size of craniotomy for placement of MCS for complex craniofacial pain, (*C*) position of motor cortex stimulators, and (*D*) postoperative radiograph showing the position of leads.

then targets such as sensory thalamic nuclei, medial posterior inferior thalamus, internal capsule, periaqueductal gray matter (PAG), and periventricular gray matter (PVG) have been used to achieve satisfactory pain relief in patients with a variety of chronic pain syndromes.[72–78] DBS of the PAG/PVG area and sensory thalamus has been shown to relieve nociceptive pain, neuropathic pain, and deafferentation pain with long-term follow-up.[79] A meta-analysis evaluating the efficacy of DBS for chronic pain reported that 56% of the patients with neuropathic pain and none with nociceptive pain achieved long-term pain control with DBS of the sensory thalamic nucleus (VPL). Fifty-nine percent of patients with nociceptive pain and 23% with neuropathic pain achieved long-term success with pain control following DBS of the PVG.[69] Overall, DBS of either PVG/PAG or sensory thalamus has been shown to be more effective in alleviating nociceptive pain (63%) than deafferentation/neuropathic pain (47%). In addition, chronic stimulation of the sensory thalamus alone (58%) has been shown to be less effective

in achieving long-term pain relief than PVG/PAG (79%) or combined PVG/PAG plus sensory thalamus/internal capsule (87%).[80] In our experience of 12 patients who underwent DBS of the sensory thalamus for chronic pain, 3 patients had TNP. These patients underwent successful trial implantation with an externalized lead for 7 days following acceptable neuropsychological assessment. Of these 3 patients, 1 had complete pain relief with 100% reduction in pain medications and the other 2 had 40% reduction in pain medications at 6 years' follow-up. Newer targets such as ventral anterior limb of the internal capsule/ventral striatum and mesial thalamic nuclei have recently been explored to achieve satisfactory pain control in these patients.[61] We prefer programming parameters with a pulse width of 60 milliseconds to avoid spillover, smaller amplitude, a rate of 50 to 100 Hz, and ventral cathodes. In addition, DBS has been shown to be effective in alleviating pain associated with failed back surgery syndromes and cluster headaches/cephalgias, and may be efficacious in conditions such as thalamic pain

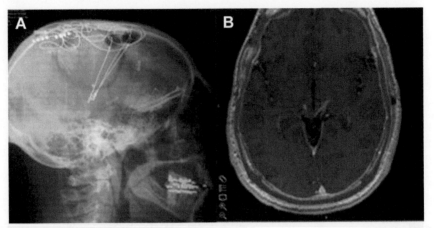

Fig. 4. (*A*) Postoperative radiograph showing the position of DBS leads in the sensory thalamus for complex craniofacial pain syndrome. (*B*) Postoperative MRI showing single lead in right sensory thalamus and 2 leads on left side (1 in sensory thalamus and 1 in centromedian-parafascicular complex).

syndromes, deafferentation pain syndromes, postherpetic neuralgia, and spinal cord injury pain.[69] DBS for complex craniofacial pain syndromes may be indicated in patients who have failed other less invasive neurmodulatory techniques. However, prospective randomized controlled studies are warranted to establish the efficacy of DBS therapy for complex craniofacial pain syndromes (**Fig. 4**).

SUMMARY

Complex craniofacial pain can be a challenging condition to manage both medically and surgically. With the technological advances and success of neurostimulation therapy in small trials there is a resurgence of interest in the role of neurostimulation therapy in managing this condition. Various surgical options for complex craniofacial pain syndromes include PFNS, ganglion stimulation, spinal cord stimulation, dorsal nerve root entry zone lesioning, MCS, and DBS. Appropriate patient selection, risks, and benefits associated with each of these therapies; presence of comorbidities; sensory deficits accompanying the area of pain; and insight into the programming parameters are key points that need to be considered in evaluating these surgical options for complex craniofacial pain syndromes. Given the reversibility and minimally invasive nature of PFNS, this modality is being explored at a rapid pace and is preferred by both patients and surgeons. To date there is a paucity of reliable evidence in the literature on the efficacy of neurostimulation therapy for chronic craniofacial pain syndromes and prospective randomized controlled trials are needed to better understand the therapy or therapies that are most beneficial. In addition, technological advances, improved understanding of the interactions of pain pathways with its affective component, and addition of novel targets will widen the horizons of neurostimulation therapy to benefit patients with complex craniofacial pain syndromes.

REFERENCES

1. Kohlmann T. Epidemiology of orofacial pain. Schmerz 2002;16(5):339–45 [in German].
2. Nguyen CT, Wang MB. Complementary and integrative treatments: atypical facial pain. Otolaryngol Clin North Am 2013;46(3):367–82.
3. Macfarlane TV, Blinkhorn AS, Davies RM, et al. Orofacial pain in the community: prevalence and associated impact. Community Dent Oral Epidemiol 2002;30(1):52–60.
4. Headache Classification Subcommittee of the International Headache Society. The international classification of headache disorders: 2nd edition. Cephalalgia 2004;24(Suppl 1):9–160.
5. Mueller D, Obermann M, Yoon MS, et al. Prevalence of trigeminal neuralgia and persistent idiopathic facial pain: a population-based study. Cephalalgia 2011;31(15):1542–8.
6. Dworkin RH. An overview of neuropathic pain: syndromes, symptoms, signs, and several mechanisms. Clin J Pain 2002;18(6):343–9.
7. Merskey H, Bogduk N. Classification of chronic pain. Descriptions of chronic pain syndromes and definitions of pain terms. 2nd edition. Seattle (WA): IASP Press; 1994.
8. Boureau F, Doubrere JF, Luu M. Study of verbal description in neuropathic pain. Pain 1990;42(2): 145–52.
9. Burchiel KJ. A new classification for facial pain. Neurosurgery 2003;53(5):1164–6 [discussion: 1166–7].

10. Feletti A, Santi GZ, Sammartino F, et al. Peripheral trigeminal nerve field stimulation: report of 6 cases. Neurosurg Focus 2013;35(3):E10.

11. Johnson MD, Burchiel KJ. Peripheral stimulation for treatment of trigeminal postherpetic neuralgia and trigeminal posttraumatic neuropathic pain: a pilot study. Neurosurgery 2004;55(1):135–41 [discussion: 141–2].

12. Frazier C, Russell E. Neuralgia of the face: an analysis of 754 cases with relation to pain and other sensory phenomena before and after operation. Arch Neurol Psychiatry 1924;11:557–63.

13. Obermann M, Holle D, Katsarava Z. Trigeminal neuralgia and persistent idiopathic facial pain. Expert Rev Neurother 2011;11(11):1619–29.

14. Eide PK, Rabben T. Trigeminal neuropathic pain: pathophysiological mechanisms examined by quantitative assessment of abnormal pain and sensory perception. Neurosurgery 1998;43(5):1103–10.

15. Sardella A, Demarosi F, Barbieri C, et al. An up-to-date view on persistent idiopathic facial pain. Minerva Stomatol 2009;58(6):289–99.

16. Fields HL, Rowbotham M, Baron R. Postherpetic neuralgia: irritable nociceptors and deafferentation. Neurobiol Dis 1998;5(4):209–27.

17. Pappagallo M, Oaklander AL, Quatrano-Piacentini AL, et al. Heterogenous patterns of sensory dysfunction in postherpetic neuralgia suggest multiple pathophysiologic mechanisms. Anesthesiology 2000;92(3):691–8.

18. Ossipov MH, Dussor GO, Porreca F. Central modulation of pain. J Clin Invest 2010;120(11):3779–87.

19. Wall PD, Sweet WH. Temporary abolition of pain in man. Science 1967;155(3758):108–9.

20. Slavin KV, Colpan ME, Munawar N, et al. Trigeminal and occipital peripheral nerve stimulation for craniofacial pain: a single-institution experience and review of the literature. Neurosurg Focus 2006;21(6):E5.

21. Weiner RL, Reed KL. Peripheral neurostimulation for control of intractable occipital neuralgia. Neuromodulation 1999;2(3):217–21.

22. Hassenbusch SJ, Stanton-Hicks M, Schoppa D, et al. Long-term results of peripheral nerve stimulation for reflex sympathetic dystrophy. J Neurosurg 1996;84(3):415–23.

23. Amin S, Buvanendran A, Park KS, et al. Peripheral nerve stimulator for the treatment of supraorbital neuralgia: a retrospective case series. Cephalalgia 2008;28(4):355–9.

24. Mobbs RJ, Nair S, Blum P. Peripheral nerve stimulation for the treatment of chronic pain. J Clin Neurosci 2007;14(3):216–21 [discussion: 222–3].

25. Magis D, Allena M, Bolla M, et al. Occipital nerve stimulation for drug-resistant chronic cluster headache: a prospective pilot study. Lancet Neurol 2007;6(4):314–21.

26. Jasper JF, Hayek SM. Implanted occipital nerve stimulators. Pain Physician 2008;11(2):187–200.

27. Reed KL. Peripheral neuromodulation and headaches: history, clinical approach, and considerations on underlying mechanisms. Curr Pain Headache Rep 2013;17(1):305.

28. Reverberi C, Bonezzi C, Demartini L. Peripheral subcutaneous neurostimulation in the management of neuropathic pain: five case reports. Neuromodulation 2009;12(2):146–55.

29. Urban BJ, Nashold BS Jr. Combined epidural and peripheral nerve stimulation for relief of pain. Description of technique and preliminary results. J Neurosurg 1982;57(3):365–9.

30. Deogaonkar M, Slavin KV. Peripheral nerve/field stimulation for neuropathic pain. Neurosurg Clin N Am 2014;25(1):1–10.

31. Kumar K, Hunter G, Demeria D. Spinal cord stimulation in treatment of chronic benign pain: challenges in treatment planning and present status, a 22-year experience. Neurosurgery 2006;58(3):481–96 [discussion: 481–96].

32. Mekhail NA, Mathews M, Nageeb F, et al. Retrospective review of 707 cases of spinal cord stimulation: indications and complications. Pain Practice 2011;11(2):148–53.

33. Slavin KV. Peripheral nerve stimulation for neuropathic pain. Neurotherapeutics 2008;5(1):100–6.

34. Popeney CA, Alo KM. Peripheral neurostimulation for the treatment of chronic, disabling transformed migraine. Headache 2003;43(4):369–75.

35. Abhinav K, Park ND, Prakash SK, et al. Novel use of narrow paddle electrodes for occipital nerve stimulation-technical note. Neuromodulation 2013; 16(6):607–9.

36. Eldrige JS, Obray JB, Pingree MJ, et al. Occipital neuromodulation: ultrasound guidance for peripheral nerve stimulator implantation. Pain Practice 2010;10(6):580–5.

37. Asensio-Samper JM, Villanueva VL, Perez AV, et al. Peripheral neurostimulation in supraorbital neuralgia refractory to conventional therapy. Pain Practice 2008;8(2):120–4.

38. Dunteman E. Peripheral nerve stimulation for unremitting ophthalmic postherpetic neuralgia. Neuromodulation 2002;5(1):32–7.

39. Lenchig S, Cohen J, Patin D. A minimally invasive surgical technique for the treatment of posttraumatic trigeminal neuropathic pain with peripheral nerve stimulation. Pain Physician 2012;15(5): E725–32.

40. Stidd DA, Wuollet AL, Bowden K, et al. Peripheral nerve stimulation for trigeminal neuropathic pain. Pain Physician 2012;15(1):27–33.

41. Surjya Prasad U, Shiv Pratap R, Mishra S, et al. Successful treatment of an intractable postherpetic neuralgia (PHN) using peripheral nerve field

stimulation (PNFS). Am J Hosp Palliat Care 2010; 27(1):59–62.

42. Yakovlev AE, Resch BE. Treatment of chronic intractable atypical facial pain using peripheral subcutaneous field stimulation. Neuromodulation 2010;13(2):137–40.

43. Oomen KP, van Wijck AJ, Hordijk GJ, et al. Effects of radiofrequency thermocoagulation of the sphenopalatine ganglion on headache and facial pain: correlation with diagnosis. J Orofac Pain 2012; 26(1):59–64.

44. Narouze SN. Role of sphenopalatine ganglion neuroablation in the management of cluster headache. Curr Pain Headache Rep 2010;14(2):160–3.

45. Ansarinia M, Rezai A, Tepper SJ, et al. Electrical stimulation of sphenopalatine ganglion for acute treatment of cluster headaches. Headache 2010; 50(7):1164–74.

46. Khan S, Schoenen J, Ashina M. Sphenopalatine ganglion neuromodulation in migraine: what is the rationale? Cephalalgia 2014;34(5):382–91.

47. Simpson BA. Spinal-cord stimulation for reflex sympathetic dystrophy. Lancet Neurol 2004;3(3):142.

48. Kumar K, Taylor RS, Jacques L, et al. Spinal cord stimulation versus conventional medical management for neuropathic pain: a multicentre randomised controlled trial in patients with failed back surgery syndrome. Pain 2007;132(1–2):179–88.

49. North RB, Kidd D, Shipley J, et al. Spinal cord stimulation versus reoperation for failed back surgery syndrome: a cost effectiveness and cost utility analysis based on a randomized, controlled trial. Neurosurgery 2007;61(2):361–8 [discussion: 368–9].

50. Simpson BA, Bassett G, Davies K, et al. Cervical spinal cord stimulation for pain: a report on 41 patients. Neuromodulation 2003;6(1):20–6.

51. Barolat G, Knobler RL, Lublin FD. Trigeminal neuralgia in a patient with multiple sclerosis treated with high cervical spinal cord stimulation. Case report. Appl Neurophysiol 1988;51(6):333–7.

52. Tomycz ND, Deibert CP, Moossy JJ. Cervicomedullary junction spinal cord stimulation for head and facial pain. Headache 2011;51(3):418–25.

53. Bullard DE, Nashold BS Jr. The caudalis DREZ for facial pain. Stereotact Funct Neurosurg 1997; 68(1–4 Pt 1):168–74.

54. Sandwell SE, El-Naggar AO. Nucleus caudalis dorsal root entry zone lesioning for the treatment of anesthesia dolorosa. J Neurosurg 2013;118(3): 534–8.

55. Delgado-Lopez P, Garcia-Salazar F, Mateo-Sierra O, et al. Trigeminal nucleus caudalis dorsal root entry zone radiofrequency thermocoagulation for invalidating facial pain. Neurocirugia (Astur) 2003;14(1):25–32 [discussion: 32].

56. Kanpolat Y, Savas A, Ugur HC, et al. The trigeminal tract and nucleus procedures in treatment of atypical

facial pain. Surg Neurol 2005;64(Suppl 2):S96–100 [discussion: S100–1].

57. Kanpolat Y, Kahilogullari G, Ugur HC, et al. Computed tomography-guided percutaneous trigeminal tractotomy-nucleotomy. Neurosurgery 2008;63(1 Suppl 1): ONS147–53 [discussion: ONS153–5].

58. Gorecki JP, Nashold BS. The Duke experience with the nucleus caudalis DREZ operation. Acta Neurochir Suppl 1995;64:128–31.

59. Monsalve GA. Motor cortex stimulation for facial chronic neuropathic pain: a review of the literature. Surg Neurol Int 2012;3(Suppl 4):S290–311.

60. Henderson JM, Lad SP. Motor cortex stimulation and neuropathic facial pain. Neurosurg Focus 2006;21(6):E6.

61. Moore NZ, Lempka SF, Machado A. Central neuromodulation for refractory pain. Neurosurg Clin N Am 2014;25(1):77–83.

62. Sharan AD, Rosenow JM, Turbay M, et al. Precentral stimulation for chronic pain. Neurosurg Clin N Am 2003;14(3):437–44.

63. Meyerson BA, Lindblom U, Linderoth B, et al. Motor cortex stimulation as treatment of trigeminal neuropathic pain. Acta Neurochir Suppl 1993;58:150–3.

64. Lima MC, Fregni F. Motor cortex stimulation for chronic pain: systematic review and meta-analysis of the literature. Neurology 2008;70(24):2329–37.

65. Raslan AM, Nasseri M, Bahgat D, et al. Motor cortex stimulation for trigeminal neuropathic or deafferentation pain: an institutional case series experience. Stereotact Funct Neurosurg 2011; 89(2):83–8.

66. Lefaucheur JP, Drouot X, Cunin P, et al. Motor cortex stimulation for the treatment of refractory peripheral neuropathic pain. Brain 2009;132(Pt 6): 1463–71.

67. Nguyen JP, Velasco F, Brugieres P, et al. Treatment of chronic neuropathic pain by motor cortex stimulation: results of a bicentric controlled crossover trial. Brain Stimul 2008;1(2):89–96.

68. Velasco F, Arguelles C, Carrillo-Ruiz JD, et al. Efficacy of motor cortex stimulation in the treatment of neuropathic pain: a randomized double-blind trial. J Neurosurg 2008;108(4):698–706.

69. Levy R, Deer TR, Henderson J. Intracranial neurostimulation for pain control: a review. Pain Physician 2010;13(2):157–65.

70. Schoenen J, Di Clemente L, Vandenheede M, et al. Hypothalamic stimulation in chronic cluster headache: a pilot study of efficacy and mode of action. Brain 2005;128(Pt 4):940–7.

71. Green AL, Owen SL, Davies P, et al. Deep brain stimulation for neuropathic cephalalgia. Cephalalgia 2006;26(5):561–7.

72. Mazars GJ. Intermittent stimulation of nucleus ventralis posterolateralis for intractable pain. Surg Neurol 1975;4(1):93–5.

73. Adams JE, Hosobuchi Y, Fields HL. Stimulation of internal capsule for relief of chronic pain. J Neurosurg 1974;41(6):740–4.

74. Hosobuchi Y, Adams JE, Rutkin B. Chronic thalamic stimulation for the control of facial anesthesia dolorosa. Arch Neurol 1973;29(3): 158–61.

75. Schvarcz JR. Chronic self-stimulation of the medial posterior inferior thalamus for the alleviation of deafferentation pain. Acta Neurochir Suppl 1980; 30:295–301.

76. Young RF, Kroening R, Fulton W, et al. Electrical stimulation of the brain in treatment of chronic pain. Experience over 5 years. J Neurosurg 1985; 62(3):389–96.

77. Hosobuchi Y, Adams JE, Linchitz R. Pain relief by electrical stimulation of the central gray matter in humans and its reversal by naloxone. Science 1977;197(4299):183–6.

78. Richardson DE, Akil H. Pain reduction by electrical brain stimulation in man. Part 1: acute administration in periaqueductal and periventricular sites. J Neurosurg 1977;47(2):178–83.

79. Levy RM, Lamb S, Adams JE. Treatment of chronic pain by deep brain stimulation: long term follow-up and review of the literature. Neurosurgery 1987; 21(6):885–93.

80. Bittar RG, Kar-Purkayastha I, Owen SL, et al. Deep brain stimulation for pain relief: a meta-analysis. J Clin Neurosci 2005;12(5):515–9.

Neurolysis, Neurectomy, and Nerve Repair/Reconstruction for Chronic Pain

CrossMark

Lindsay J. Lipinski, MD, Robert J. Spinner, MD*

KEYWORDS

- Neurectomy • Neurolysis • Nerve repair/reconstruction • Neuropathy

KEY POINTS

- Careful examination, including detailed sensory and motor findings and the presence of percussion tenderness, assists in the localization of nerve injury and the potential site of intervention.
- In our experience, the presence of at least 3 supportive features (history, physical examination, electrophysiologic studies, imaging findings, and diagnostic blocks) should support the diagnosis of neuropathic pain before operative intervention is considered.
- Nerve-related procedures, including neurolysis/decompression, neurectomy, and nerve repair/reconstruction, are considered first-line interventions.
- Nerve decompression/neurolysis should be considered in the setting of entrapment or significant scarring that may impair nerve transmission and cause pain.
- Neurectomy can be considered for sensory nerves when numbness is an acceptable trade-off for painful dysesthesias, or after failed neurolysis of a sensory nerve.
- Nerve repair/reconstruction is generally performed with the goal of regaining motor function but also plays a role in improving neuropathic pain by directing axons past the neuroma.

INTRODUCTION

An estimated 6% to 8% of the population has chronic neuropathic pain.[1,2] Causes vary widely, including diabetic neuropathy, postherpetic neuralgia, human immunodeficiency virus neuropathy, chemotherapy-induced neuropathy, complex regional pain syndrome, phantom limb pain, multiple sclerosis, and pain related to spinal cord injury or stroke. Most of these pain syndromes are managed medically. In a neurosurgical practice, patients may present with pain identifiable to a particular nerve distribution, and occasionally more than one distribution. In such patients, surgical intervention may play a role.

Pain is a frequent complaint after peripheral nerve damage. Nerve injury can occur idiopathically or in relation to a specific injury or intervention. This pain is often chronic and can significantly affect quality of life. The pathophysiology of neuropathic pain is poorly understood, but multiple mechanisms, including compression, transection, contusion, stretch, and crush injuries to nerves, can play an inciting role. Treatment options vary widely and correlate with the suspected mechanism of injury. Treatment should begin with the least invasive option and progress toward surgical intervention after the failure of reasonable conservative management trials.

This article provides an overview of the indications for, techniques of, and potential complications related to first-line nerve-related procedures, including neurolysis, neurectomy, and nerve repair/reconstruction in the setting of peripheral nerve pain from a postganglionic source. We find that stimulation (central nervous system [CNS] or peripheral nervous system [PNS]) represents a

Department of Neurologic Surgery, Mayo Clinic, Rochester, MN, USA
* Corresponding author. Mayo Clinic, Gonda 8-214, Rochester, MN 55905.
E-mail address: spinner.robert@mayo.edu

Neurosurg Clin N Am 25 (2014) 777–787
http://dx.doi.org/10.1016/j.nec.2014.07.002
1042-3680/14/$ – see front matter © 2014 Elsevier Inc. All rights reserved.

secondary procedure in these cases. For completeness, other techniques used in the treatment of other types of pain, such as dorsal root entry zone (DREZ) lesion, myelotomy, cordotomy (complex ablative procedures) and intrathecal drug delivery, are discussed elsewhere in this issue.

DIAGNOSIS

Establishing the diagnosis of neuropathic pain in a timely fashion is helpful in management, because sensitization and the development of related pain behaviors may be difficult to address. Diagnosis is often established by history and physical examination supported by electrophysiologic and imaging studies as well as diagnostic blocks. With peripheral nerve disorders, pain is referred along the distribution of the injured nerve. Therefore, a detailed understanding of the anatomic course of the nerve, including its motor, sensory, and autonomic supply, is key.

History typically includes precise descriptions of the distribution of motor, sensory, and autonomic changes. Assessing the quality of pain, as well as additional pain generators (inflammation of an adjacent muscle or joint), is necessary. Palliative and provocative positions are helpful. Occupational and recreational activities and medical comorbidities should be determined. A full list of current and past medications (and dosages) should be obtained.

A detailed neurologic examination is performed, including testing motor, sensory, pain, and when necessary autonomic fibers. Decreased sensation, hypersensitivity, or allodynia in the distribution of, versus beyond, a single nerve territory is sought. Percussion of the skin over a nerve at the site of an injury may evoke tingling or pain in the distribution of the nerve (percussion tenderness). This examination technique is particularly useful because it assists in localization of injury. This phenomenon is thought to occur because of disrupted or sensitized nerve fibers at the point of injury and may be seen in both traumatic injuries and compression syndromes. The Tinel sign indicates distal migration of the axonal cone; progression of the Tinel sign over time indicates ongoing nerve regeneration and suggests recovery. The Tinel sign is limited to nerves with sensory components, and generally is not present in purely motor nerves.

Adjunct testing, such as electrophysiologic studies, and magnetic resonance imaging (MRI) or ultrasonography may be useful in confirming the diagnosis; however, normal studies do not exclude pain of peripheral nerve origin. Electromyogram (EMG)/nerve conduction study may be normal because these tests do not measure pain fibers. However, abnormalities may be present, and indicate motor or sensory dysfunction, which can be interpreted in the context of pain in that nerve's distribution. High-resolution imaging (MRI or ultrasonography) may show an enlarged nerve: MRI may show hyperintensity of the nerve on T2-weighted images; ultrasonography may show focal thickening at the site of injury or entrapment.

Nerve blocks may play a role in the establishment of the diagnosis. In our practice, blocks are generally done for diagnostic purposes and can be performed by the surgeon, radiologist, or pain specialist, typically with image guidance. Blocks are performed with local anesthetic at a site distant from and proximal to the suspected site of injury. Interpretation of the block can be complex. A positive response is helpful but nonspecific. We appreciate the benefit of, but seldom use, dilute blocks or placebos as part of our routine practice.

All of this information must be used in tandem to make the diagnosis and determine the yield of surgical management and a specific operative intervention. We try to have 3 or more diagnostic features (history, physical, electrophysiologic studies, imaging, diagnostic blocks) that support the diagnosis before considering or prognosticating on an operative intervention.

THERAPEUTIC OPTIONS

Management options vary widely depending on the acuity of the pain, the mechanism of the injury, the nerve involved (ranging from a small cutaneous nerve to a single major nerve to multiple major nerves), and physiologic and psychosocial factors of the individual patient. Options range from physical therapy, to pharmacotherapy, to surgical treatment directed at specific nerves (as described in this article). Intervention should be considered in tiers ranging from the least invasive to more invasive, and should be tailored to the individual patient.

Nonoperative

Once the diagnosis of pain originating from a peripheral nerve is made, initial management of neuropathic pain is almost always nonoperative. A multidisciplinary approach including consultation with a pain management specialist may also be of use. In many cases, pain improves with time and/or nerve regeneration, and a course of pain management and observation is therefore indicated. Pharmacotherapy for pain includes a wide range of medication classes, including antidepressants, anticonvulsants, and analgesics. Rehabilitation plays a role, including physical therapy, massage, and alternative holistic therapies such as acupuncture. Psychosocial intervention such as counseling, biofeedback, relaxation therapy, and support groups may prove useful. Desensitization techniques have been recommended for treatment of painful neuromas.[3] Depending on the cause of the pain, management options such as bracing or activity modification/cessation (eg, carpal tunnel syndrome), weight reduction (eg, meralgia paresthetica), steroid injections, or transcutaneous electric nerve stimulation may be indicated. Detailed descriptions of such management options are described elsewhere in this issue. Effectiveness of nonoperative interventions varies widely but successful nonsurgical management is typically preferable to an invasive procedure. Patient selection is paramount to outcome.

Operative

Decompression/neurolysis

Neurolysis can be considered in the case of entrapment or in the case of traumatic or iatrogenic injury causing neuroma-in-continuity. Compressive injuries occur when nerves are subjected to repetitive low-impact forces, leading to structural and functional damage. Points of compression may be static because of entrapment within a rigid fibro-osseous tunnel, or scarring in or apart from a tunnel. Compression may also be caused by dynamic factors, such as within an anatomic narrowing of the nerve from muscular contraction or angulation during positioning. These mechanisms can interrupt microvascular blood flow and lead to ischemia and edema. On a microscopic level, compressive forces can also alter axonal transport, aggravating nerve dysfunction. Freeing the nerve at the point of compression or modification of the environment around the nerve may improve nerve function and decrease pain symptoms.

The technique of decompression is commonly applied to many peripheral nerves, including the median nerve at the carpal tunnel, and the ulnar nerve at the cubital tunnel. Surgical technique involves releasing the compressive structure to free the nerve, or unroofing the nerve from a compressive ligament. Neurolysis in our context refers to external neurolysis (circumferentially). Dissection outside the epineurium is performed to free the nerve from points of compression, strangulation, or tethering in order to mobilize the nerve. Neurolysis for entrapment syndromes is commonly performed for the peroneal nerve at the fibular neck, or the tibial nerve at the tarsal tunnel. It is also performed commonly for neuromas-in-continuity, such as those following injury to a mixed motor and sensory nerve. Neurolysis of a nerve from scar is applied to nerves that have experienced injury and altered signaling caused by focal changes in the environment. Internal neurolysis, or interfascicular dissection, tends to be performed when treating a nerve injury that is affecting a portion of the cross section of the nerve or when removing an intraneural tumor (with preservation of as many fascicles as possible).

The surgical technique of neurolysis involves first obtaining proximal and distal control of the normal nerve by identifying and mobilizing it above and below the site of injury through as generous an incision as is necessary. Next the dissection is performed toward the site of the disorder by carefully releasing the nerve from any exterior scar, points of tethering, or abnormalities in its course; it is thought that altering this environment may improve nerve function. Ensuring a good vascularized bed is important. Vascularized flaps (eg, fat) or tissue coverage may be used to achieve this goal, especially in revision cases. Early active movement after surgery may promote nerve gliding (ie, decrease adhesion formation), which has been associated with more favorable outcomes.

> Case example 1: a 79-year-old right hand–dominant retired mechanic presented after 2 previous carpal tunnel surgeries to the left hand. The diagnosis of recurrent median nerve entrapment at the wrist/palm was confirmed on clinical presentation, including median distribution of weakness, sensory loss, and provocative maneuvers, and on EMG. He had experienced transient (2–3 months) improvement after the first surgery and 5-year symptom relief after a revision surgery. MRI was performed at the time of his second recurrence and showed a flattened nerve with T2 hyperintensity of the nerve in the distal carpal tunnel. At reoperation, the proximal most portion of the transverse carpal ligament appeared to have reconstituted. Scarring was dense proximally and a limited epineurotomy was performed (**Fig. 1**). Although a vascularized fat flap had been considered before surgery, the operative bed seemed favorable so this was not performed. One year later, the patient had complete relief of his pain symptoms with improved 2-point discrimination (>15 mm to 8 mm) and strength in abductor pollicis brevis (Medical Research Council, 0–3/5).
> This case shows that neurolysis occurs at points of both entrapment and of prior scar. Initial carpal tunnel surgery is performed for

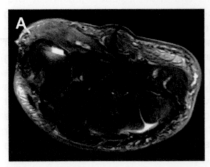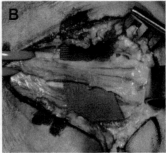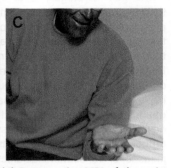

Fig. 1. Multiple revised median nerve decompression at the carpal tunnel. (*A*) Preoperative MRI of the wrist showed the prior scar over the midline palm, compressing the median nerve within the carpal tunnel. (*B*) The median nerve after decompression and neurolysis, showing marked flattening and venous congestion. (*C*) The patient at 1-year follow-up, happy with his outcome: pain relief and improved motor function.

compression, but in revision surgeries it is important to consider that the nerve is now freed both from points of the original spontaneous compression and from reentrapment from scar from the prior surgery. Although the likelihood of success may be lower in reoperations, excellent outcomes are still possible; in these cases, the goal of further surgery is often to improve pain more than function.

As shown in this case, reoperation using a primary nerve-related procedure is generally attempted if the first operation was not done by us, a surgeon known to us, or a peripheral nerve specialist. If such were the case, then we would consider other measures (eg, a secondary procedure, such as stimulation).

Case example 2: a 34-year-old right-handed female police officer presented with a history of medial elbow pain and numbness and tingling into her ulnar 1.5 digits. Her pain initially began after a trauma with a nondisplaced radial head

fracture. After rehabilitation, the symptoms improved, but recurred again approximately 6 months later after an altercation while a person was being apprehended. Examination revealed guarding and tenderness at the medial elbow in the retrocondylar groove, but normal strength and sensation in the limb. Electrophysiologic testing was normal as well. In view of the negative neurologic examination and electrophysiologic testing, her local surgeons did not consider operative intervention; they thought that the persistent symptoms were related to worker's compensation issues. She was referred with a diagnosis of complex regional pain syndrome. We were impressed by the consistent and reproducible percussion tenderness directly over the ulnar nerve and the positive elbow flexion test. Ultrasonography showed a focally swollen nerve at the cubital tunnel, and MRI showed increased T2 signal in the ulnar nerve at the cubital tunnel. Ultrasonography showed a focally swollen nerve at the cubital tunnel (**Fig. 2**). An ultrasonography-guided block with local anesthetic was

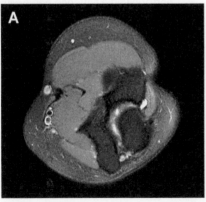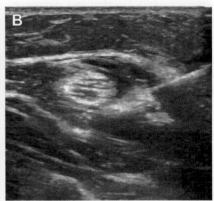

Fig. 2. Preoperative imaging of the ulnar nerve at the cubital tunnel. (*A*) MRI shows focal hyperintensity of the ulnar nerve within the cubital tunnel. (*B*) Ultrasonography shows focal swelling of the nerve within the cubital tunnel.

performed 7 cm above the elbow with temporary complete relief of her symptoms. She underwent ulnar nerve in situ decompression at the elbow (a simple, small approach but an effective option for ulnar neuropathy). She had excellent pain relief and returned to work 8 weeks after surgery. At follow-up 6 months after surgery, she had complete pain relief.

This case shows several interesting points. First, although the examination may not show neurologic loss from a more severe compressive syndrome, she still displayed elements suggesting nerve irritation. The focal findings on her examination correlated with the imaging and supported the notion that operative intervention could play a role. Second, the nerve block had great utility in predicting a favorable response to nerve decompression. We have found imaging (and diagnostic blocks) to be helpful in providing additional information to our armamentarium when evaluating patients with nonclassic conditions, such as EMG-negative entrapment syndromes, in whom surgery is being considered after a failed course of nonoperative treatment.

The link between complex regional pain syndrome and nerve compression is being investigated. Some studies have shown hastened recovery in patients with this diagnosis who also have clinical and electrophysiologic evidence of nerve compression,[4] despite historical arguments against intervention in these patients. Studies like this may help to explain the neurogenic phenomenon in this poorly understood syndrome, and decompression/neurolysis may play a larger role in the future.

Neurectomy

Neurectomy can be considered in patients who have pain in the distribution of purely sensory nerves. In this case, the goal of the surgery is for the patient to exchange painful dysesthesias for hypesthesia (an area of numbness) in the distribution of the nerve. The numbness is permanent but, over 1 year, diminishes to some extent as other overlapping, neighboring nerves fill in at the edges of the territory. The diagnostic block helps predict the zone of the anticipated permanent numbness and allows the patient to experience the feeling in advance; this can be an odd sensation to some. Neurectomy of a sensory nerve, despite being a more permanent step than neurolysis, can be considered as an alternative primary procedure to it or it can be performed after a failed neurolysis or nerve reconstruction. In addition,

repeat neurectomy can also be considered if the original procedure was thought to be suboptimally performed.

Patients with sensory neuropathies in this category typically have experienced focal trauma or iatrogenic nerve injury. Nerves amenable to neurectomy (understanding the trade-off for cutaneous numbness) include such sensory nerves as the saphenous nerve; sural nerve; superficial radial nerve; and most cutaneous nerves of the arm, forearm, thigh, leg and trunk. On rare occasions, neurectomy can be considered for mixed motor nerves; however, the treatment plan must take into account whether or not the function of the nerve can be sacrificed or cannot be reconstructed. Joint denervation can also be done for chronic joint pain by performing neurectomies of articular branches.

Both stump (eg, amputation) neuromas and neuromas-in-continuity may be responsible for pain syndromes, but pain may also be generated from a nerve that does not show visible abnormality. Neuromas form as a tangle of regenerating axons and Schwann cells without an end destination. Primary repair of an injured nerve may be the preferred method to minimize neuroma formation, but this is often not feasible because of traumatic or surgical amputation or in noncritical sensory nerves whereby repair is not considered. Numerous methods have been studied in such scenarios to prevent neuroma formation, including physiologic and mechanical barriers and techniques, such as resection and/or relocation into muscle or bone, without success.[5,6] Therefore neuroma formation is inevitable and the technique involved resection and/or relocation and implantation into muscle or bone to guide axonal growth.

The preferred technique for neurectomy is controversial as well. We prefer to do the surgery under general anesthesia so as to maximize the comfort of the surgery. Others use peripheral nerve blocks as well. Identifying stumps can be challenging, especially given altered planes of dissection from scar. The surgeon must be comfortable finding the nerve in areas in which the nerve may not be typically identified. A lengthier incision may be helpful. Ultrasonography can assist the surgeon in localizing the nerve. Surgery entails sharp transection of the proximal stump, and relocating and implanting it into a muscle, away from a joint. This technique allows the nerve to form a new neuroma deep, away from scar and frequent movement. We do not implant proximal stumps into bone.

Case example 3: a 73-year-old retired woman presented with a 1-year history of left lateral thigh pain with insidious onset after a lumbar surgery for which she was positioned prone. The pain was burning and prickly in nature and extended from the anterior superior iliac spine region laterally to the knee. She was unable to sit for any prolonged period because this exacerbated her pain. She had failed conservative therapy. On examination she had hypersensitivity over the described distribution in the lateral thigh. Percussion medial to the anterior superior iliac spine reproduced her radiating pain. She had normal strength and a preserved knee deep tendon reflex. Diagnostic block was successful (for several hours). She wished to proceed with operative intervention. Neurolysis versus neurectomy was discussed with the patient and, given the risk of recurrence with neurolysis, she elected neurectomy. At the time of surgery, a pseudoneuroma was seen at the site where the nerve exits the inguinal ligament (**Fig. 3**). The ligament was opened partially and the nerve was transected. It was allowed to retract into the pelvis. After surgery she had relief of the dysesthesias and was able to tolerate sitting upright.

In meralgia paresthetica, neurolysis or neurectomy of the lateral femoral cutaneous nerve can be performed, and the literature supports both options[7,8] (perhaps even favoring neurectomy in small series).

Case example 4: a 56-year-old woman presented with debilitating left knee pain following a total knee arthroplasty performed 5 years earlier. She underwent multiple surgical interventions for her pain, including multiple revisions of the knee replacement, a wedge resection of the area of her focal pain, and spinal cord and peripheral nerve stimulation with only transient response. On examination, she had normal neurologic function. There was percussion tenderness in the distal third of the midthigh anteriorly that reproduced her pain. Ultrasonography showed a neuroma corresponding with the point of maximal tenderness. A block with local anesthesia provided her with temporary relief. During surgery, a proximal nerve stump of the anterior femoral cutaneous nerve was identified at the area of percussion tenderness (**Fig. 4**). The neuroma was resected and the stump was resected and implanted into the quadriceps muscle. The nonfunctioning peripheral nerve leads were also removed. At 3-month follow-up, her pain had improved by 80%.

This case shows that a cutaneous nerve was likely transected during her initial surgery, which led to the development of a painful stump neuroma. The type of pain can be difficult to diagnose in this clinical setting to be neurogenic, but careful examination (including percussion tenderness) and appropriate imaging are clues to the diagnosis.

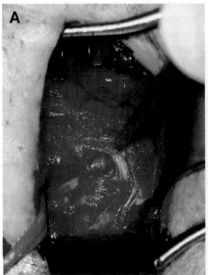
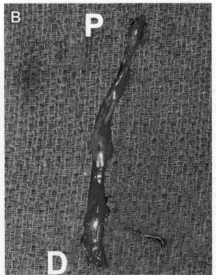

Fig. 3. Intraoperative findings in a patient with meralgia paresthetica. (*A*) The lateral femoral cutaneous nerve in situ, with a visible pseudoneuroma just below the level of the inguinal ligament (seen to the right of the nerve). Such findings can develop in patients with compressive syndromes, particularly with a stiff inguinal ligament. (*B*) The neurectomy specimen, showing focal abnormality thought to be responsible for the patient's symptoms. D, distal; P, proximal.

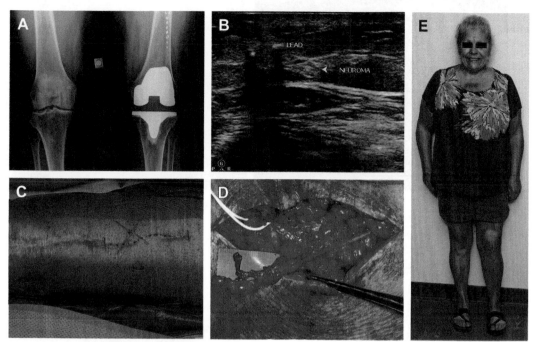

Fig. 4. Painful anterior femoral cutaneous neuroma after total knee arthroplasty. (*A*) Postarthroplasty radiograph with satisfactory positioning of hardware. A lead from the peripheral nerve stimulator is visible superior to the left knee replacement. (*B*) Ultrasonography shows a subcutaneous neuroma (*arrowhead*) of the anterior femoral cutaneous nerve in close proximity to the nerve stimulator lead. (*C*) Preoperative marking of the patient's point of maximal tenderness corresponding with the location of the neuroma. (*D*) The stump neuroma at the location marked in C. (*E*) Clinical photograph 6 months after surgery showing her pain relief.

Case example 5: a 58-year-old woman who had undergone left forequarter amputation for necrotizing fasciitis presented with pain at her previous surgical site. She had a complicated course following her amputation but, once recovered, she developed phantom limb pain controlled by spinal cord stimulation as well as focal pain at an area of nonhealing within the shoulder scar (**Fig. 5**). This localized pain prevented her from wearing her prosthesis. Ultrasonography revealed the neuromas at the proximal stumps of the supraclavicular brachial plexus as well as suture material within neural tissue near the skin. Surgical exploration was performed and neuromas of the upper trunk and its divisions were most prominent. Neuromas extended to the surface of the incision. Foreign body reaction was present at the area of nonhealing. The nerve stumps were recut sharply and a full-thickness bed was created to create a blanket protecting the new nerve stumps in a deeper location. Six months after surgery, her phantom pain was mild at night but readily controllable. The superficial, more problematic pain had resolved completely. She was able to wear her prosthesis without discomfort.

This case shows the importance of stump implantation after neurectomy. In this patient after limb amputation, the stumps had previously remained close to, perhaps even incorporated into, the skin closure. This proximity of the stump neuromas to the skin caused significant hypersensitivity and pain. Although the stumps were reresected, the key to the success of the procedure was to create a vascularized fat flap as a protective layer between the incision and the nerve endings.

Case example 6: a 61-year-old woman with a prior injury to the distal humerus with a known nonunion presented with painful dysesthesias of the posterior forearm. She had been initially treated with open reduction internal fixation (ORIF) and this was revised 6 months later with plate fixation; her hypersensitivity started after the revision surgery. On examination, her hypersensitivity corresponded with the distribution of the posterior cutaneous nerve of the forearm. She underwent total elbow arthroplasty and exploration of the nerve with neurectomy at the same time (**Fig. 6**). She had immediate pain relief in the forearm

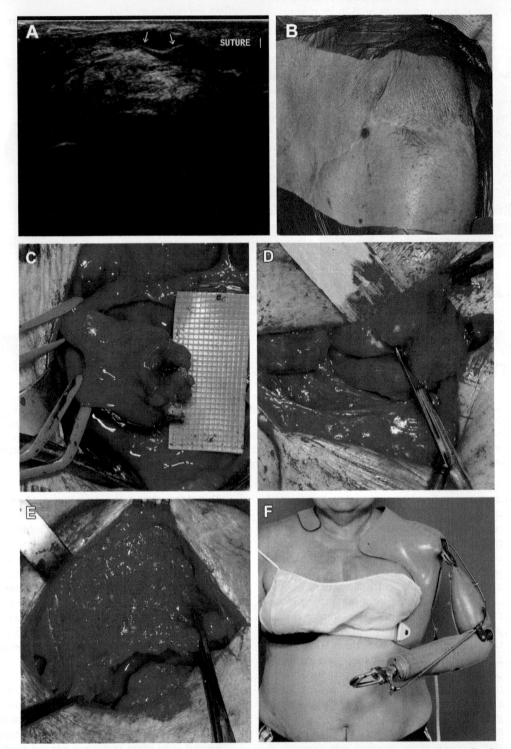

Fig. 5. Painful brachial plexus neuromas after forequarter amputation. (*A*) Preoperative ultrasonography showing the nerve stumps with suture visible (*arrows*). (*B*) Note the area of the nonhealing skin wound at the site of the prior amputation, consistent with the patient's point of maximal tenderness. (*C*) The plexus stump dissected from the skin with a piece of suture visible. (*D*) Neuromas are resected. (*E*) The nerve stumps are covered with a vascularized fat flap for protection. (*F*) The patient wearing her prosthesis 6 months after the stump neurectomy.

(pain was replaced by numbness) that persisted at 6-month follow-up.

Nerves that are not typically affected by compressive syndromes may be injured iatrogenically during surgical procedures. This pain may respond to conservative management, but also may persist or worsen and require intervention.

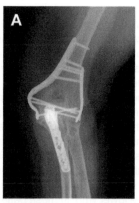
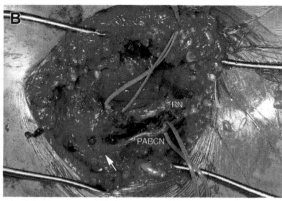

Fig. 6. Posterior antebrachial cutaneous neuroma-in-continuity. (*A*) Preoperative radiograph shows the previous ORIF. (*B*) At operation, distal scarring (*arrow*) of the posterior antebrachial cutaneous nerve (PABCN) was seen. Neurectomy of the PABCN was done. The radial nerve (RN) was neurolysed.

Nerve repair/reconstruction

Nerve repair or reconstruction can be considered in patients with intractable pain from a nerve injury. In certain circumstances, in an injury in which there exists a focal neuroma-in-continuity or when proximal and distal stumps are in close proximity, direct repair can be accomplished. In contrast, with longer gaps, nerve grafts or a biological or synthetic nerve conduit may be used. These techniques can be used to guide or direct neurite growth across the suture line, perhaps decreasing the risk of a patient developing a painful neuroma.

Case example 7: a 57-year-old man who underwent resection of an infected sebaceous cyst from the posterior cervical triangle presented with pain that developed immediately after surgery. The patient became aware of shoulder weakness several weeks after the surgery when he noted the inability to elevate his arm over his head. Examination showed severe trapezius weakness, scapular winging, and decreased shoulder abduction. EMG showed no motor units in the trapezius. He underwent exploration of the prior wound. Proximal and distal stumps of the spinal accessory nerve were identified and repaired primarily after excision of the injured ends (**Fig. 7**). One year after surgery, he had considerable improvement in both pain and function.

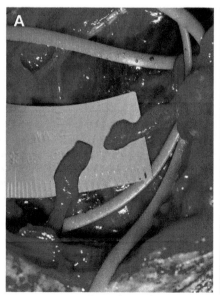
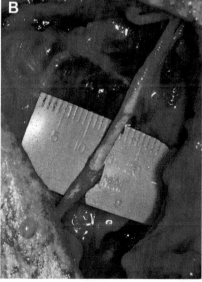

Fig. 7. Iatrogenic spinal accessory nerve transection and repair. (*A*) A grossly transected spinal accessory nerve. The great auricular nerve is also in a blue vasoloop and is used as a landmark. (*B*) Coaptation after resection of injured proximal and distal stumps. The nerve was able to be repaired primarily without tension. One year after surgery the patient had improvement in shoulder abduction and relief of pain.

Although nerve reconstruction is routinely done to restore motor function, it may be used to address pain. In addition to the well-known motor fibers of the spinal accessory nerve, this nerve also contains pain fibers. As shown in this patient, nerve transection with significant pain can improve within a short time after surgery. Reconstruction in cases in which there is nerve transection can be accomplished via direct repair or by grafting. Direct repair is generally preferred if the repair can be performed without tension on the nerve. If that is not able to be accomplished based on the extent of injury, a sensory nerve graft (such as sural nerve) or a nerve conduit can be used to bridge gaps. Care should be taken using a donor nerve in a patient who already has neuropathic pain because there is, anecdotally, increased risk for the patient to develop another site for pain.

In cases of neuroma-in-continuity, if a reasonable time frame for recovery has been reached without improvement, the neuroma can be resected alone or resected with repair of the nerve. As previously discussed, nerve reconstruction typically does not have to be performed in sensory nerves and the neuroma can be resected with implantation of stumps into muscle. However, if nerve repair is chosen, resection of the neuroma should proceed by sequentially sectioning the nerve ends until normal fascicles are visualized on both sides, and primary repair or grafting is performed.

In particular clinical settings, other nerve reconstruction techniques have been described: end-to-side coaptation of a neuroma into a neighboring sensory nerve has been performed with reasonable results,[9] and end-to-end neurorrhaphy of 2 nerves following recurrent neuromas after limb amputation.[10]

Brachial plexus injuries are commonly associated with significant pain. Multiple mechanisms for this pain have been proposed,[11,12] although the pain is neuropathic. Postganglionic pain often responds to resection of the ruptures or neuromas-in-continuity and grafting techniques. In contrast, preganglionic pain may respond to DREZ lesions (see the article elsewhere in this issue). Limb amputation does not improve pain from root avulsions.

CLINICAL OUTCOMES
Decompression

Results from simple decompression are beneficial overall, and usually excellent in patients with common nerve compression syndromes. In carpal tunnel decompression, pain relief occurs in 87% of patients.[13] Meta-analyses of ulnar decompression at the elbow cite clinical improvement rates of approximately 70%.[14] With regard to entrapment of the lateral femoral cutaneous nerve, success rates with decompression are as high as 88% in meta-analyses.[7] Less common entrapments have fewer outcome studies available to support intervention, although success rates are generally good if the history, clinical, radiologic, and electrophysiologic studies support the diagnosis. Although controversial, recent evidence has shown benefit for pain control in selected patients with diabetic neuropathy in the lower limb; in these patients decompression of several tunnels (tarsal and plantar tunnels, fibular tunnel, deep peroneal nerve on dorsal foot) may be done singly or in combination.

Neurectomy

Neurectomy is patient and case specific and therefore large studies are generally readily available. Published case series have variable results.[15,16] In the case of meralgia paresthetica, neurectomy has been reported to have a 94% rate of improvement.[7] For painful neuromas good/excellent outcomes are between 64% and 75% with traditional resection and reimplantation techniques.[17–20] Overall, results decrease with careful long-term follow-up.

Nerve Repair/Reconstruction

Long-term outcome of nerve repair generally focuses on motor recovery, and therefore it is difficult to quantify pain improvement. More research is needed in pain relief with reconstruction procedures and novel neurorrhaphy procedures.

COMPLICATIONS AND CONCERNS

The most common complication relates to failed surgery. Inappropriate patient selection may account for treatment failure, which shows the need for detailed preoperative evaluation. A lengthy discussion of outcomes and expectations should therefore take place. Patients with chronic pain often require multidisciplinary treatment. In straightforward cases, simple decompression or neurolysis can make a significant impact on quality of life. However, the risk of failing to improve or worsening symptoms should be explained before surgery, given that complex pain syndromes may lead to a cycle of worsening symptoms after any sort of intervention. If pain is not improved after the initial surgery, it is unlikely that subsequent surgeries will be successful, and further attempts may have diminishing returns.[21]

In cases in which sensory loss occurs (as in neurectomy), patients must be instructed to be conscientious about care of these areas, inspecting them frequently for any evidence of unnoticed injury.

Recurrent neuromas after neurectomy are unavoidable; the goal is to prevent the formation of painful neuromas. Therefore, careful implantation of the nerve stumps to allow them to be seated in a deep plane gives a layer of protection.

Early dysesthetic neuropathic pain is common in patients who undergo neurolysis or neurectomy in the immediate postoperative period, which typically but not always resolves over several days to weeks. Desensitization strategies may be useful in these cases.

SUMMARY

Peripheral nerve pain from a postganglionic source can be a complex issue for the neurosurgeon. Our suggested algorithm progresses from least invasive to most invasive therapy.

- Nonoperative measures: physical therapy, pharmacotherapy, and so forth.
- Operative interventions:
  1. Primary nerve–relative procedures: neurolysis, neurectomy (simple ablative), and nerve repair/reconstruction.
  2. Secondary procedures: stimulation (CNS/PNS).

REFERENCES

1. Torrance N, Smith BH, Bennett MI, et al. The epidemiology of chronic pain of predominantly neuropathic origin. Results from a general population survey. J Pain 2006;7(4):281–9.
2. Bouhassira D, Lanteri-Minet M, Attal N, et al. Prevalence of chronic pain with neuropathic characteristics in the general population. Pain 2008;136(3):380–7.
3. Whipple RR, Unsell RS. Treatment of painful neuromas. Orthop Clin North Am 1988;19(1):175–85.
4. Placzek JD, Boyer MI, Gelberman RH, et al. Nerve decompression for complex regional pain syndrome type II following upper extremity surgery. J Hand Surg Am 2005;30(1):69–74.
5. Mathews GJ, Osterholm JL. Painful traumatic neuromas. Surg Clin North Am 1972;52(5):1313–24.
6. Burchiel KJ, Ochoa JL. Surgical management of posttraumatic neuropathic pain. Neurosurg Clin N Am 1991;2(1):117–26.
7. Khalil N, Nicotra A, Rakowicz W. Treatment for meralgia paraesthetica. Cochrane Database Syst Rev 2012;(12):CD004159.
8. de Ruiter GC, Wurzer JA, Kloet A. Decision making in the surgical treatment of meralgia paresthetica: neurolysis versus neurectomy. Acta Neurochir (Wien) 2012;154(10):1765–72.
9. Aszmann OC, Moser V, Frey M. Treatment of painful neuromas via end-to-side neurorraphy. Handchir Mikrochir Plast Chir 2010;42(4):225–32 [in German].
10. Barbera J, Albert-Pamplo R. Centrocentral anastomosis of the proximal nerve stump in the treatment of painful amputation neuromas of major nerves. J Neurosurg 1993;79(3):331–4.
11. Bertelli JA, Ghizoni MF. The possible role of regenerating axons in pain persistence after brachial plexus grafting. Microsurgery 2010;30(7):532–6.
12. Bertelli JA, Ghizoni MF. Pain after avulsion injuries and complete palsy of the brachial plexus: the possible role of nonavulsed roots in pain generation. Neurosurgery 2008;62(5):1104–13 [discussion: 1113–4].
13. Spinner R. Median nerve. In: Kim D, Midha R, Murovic JA, et al, editors. Kline and Hudson's nerve injuries. 2nd edition. Philadelphia: WB Saunders; 2008. p. 139.
14. Caliandro P, La Torre G, Padua R, et al. Treatment for ulnar neuropathy at the elbow. Cochrane Database Syst Rev 2012;(7):CD006839.
15. Nikolajsen L, Black JA, Kroner K, et al. Neuroma removal for neuropathic pain: efficacy and predictive value of lidocaine infusion. Clin J Pain 2010;26(9):788–93.
16. Guse DM, Moran SL. Outcomes of the surgical treatment of peripheral neuromas of the hand and forearm: a 25-year comparative outcome study. Ann Plast Surg 2013;71(6):654–8.
17. Novak CB, van Vliet D, Mackinnon SE. Subjective outcome following surgical management of lower-extremity neuromas. J Reconstr Microsurg 1995;11(3):175–7.
18. Novak CB, van Vliet D, Mackinnon SE. Subjective outcome following surgical management of upper extremity neuromas. J Hand Surg Am 1995;20(2):221–6.
19. Sood MK, Elliot D. Treatment of painful neuromas of the hand and wrist by relocation into the pronator quadratus muscle. J Hand Surg 1998;23(2):214–9.
20. Herbert TJ, Filan SL. Vein implantation for treatment of painful cutaneous neuromas. A preliminary report. J Hand Surg 1998;23(2):220–4.
21. Vernadakis AJ, Koch H, Mackinnon SE. Management of neuromas. Clin Plast Surg 2003;30(2):247–68, vii.

Peripheral Nerve/Field Stimulation for Chronic Pain

Erika A. Petersen, MD[a], Konstantin V. Slavin, MD[b],*

KEYWORDS

- Peripheral nerve stimulation • Peripheral nerve field stimulation • Neuropathic pain
- Neuromodulation

KEY POINTS

- Peripheral nerve stimulation (PNS) offers a reversible, adjustable, and testable means of treating focal neuropathic pain.
- Peripheral nerve field stimulation (PNfS) provides a similar treatment of painful areas that may involve fine branches of terminal nerves.
- The number of clinical conditions that may benefit from PNS or PNfS continues to increase.
- Studies are ongoing to develop further evidence in support of PNS and PNfS.

INTRODUCTION: NATURE OF THE PROBLEM

Patients with refractory severe chronic, focal neuropathic pain (eg, posttraumatic neuropathy, complex regional pain syndromes, postherpetic neuralgia affecting 1 or 2 dermatomes) may benefit from peripheral nerve stimulation (PNS), a low morbidity treatment modality for patients who have failed medical management. PNS involves the placement of a stimulating electrode over a named peripheral nerve (eg, occipital, genitofemoral) to elicit paresthesias along the innervated territory. This technique was first described in 1966 by Wall and Sweet[1] and then used in selected centers worldwide, but it did not gain traction as a treatment option until the description by Weiner and Reed[2] of a percutaneous PNS technique in 1999 when it was used in a series of patients with occipital neuralgia. The lower invasiveness (as compared with an open exploration of the nerve and direct application of an electrode) resulted in an easier trial for patients. This percutaneous technique led to an expansion of the number of physicians offering the procedure beyond surgeons (neurosurgeons, orthopedic surgeons, and plastic surgeons) to include anesthesiologists and other pain management specialists. The introduction of an ultrasound-guided technique further advanced the accessibility of the procedure, translating the common use of ultrasound localization for regional anesthesia to electrode placement technique.[3] PNS has been applied to various named nerves throughout the body, including occipital, supraorbital, infraorbital, radial, ulnar, median, tibial, peroneal, and sciatic nerves.

Peripheral nerve field stimulation (PNfS), sometimes referred to as subcutaneous neurostimulation or targeted subcutaneous stimulation,[4] involves positioning of one or more electrodes within the region of maximal pain, where small distal branches of nerves are targeted within the subcutaneous space. Field stimulation produces

[a] Department of Neurosurgery, University of Arkansas for Medical Sciences, 4301 West Markham, Slot 507, Little Rock, AR 72205, USA; [b] Department of Neurosurgery, University of Illinois at Chicago, M/C 799, 912 South Wood Street, Chicago, IL 60612, USA
* Corresponding author.
E-mail address: kslavin@uic.edu

Neurosurg Clin N Am 25 (2014) 789–797
http://dx.doi.org/10.1016/j.nec.2014.07.003
1042-3680/14/$ – see front matter © 2014 Elsevier Inc. All rights reserved.

paresthesias along a diffuse painful area that may not correlate with one specific dermatome or otherwise be well defined. Body regions rather than nerves are used to describe the PNfS (eg, low back, trunk, joint).

The use of spinal cord stimulation (SCS) combined with PNfS has been referred to as "hybrid" stimulation,[5] spinal-peripheral neurostimulation,[6] and triangular stimulation.[7] This technique has been shown to achieve broader coverage of axial back pain than either SCS or PNfS individually.[8]

INDICATIONS

Many of the conditions addressed by PNS also respond with other neuromodulation techniques, including spinal cord stimulation. However, because of the relatively simple nature of the procedure and its low invasiveness, PNS and/or PNfS may be preferable to more central neuromodulatory procedures. It should be noted that the devices used for PNS or PNfS are those approved for other interventions, such as spinal cord stimulation, and are used "off-label" in the United States, although in many other countries both PNS and PNfS are among approved uses for these devices. Current indications for PNS/PNfS include the following:

- Neuropathic pain disorders
  - Posttraumatic neuralgia
  - Postsurgical neuropathic pain
  - Occipital neuralgia or cervicogenic occipital pain
  - Postherniorrhaphy inguinal neuralgia
  - Genitofemoral neuralgia
  - Postherpetic neuralgia
  - Coccygodynia
- Complex regional pain syndrome, especially type II
- Cephalgias
  - Migraine, both chronic and transformed
  - Hemicrania continua
  - Cluster headaches
  - Chronic daily headaches
  - Cervicogenic and occipital headaches
- Axial pain syndromes
- Emerging indications
  - Musculoskeletal pain
  - Fibromyalgia

SURGICAL TECHNIQUE

PNS can be performed using either an open or a percutaneous technique. In most cases, fluoroscopy is being used to guide electrodes in relation to bony landmarks. Because fluoroscopy does not visualize the nerves and vessels, other means of image guidance, such as ultrasound, may be a useful adjunct to ensure optimal electrode positioning and help to avoid nearby vessels.[9] In PNfS, a careful identification of the region of pain guides placement of the electrodes. Marking the region based on the patient report before electrode placement facilitates the optimal position at the site of maximal pain and also serves as an avenue to discuss pain improvement expectations for the procedure. The optimal number and type of leads to use vary based on location and dimensions of painful area.

A choice of cylindrical electrodes and paddles is available to the implanting surgeon. Cylindrical leads are conducive to placement through a percutaneous approach. Narrow paddle electrodes may also be introduced percutaneously as anatomy allows. An open approach permits the direct application of either a cylindrical or a paddle electrode along the target nerve. Because the open approach may be associated with a higher risk of perineural fibrosis, it is performed less frequently.[10]

Preoperative Planning

Patients may experience suboptimal results from PNS if the therapy is used in a pain syndrome that has low likelihood of response. A thorough history and physical examination including a detailed pain history should confirm the patient's diagnosis and prior treatments attempted and their outcomes. A scale of disability such as the Pain Disability Index[11] can assess the degree to which the patient's quality of life is affected. The distribution of the pain should be clearly defined.

Inclusion criteria

- Patients should have chronic, severe, disabling neuropathic pain refractory to other treatments, including medications, nerve blocks, trigger point injections, physical therapy, and so on.
- Sensory aberrations or loss in the distribution of pain may increase the chances of a trial failure.
- Local anesthetic block may confirm which nerve is affected, but is not predictive of PNS success.
- Similarly, transcutaneous electrical nerve stimulation (TENS) use may suggest a region amenable to PNfS, but TENS does not have a clear predictive value.[12]
- Focal areas within the territory of a single peripheral nerve are most amenable to PNS,

whereas larger and irregular regions may be treated with PNfS.

- Disorder-specific selection criteria may also be relevant.

Exclusion criteria

- Patients with active infectious processes or severely immunocompromised
- Patients taking anticoagulant medications that cannot be stopped for the perioperative period, or those with bleeding disorders
- Cognitive impairment that limits the patient's ability to use the device effectively or to cooperate with lead placement
- Patients with untreated psychiatric disease (including depression anxiety and personality disorders)
- Malingering
- Patients with larger areas of pain that may not be covered using a reasonable number of implanted electrodes may still be considered candidates for SCS or other neuromodulatory alternatives.

Neuropsychological evaluation

A pretrial psychological screening is recommended to identify any psychosocial issues that may adversely impact the therapy. This screening may include cognitive impairment or dementia, substance abuse, untreated anxiety or depression, or unrealistic expectations related to the stimulator.[13]

Trial stimulator

The trial involves placement of electrode leads along the target nerve or region. The leads are externalized, and the patient tests the stimulation for a time period ranging from 2 to 14 days. The surgical technique for the placement of the trial and permanent electrode leads is similar but while trial leads are usually sutured to the skin at the site of their exit, permanent leads are sutured to the fascia.

Preparation and Patient Positioning

- May be performed with conscious sedation, which keeps patients comfortable while the electrodes are being placed, but also permits for intraoperative testing of the positioned electrode
- Expose the entire neuropathic area to allow direct access
- Use of fluoroscopy and/or ultrasound to confirm electrode location
- Perioperative antibiotics

Surgical Approach

- The patient is positioned with optimal access to the target area. Positioning should also take into consideration optimal fluoroscopic images of the target site.
- Standard surgical preparation and draping are performed with the entire planned path of the electrode visible in the field.

Surgical Procedure for Percutaneous Lead Placement

Step 1: Skin is infiltrated with local anesthetic at the entry point and then a small entry incision is made (**Fig. 1**).

Step 2: A Tuohy needle is advanced in the subcutaneous space overlying the nerve. The trajectory of the needle may be in parallel to the target nerve or at an angle to it. PNfS electrodes may be arranged in various ways to achieve best coverage for the entire area of pain.

Step 3: The inner stylet of the Tuohy needle is withdrawn, and a guidewire is advanced. Fluoroscopic images are obtained to follow the guidewire's trajectory.

Step 4: The Tuohy needle is withdrawn, and a plastic cannula is advanced over the guidewire.

Step 5: The guidewire is withdrawn.

Step 6: The electrode lead is threaded through the cannula and its position is confirmed. The cannula is withdrawn.

Step 7: The electrode lead is connected to a temporary testing cable. The patient's sedation is lightened to enable testing. The patient reports the paresthesias perceived. The optimal stimulation coverage can be ascertained by changing the combination of anode and cathode contacts and varying amplitude, frequency, and pulse width. If these alterations do not result in optimal coverage of the target area, then the electrode lead can be repositioned.

Step 8: Once optimal electrode position is confirmed, the electrode is secured at the entry site with a single stitch. The site is further dressed with a sterile occlusive dressing. The externalized trial electrode is connected to the trial stimulator system. Further programming of the stimulator is performed postoperatively. Fluoroscopic images or plain radiographs should be obtained to document final electrode position.

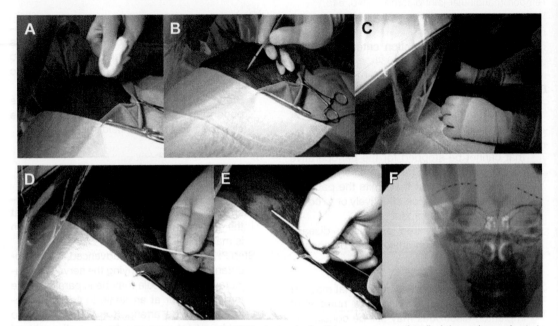

Fig. 1. Surgical steps for the introduction of a PNS electrode (in this case, supraorbital). (*A*) Local anesthetic infiltrated at the entry point at the purple mark. (*B*) A small "stab" incision is made at the entry point. (*C*) Tuohy needle is advanced. (*D*) After the guidewire is advanced, the plastic cannula is introduced. (*E*) The lead is threaded into position through the plastic cannula. (*F*) Fluoroscopic image shows lead position.

Step 9: These steps are repeated for each additional electrode planned. For most PNSs, 1 or 2 electrodes are used. For PNfS, multiple electrodes may be needed to provide adequate coverage.

Operative Tricks and Tips

Incisions and lead positioning depend on the indication and the target region:

- Face: incisions are usually behind the hairline. Leads should not be too close to the orbit to avoid twitching
- Axial: electrodes are used to "frame" the pain area with the goal of maximizing coverage
- Extremity: the electrodes should cross as few joints as possible to minimize fracture and migration risk. Anchoring is essential in high-mobility areas
- Ilioinguinal: using ultrasound improves positioning of the electrode along the nerve

Careful attention should be paid to electrode depth; if too superficial, there is high erosion risk, and if too deep, stimulation provokes muscle contraction and poor paresthesias.

Immediate Postoperative Care

- Trial period of 2 to 14 days. Patients are asked to go about their daily routine to test the PNS system's effectiveness. Periodic adjustment of the stimulator settings may be required to attain optimal relief.
- Patients should keep the externalized cables clean and dry, which may necessitate sponge bathing instead of showering.
- Patients should refrain from sudden and strenuous movements that might cause the lead to dislodge.
- Although there is scarce evidence to support the practice, some surgeons prescribe a regimen of oral antibiotics for the duration of the outpatient stimulation trial.
- A trial may be considered successful if a patient experiences more than 50% improvement in pain severity. Furthermore, the patient should express satisfaction with the quality and degree of pain relief.
- Patients with a failed trial should not proceed to permanent system implantation.

Permanent stimulator

The steps for implantation of the permanent system are similar. Most often, this procedure is performed under general anesthesia using fluoroscopy to ensure that lead placement is identical to the trial leads. General anesthesia permits better patient comfort, especially during tunneling of the cables to the generator site. Preparation and positioning are similar, with careful attention to accessing the generator site and the ability to tunnel the leads between electrode site and generator pocket.

Surgical Approach

- The patient is positioned with optimal access to the target area. Positioning should be performed to allow optimal fluoroscopic images of the target site and to facilitate tunneling to the generator pocket.
- Standard surgical preparation and draping are performed with the entire planned path of the electrode visible in the field.

Surgical Procedure for Percutaneous Lead Placement

Steps 1 through 6: identical to the trial procedure.

Step 7: The electrode is anchored to the fascia. This step can be performed using a nonabsorbable stitch or with commercially available anchors. A strain-relief loop (**Fig. 2**) can minimize risk of lead migration or fracture due to device kinking.

Step 8: The subcutaneous pocket is prepared for the implantable pulse generator (IPG). Gluteal, abdominal, axillary, and infraclavicular sites may be considered depending on their proximity to the lead site.

Step 9: The leads are tunneled from the anchor site to the IPG pocket. Depending on the course, extension cables may be required. The leads are connected to the IPG (**Figs. 3** and **4**).

Step 10: An impedance check is performed on the system to assess technical function of the system.

Step 11: Antibiotic irrigation is performed at the incision sites, and then the incisions are closed and dressed.

Immediate Postoperative Care

- Most PNS implants are performed as outpatient procedures. Patients are discharged home from the recovery room.
- Periodic adjustment of the stimulator settings may be required to attain optimal relief. Patients may be given some degree of control over the device depending on their level of comfort interacting with the technology.
- Patients are reminded to refrain from strenuous and vigorous activities for several weeks after PNS system implantation to allow the tissue to heal and to minimize the risk of lead migration.

REHABILITATION AND RECOVERY

- For most patients, the benefit of PNS is immediate. Patients may be able to wean off their medications if pain relief from stimulation is sufficient. A gradual taper of medications in

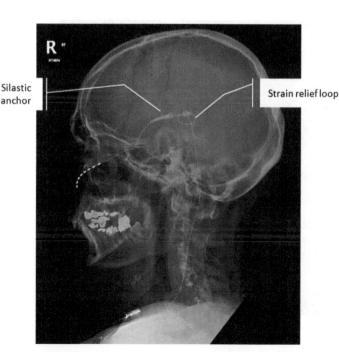

Fig. 2. Lateral radiograph shows the course of an infraorbital PNS electrode. Note the radio-opaque anchor device and the strain relief loop.

Silastic anchor

Strain relief loop

R

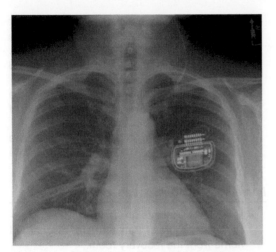

Fig. 3. Anteroposterior radiograph shows the course of the lead down to the IPG in the generator pocket.

coordination with the patient's prescribing physicians is recommended.

- Patients may benefit from periodic adjustments of the device's stimulation settings. These "tune-ups" may provide improved pain relief or eliminate extraneous paresthesias.
- Should the patient notice a change in the quality of stimulation or in the degree of pain relief, interrogation of the system should be

performed. If there are no electrical faults, then adjustment of the stimulation parameters may reestablish adequate function. In some cases, a "holiday" period in which the stimulator is turned off can lead to a resumption of effective stimulation when the device is reactivated.

- The most common complications include infection, lead erosion, migration of the lead, or mechanical issues with the device (**Table 1**). Pain at the site of the generator or lead site occurs in some patients. Neural injury is relatively rare. Patients should be counseled on these risks and of the warning signs that should lead them to seek immediate assistance.
- Most of the electrodes, extensions, and IPGs used in PNS are not magnetic resonance imaging (MRI) compatible, and lead heating, device damage, or unintentional stimulation may occur. Medtronic (Minneapolis, MN, USA) manufactures spinal cord stimulation electrodes and generators that are conditionally safe for MRI scanning,[14] and Boston Scientific (Natick, MA, USA) has a Conformité Européenne (CE) mark approval for head-only imaging in Europe.[15] However, these devices have not been assessed for MRI safety if implanted outside the spinal canal (ie, off-label PNS/PNfS applications). Device manufacturers provide up-to-date information on MRI

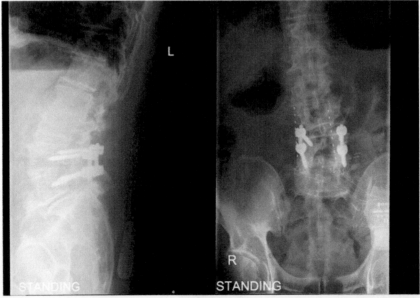

Fig. 4. Lateral and anteroposterior radiographs show the position of 2 PNfS electrodes to address low back pain.

Table 1
Common complications in PNS and PNfS

	PNfS	PNS
Infection	4.4%[40]	3.6%–17.9%[39]
Erosion	2.2%[40]	4.5%[26]–50%[37]
Migration	15.6%[40]	9%[38]–25%[39]
Mechanical failure (fracture, short circuit, etc)	11%[26]	3.6%[39]
Lack of efficacy	4.7%[12]–17%[40]	21%[39]

Data from Refs.[10,36–40]

Table 3
Prospective trials of PNS for migraine

Author		N	Result
Saper et al,[41] 2011	ONSTIM	66	39% responder rate to adjustable ONS
Lipton et al,[42] 2009	PRISM	132	No statistically significant reduction in headache days with ONS vs sham
Silberstein et al,[43] 2012		157	Reduction in headache days and MIDAS score with ONS

safety that can be accessed by patients, MRI technicians, and physicians.

CLINICAL RESULTS IN THE LITERATURE

Despite the longevity of the therapy, few well-designed prospective studies of PNS and PNfS exist. A handful of prospective multicenter controlled studies of PNfS and PNS have been completed (**Tables 2** and **3**). One of the challenges in controlled trials is the lack of blinding, because active stimulation is always associated with paresthesias. In some study designs, low-amplitude and high-amplitude stimulation substituted for the usual sham and active groups to address this limitation.[16] Nevertheless, most published experience is in the form of single-center retrospective series[17–34] and case reports.[35]

Table 2
Prospective trials of PNfS for chronic back pain

Condition/ Series	N	Result
Mironer et al,[8] 2011	40	79% of patients opted for combined SCS and PNfS during externalized trial; >90% experienced successful trials
McRoberts et al,[40] 2013	44	75% of patients experienced successful trials; VAS score and patient pain reports remained stable in 69% of patients at 1 y
Kloimstein et al,[12] 2014	118	Up to 75% of patients have maintained relief at 6 mo

SUMMARY

PNS and PNfS are effective techniques for the management of chronic neuropathic pain disorders and other pain syndromes. The success of the therapy hinges on appropriate candidate selection and optimal placement of the leads for most effective stimulation. Although PNS and PNfS carry lower risk of complications than other neuromodulation procedures, infection, lead erosion, and mechanical issues with the device are possible. Patients with suboptimal outcomes may have unrealistic expectations for the device. An ongoing dialogue between the implanting surgeon and the patient about the risks and benefits and their expectations for pain relief should be part of the patient preparation process. Improvements are expected in pain relief and device-related comfort for patients as new devices are developed.

REFERENCES

1. Wall PD, Sweet WH. Temporary abolition of pain in man. Science 1967;155:108–9.
2. Weiner RL, Reed KL. Peripheral neurostimulation for control of intractable occipital neuralgia. Neuromodulation 1999;2:217–21.
3. Huntoon MA, Burgher AH. Ultrasound-guided permanent implantation of peripheral nerve stimulation (PNS) system for neuropathic pain of the extremities: original cases and outcomes. Pain Med 2009;10: 1369–77.
4. Levy RM. Differentiating the leaves from the branches in the tree of neuromodulation: the state of peripheral nerve field stimulation. Neuromodulation 2011;14:201–5.
5. Lipov EG. 'Hybrid neurostimulator': simultaneous use of spinal cord and peripheral nerve field

stimulation to treat low back and leg pain. Prog Neurol Surg 2011;24:147–55.

6. Mironer YE, Monroe TR. Spinal-peripheral neurostimulation (SPN) for bilateral posthernorraphy pain: a case report. Neuromodulation 2013;16:603–6.

7. Navarro RM, Vercimak DC. Triangular stimulation method utilizing combination spinal cord stimulation with peripheral subcutaneous field stimulation for chronic pain patients: a retrospective study. Neuromodulation 2012;15:124–31.

8. Mironer YE, Hutcheson JK, Satterthwaite JR, et al. Prospective, two-part study of the interaction between spinal cord stimulation and peripheral nerve field stimulation in patients with low back pain: development of a new spinal-peripheral neurostimulation method. Neuromodulation 2011;14:151–5.

9. Chan I, Brown AR, Park K, et al. Ultrasound-guided, percutaneous peripheral nerve stimulation: technical note. Neurosurgery 2010;67(3 Suppl Operative): ons136–9.

10. Slavin KV. Technical aspects of peripheral nerve stimulation: hardware and complications. Prog Neurol Surg 2011;24:189–202.

11. Tait RC, Pollard CA, Margolis RB, et al. The pain disability index: psychometric and validity data. Arch Phys Med Rehabil 1987;68:438–41.

12. Kloimstein H, Likar R, Kern M, et al. Peripheral nerve field stimulation (PNFS) in chronic low back pain: a prospective multicenter study. Neuromodulation 2014;17:180–7.

13. Campbell CM, Jamison RN, Edwards RR. Psychological screening/phenotyping as predictors for spinal cord stimulation. Curr Pain Headache Rep 2013; 17:307.

14. Available at: https://professional.medtronic.com/wcm/groups/mdtcom_sg/@mdt/@neuro/documents/documents/scs-mri-guidelines-us.pdf. Accessed April 29, 2014.

15. Available at: http://news.bostonscientific.com/index.php?s=24889&item=132247. Accessed April 29, 2014.

16. Wilbrink LA, Teernstra OP, Haan J, et al. Occipital nerve stimulation in medically intractable, chronic cluster headache. The ICON study: rationale and protocol of a randomised trial. Cephalalgia 2013; 33:1238–47.

17. Al-Jehani H, Jacques L. Peripheral nerve stimulation for chronic neurogenic pain. Prog Neurol Surg 2011; 24:27–40.

18. McRoberts WP, Roche M. Novel approach for peripheral subcutaneous field stimulation for the treatment of severe, chronic knee joint pain after total knee arthroplasty. Neuromodulation 2010;13: 131–6.

19. Paicius RM, Bernstein CA, Lempert-Cohen C. Peripheral nerve field stimulation in chronic abdominal pain. Pain Physician 2006;9:261–6.

20. Cairns KD, McRoberts WP, Deer T. Peripheral nerve stimulation for the treatment of truncal pain. Prog Neurol Surg 2011;24:58–69.

21. Hegarty D, Goroszeniuk T. Peripheral nerve stimulation of the thoracic paravertebral plexus for chronic neuropathic pain. Pain Physician 2011;14: 295–300.

22. Burgher AH, Huntoon MA, Turley TW, et al. Subcutaneous peripheral nerve stimulation with inter-lead stimulation for axial neck and low back pain: case series and review of the literature. Neuromodulation 2012;15:100–7.

23. Yakovlev AE, Resch BE. Treatment of chronic intractable hip pain after iliac crest bone graft harvest using peripheral nerve field stimulation. Neuromodulation 2011;14:156–9.

24. Patil AA, Otto D, Raikar S. Peripheral nerve field stimulation for sacroiliac joint pain. Neuromodulation 2014;17:98–101.

25. Ellens DJ, Levy RM. Peripheral neuromodulation for migraine headache. Prog Neurol Surg 2011;24: 109–17.

26. Slavin KV, Colpan ME, Munawar N, et al. Trigeminal and occipital peripheral nerve stimulation for craniofacial pain: a single-institution experience and review of the literature. Neurosurg Focus 2006;21(6):E5.

27. Krutsch JP, McCeney MH, Barolat G, et al. A case report of subcutaneous peripheral nerve stimulation for the treatment of axial back pain associated with postlaminectomy syndrome. Neuromodulation 2008; 11:112–5.

28. Stidd DA, Wuollet AL, Bowden K, et al. Peripheral nerve stimulation for trigeminal neuropathic pain. Pain Physician 2012;15:27–33.

29. Perini F, De Boni A. Peripheral neuromodulation in chronic migraine. Neurol Sci 2012;33(Suppl 1): S29–31.

30. Mammis A, Gudesblatt M, Mogilner AY. Peripheral neurostimulation for the treatment of refractory cluster headache, long-term follow-up: case report. Neuromodulation 2011;14:432–5.

31. Plazier M, Vanneste S, Dekelver I, et al. Peripheral nerve stimulation for fibromyalgia. Prog Neurol Surg 2011;24:133–46.

32. Al Tamimi M, Davids HR, Barolat G, et al. Subcutaneous peripheral nerve stimulation treatment for chronic pelvic pain. Neuromodulation 2008;11:277–81.

33. Sator-Katzenschlager S, Fiala K, Kress HG, et al. Subcutaneous target stimulation (STS) in chronic noncancer pain: a nationwide retrospective study. Pain Pract 2010;10:279–86.

34. Desai M, Jacob L, Leiphart J. Successful peripheral nerve field stimulation for thoracic radiculitis following Brown-Sequard syndrome. Neuromodulation 2011; 14:249–52.

35. Goroszeniuk T, Pang D. Peripheral neuromodulation: a review. Curr Pain Headache Rep 2014;18:412.

36. Mobbs RJ, Nair S, Blum P. Peripheral nerve stimulation for the treatment of chronic pain. J Clin Neurosci 2007;14:216–23.

37. Verrills P, Rose R, Mitchell B, et al. Peripheral nerve field stimulation for chronic headache: 60 cases and long-term follow-up. Neuromodulation 2014;17:54–9.

38. Melvin EA Jr, Jordan FR, Weiner RL, et al. Using peripheral stimulation to reduce the pain of C2-mediated occipital headaches: a preliminary report. Pain Physician 2007;10:453–60.

39. Falowski S, Wang D, Sabesan A, et al. Occipital nerve stimulator systems: review of complications and surgical techniques. Neuromodulation 2010; 13:121–5.

40. McRoberts WP, Wolkowitz R, Meyer DJ, et al. Peripheral nerve field stimulation for the management of localized chronic intractable back pain: results from a randomized controlled study. Neuromodulation 2013;16:565–75.

41. Saper JR, Dodick DW, Silberstein SD, et al, ONSTIM Investigators. Occipital nerve stimulation for the treatment of intractable chronic migraine headache: ONSTIM feasibility study. Cephalalgia 2011;31:271–85.

42. Lipton RB, Goadsby PJ, Cady RK, et al. PRISM study: occipital nerve stimulation for treatment-refractory migraine [abstract PO47]. Cephalalgia 2009;29(1 Suppl 1):30.

43. Silberstein SD, Dodick DW, Saper J, et al. Safety and efficacy of peripheral nerve stimulation of the occipital nerves for the management of chronic migraine: results from a randomised, multi-center, double blinded, control study. Cephalalgia 2012;32:1165–79.

Chronic Pain Rehabilitation

Manu Mathews, MD*, Sara Davin, PhD

KEYWORDS

- Chronic pain • Interdisciplinary pain rehabilitation • Multidisciplinary • Rehabilitation

KEY POINTS

- Pain is a multidimensional experience that has an impact on a person's ability to function.
- Functional restoration is the cornerstone of a good chronic pain management strategy.
- Interdisciplinary treatment has been well established in the literature as the most effective approach, with improvements in pain, mood, and function.
- Opioid discontinuation undertaken as a part of an interdisciplinary treatment approach often leads to improvement in pain mood and function.

INTRODUCTION

Pain is a multidimensional experience that often expresses itself as reduced quality of life and functional ability. The biopsychosocial model of the assessment and management is increasingly considered to be the best model. Interdisciplinary pain rehabilitation programs have been shown to be very effective in improving pain mood and function in patients with chronic pain.[1] A meta-analysis of 65 studies of multidisciplinary pain rehabilitation showed significant improvement in function.[2] Another study of 27 randomized controlled trials (RCTs) demonstrated greater effectiveness of this approach compared with no treatment, standard treatments, or nonmultidisciplinary treatment.[3]

This improvement has been shown to persist for up to 13 years.[4]

Although these programs are more resource intensive initially, interdisciplinary pain rehabilitation programs (IPRPs) have been shown to be effective in reducing the use of pharmacologic treatment, surgeries, implantable pain devices, and physical therapy. Among all pain-related treatments, this is the only approach that has consistently been shown to be associated with return to work, reduction in hospitalizations over a 10-year period, and meaningful, sustained improvement in pain and function.

This article will discuss the approach and principles of chronic pain rehabilitation in an inter- or multidisciplinary environment. It will also highlight the common practices across some of the chronic pain rehabilitation programs in the United States.

COMPONENTS OF IPRPs

There is no consensus about what constitutes IPRPs. The terms interdisciplinary and multidisciplinary may be used interchangeably. Generally, these programs consists of providers from multiple backgrounds, including pain medicine, other medical backgrounds, psychologists, physical therapists, occupational therapists, addiction counselors, vocational rehabilitation specialists, and others, working together on a common treatment plan for every patient. This coordination and common treatment goal setting differentiate these programs from routine fragmented or unimodality care. The duration of programming can vary. Although patients in some programs are in rehabilitation 8 to 9 hours a day for 3 to 4 weeks, in others, patients attend 3 to 4 hours, a few days a week, for a few months. Often, patients are treated in groups.

Pain Medicine and Rehabilitation, Cleveland Clinic, 10524 Euclid Avenue, Cleveland, OH 44195, USA
* Corresponding author.
E-mail address: Mathews.manu@gmail.com

Neurosurg Clin N Am 25 (2014) 799–802
http://dx.doi.org/10.1016/j.nec.2014.07.004
1042-3680/14/$ – see front matter © 2014 Elsevier Inc. All rights reserved.

The primary approach is addressing the factors that lead to disability and suffering. Pain behaviors are discouraged, and wellness behaviors are encouraged. Patients are usually in a stage of acceptance of their pain. The treatment is based on the physical and psychological needs of the individual patient. The flavor of the program can vary depending on the expertise of the providers. Although some providers may be pharmacologically biased, others may lean more toward psychological or physical therapy techniques. Nevertheless, the presence of all of these approaches in a coordinated fashion is common to all such programs.

PSYCHOLOGICAL FACTORS THAT AFFECT PAIN
Pain Catastrophizing

Multiple studies have shown that catastrophization leads to a heightened pain experience and is associated with poorer treatment outcomes. Catapstophizing is considered to be attribution of magnified negative meaning to the experience of pain. For example: "my nerves are being pulled," or "my back was broken" may be used to describe sciatica or back pain, respectively. Catastrophization can be contagious. Catastrophization by family members has been associated with the same in adults and children.[5]

Mood and Affect States

Like depression, anxiety and anger have been shown to impact the pain experience and treatment outcomes.[6] Thirty percent to 60% of patients with chronic pain have comorbid depression or anxiety.[7]

Acceptance is an important part of chronic pain rehabilitation. Patients entering these programs do better when they accept their pain and are looking to work on managing their lives better, reducing its effect on their function and moving away from a sick role to take on more appropriate role with their families, work, and friends.[8] Patients who are looking for more tests and surgeries to cure their pain may not be appropriate candidates for treatment in this environment.

Interestingly, the only imaging correlate with poor outcome was moderate-to-severe Modic changes of the vertebral end plate, which were weakly associated with an adverse outcome.[9]

PSYCHOLOGICAL MANAGEMENT
Principles of Chronic Pain Rehabilitation

Behavior modification
Behavioral modification and cognitive restructuring are concepts at the core of pain rehabilitation. These principles are applicable to the patient and their families. The basis of behavior modification is operant conditioning. Behavior rewarded is behavior repeated (Skinner), and unrewarded behaviors tend to get extinguished. By converse analogy, most behaviors can be explained by looking for the incentives driving them. Pain-related behaviors like somatic conversation, wearing dark glasses, reclining, avoiding social contacts, and moaning can be replaced with wellness behaviors by changing the incentives.

Behavior modification in chronic pain rehabilitation occurs in the context of patients' interactions with their treating team, including psychotherapists, nurses, physicians, and physical and occupational therapists.

Education
Education is the cornerstone of treating chronic pain. Helping the patient to differentiate between hurt and harm and addressing fear avoidance is an important first step of the treatment process. Patients often carry the acute pain construct with them while living with chronic pain and believe that they need to protect their body to avoid further damage. The experience of increased pain with movement leads to splinting of the body or part of it in the hope of recovery and the desire to limit perceived damage. This may often also be encouraged by health care providers who may be fearful of having patients push through their chronic pain in fear of structural damage. The failure to re-educate and rescind postoperative instructions may lead to the patient continuing with significant restrictions for many years, leading to deconditioning and deterioration (patient continuing to follow a 5 lb carrying restriction 5 years following spine surgery despite a solid fusion).

The treating team can play a critical role in identifying the misinformation and re-educating the patient and his or her family. Education can lead to a perception of increased control of disease, resolution of depression, and promotion of health-promoting activities like exercise and relaxation.

Education includes not only the patient, but also his or her family. There is ample evidence that patients do better when families are engaged in the rehabilitation process.[10,11] Families may respond to the patient's pain and disability in a few different ways. Some respond by enabling them: protecting them, taking over their responsibilities, lowering expectations in terms of work, chores, financial role fulfillment, and intimacy. Others may become angry and reject the patient, questioning the credibility of the patient's experience. Interestingly, both these approaches typically lead to the patient being isolated and left out of family gatherings and recreational activities.

Evidence suggests that rewarding pain behaviors by families will lead to an increase in them, and ignoring them while encouraging activity can lead to a reduction. Overprotecting and suggesting rest will lead to a poorer outcome. Families are recommended to support and validate the patient's experience and move away from the role of a caretaker or nurse and return to a more appropriate relational role (spouse, child).

Cognitive Behavioral Therapy

One's thoughts, behaviors, and feelings are inter-linked. Maladaptive thoughts can lead to negative feelings. Cognitive behavioral therapy (CBT) is a modality of therapy that is designed to address this maladaptive pattern. The core focus on CBT is to address maladaptive thoughts and beliefs about the pain experience to enable the patient to change the behaviors related to it.

CBT has one of the most robust outcomes in chronic pain management. Multiple studies have shown improvement in pain, mood, and function lasting up to 5 years. CBT forms one of the core therapies of chronic pain rehabilitation.

Relaxation Training, Guided Imagery, and Biofeedback

The role of anxiety and stress in the pain experience is well known. The experience of pain is amplified by stress and emotional distress. Relaxation training can take various forms like progressive muscle relaxation, guided imagery, and deep breathing and biofeedback. Biofeedback is a method of monitoring physiologic parameters including heart rate, sweating, muscle tension, and brain activity. Studies have shown inconsistent efficacy of biofeedback to improve pain and function, although there is an understanding that provider skill is an important factor in outcome.

Addressing Affective States

Depression and anxiety are conditions that are over-represented in the chronic pain population compared with the general population, with a prevalence of both conditions between 30% and 50%. A systematic review concluded that depression is more likely to be a result of chronic pain, although chronic pain may develop in those with a predisposition to depression. CBT has been shown to be effective in treating mild-to-moderate depression and when combined with antidepressants, it is more effective than antidepressants alone in moderate depression.

Pharmacologic Strategies

The pharmacologic management of depression has been described in the chapter on multi-modality treatment of pain. Various tricyclic antidepressants and serotonin nor-epinephrine reuptake inhibitors have been shown to be effective in the management of chronic pain. Often, a combination of antidepressants (with an analgesic effect), anti-epileptics, and other agents including tricyclics, is used to achieve adequate analgesia.

Opioids

Opioids can be a useful modality of treatment in pain rehabilitation. Many patients who are referred to pain rehabilitation programs have often failed opioid therapy. Over the past few years, evidence has emerged that discontinuation of opioids in interdisciplinary pain rehabilitation environment resulted in improvement in pain mood and function that is sustained over time.[12] IPRPs provide an ideal environment for the discontinuation of opiates in patients with chronic pain, as the concurrent use of physical and occupational therapy, psychological strategies to improve pain coping, and reconditioning replaces the opiates as the coping strategy and avoids the relapse that is seen so often in patients who only undergo detoxification.

Physical and Occupational Therapy

Active modalities increase flexibility, endurance, and strength. Psychological techniques can be used to help patients tolerate exercises better and self-regulate exercise-induced pain.

Occupational and Vocational Therapy

Return to home, work, and leisure activities is important to prevent relapse of pain behaviors. Patients who have vocational goals to accomplish tend to do better in the long term.

SUMMARY/DISCUSSION

IPRPs have the most evidence in literature for sustained pain and function improvement. The initial expenses and unfavorable reimbursement environment have made their availability scarce. As medicine moves to a more evidence- and outcomes-based practice, the expansion of these programs is inevitable.

REFERENCES

1. Gatchel RJ, Okifuji A. Evidence-based scientific data documenting the treatment and cost-effectiveness of

comprehensive pain programs for chronic nonmalignant pain. J Pain 2006;7(11):779–93.

2. Flor H, Fydrich T, Turk DC. Efficacy of multidisciplinary pain treatment centers: a meta-analytic review. Pain 1992;49:221–30.

3. Scascighinil L, Toma V, Dober-Spielmann S, et al. Multidisciplinary treatment of chronic pain: a systematic review of interventions and outcomes. Rheumatology 2008;47:670–8.

4. Patrick LE, Altamaier EM, Found EM. Long-term outcomes in multidisciplinary treatment of chronic low back pain: results of a 13-year follow-up. Spine 2004;29(8):850–5.

5. Langer LS, Romano JM, Mancl L, et al. Parental catastrophizing partially mediates the association between parent-reported child pain behavior and parental protective responses. Pain Res Treat 2014;2014:751097.

6. Fernandez E, Turk DC. The scope and significance of anger in the experience of chronic pain. Pain 1995;61(2):165–75.

7. Stewart SH, Asmundson GJ. Anxiety sensitivity and its impact on pain experiences and conditions: a state of the art. Cogn Behav Ther 2006;35(4): 185–8.

8. McCracken ML, Vowles KE, Eccleston C. Acceptance-based treatment for persons with complex, long standing chronic pain: a preliminary analysis of treatment outcome in comparison to a waiting phase. Behav Res Ther 2005;43(10):1335–46.

9. Carragee EJ, Alamin TF, Miller JL, et al. Discographic, MRI and psychosocial determinants of low back pain disability and remission: a prospective study in subjects with benign persistent back pain. Spine J 2005;5(1):24–35.

10. McCracken LM. Social context and acceptance of chronic pain: the role of solicitous and punishing responses. Pain 2005;113:155–9.

11. Raichle KA, Romano JM, Jensen MP. Partner responses to patient pain and well behaviors and their relationship to patient pain behavior, functioning, and depression. Pain 2011;152(1):82–6.

12. Murphy JL, Clark EM, Banou E. Opioid cessation and multidimensional outcomes after interdisciplinary chronic pain treatment. Clin J Pain 2013; 29(2):109–17.

Multimodal Treatment of Pain

Manu Mathews, MD

KEYWORDS

- Chronic pain • Physical therapy • Occupational therapy • Cognitive behavioral therapy • Tai chi
- Yoga

KEY POINTS

- Pain is a multidimensional experience and its management should account for this.
- Although some of the unimodal therapies can be effective in selected groups of patients, practitioners often find it necessary to use a combination of various pharmaceutical agents, physical approaches, and psychological approaches to bring about optimum outcomes.
- Especially in cases in which pain has led to significant functional impairment, it is important to fully evaluate the psychological factors in addition to the anatomic disorder.
- The effect of other medical conditions on the patient should not be ignored.

INTRODUCTION

Spinoza said that pain is a localized form of sorrow. It is rare for chronic pain to occur as an isolated phenomenon. This complex disorder lends itself better to a biopsychosocial model of assessment and treatment. Despite efforts over the past 3 decades to address chronic pain from mostly a biological perspective, chronic pain may not be managed any better now than it was a decade ago.[1]

The principles of chronic pain rehabilitation are discussed elsewhere in this issue. This article discusses some of these modalities in greater detail. It is important to address chronic pain in every patient from a variety of different angles and use more than 1 treatment approach wherever indicated. The risk of suboptimal outcome is greatly increased if the obvious comorbidities are ignored.

PATIENT EVALUATION OVERVIEW

Effective management starts with a thorough evaluation, especially in the management of chronic pain. It is increasingly clear that multiple factors affect chronic pain treatment outcomes. Although

many aspects of such an evaluation are standard in most medical evaluations, a good pain evaluation has some key variations (**Box 1**). The emphasis is on assessing the biological, psychological, and social aspects of the history, and diagnosis should include these multiple domains.[2]

PHARMACOLOGIC TREATMENT OPTIONS

Pharmacologic interventions encompass the most widely used modality in the treatment of chronic pain. The choice of the pharmacologic approach should be based on the diagnosis. A variety of classes of agents are available and the salient features of some of them are discussed here.

Nonsteroidal Antiinflammatory Agents

Nonsteroidal antiinflammatory agents act by inhibition of the cyclooxygenase (COX) enzymes and exert both central and peripheral effects.[3] There is no risk of physiologic tolerance, but caution needs to be exercised when these agents are prescribed to patients with renal, cardiac, and gastrointestinal disease and in the elderly. Although the COX-2 inhibitors are purported to have a lower

Pain Medicine and Rehabilitation, Cleveland Clinic, 9500 Euclid Avenue, Cleveland, OH 44195, USA
E-mail address: mathews.manu@gmail.com

Neurosurg Clin N Am 25 (2014) 803–808
http://dx.doi.org/10.1016/j.nec.2014.07.005
1042-3680/14/$ – see front matter © 2014 Elsevier Inc. All rights reserved.

> **Box 1**
> **Pain evaluation**
>
> - Detailed pain history:
>   - Standard format that includes onset and progression of symptoms.
>   - A detailed evaluation of all the pain-related complaints in the format mentioned earlier because presence of other pain syndromes may affect treatment outcomes (multifocal pain being a predictor of poor outcome from knee surgery).
>   - The presence of other pain syndromes may change the diagnosis: for example, a patient presenting with spine pain may have fibromyalgia.
> - Complete list of current medications including over-the-counter and herbal products:
>   - Medication-induced phenomena like opiate-induced hyperalgesia or medication overuse headaches from over-the-counter analgesics are common.
>   - Interaction of herbal products with pharmaceutical agents (especially methadone, antidepressants).
>   - Pattern of analgesic use, evaluation of red flags that suggest loss of control, use despite consequences.
> - Past treatments and response:
>   - For example, pharmacologic, interventional, surgical, and physical and occupational therapy modalities.
> - Functional/disability status:
>   - Evaluated with activity and occupational history, quality-of-life scales, or functional measures like the Oswestry Disability Index or Roland Morris Disability Questionnaire, Pain Disability Index, etc. These tools can help assess treatment outcomes.
> - Assessment of mood and other psychiatric symptoms:
>   - For example, depression, anxiety, substance abuse history, self-injurious behavior.
> - Social and developmental history:
>   - For example, current and past relationships and their current roles; history of neglect, abuse, physical and sexual trauma.
> - Psychiatric history:
>   - Diagnosis, hospitalization, current mood state, self-injurious behavior, past and current substance use history.
> - Physical:
>   - Comprehensive multisystem examination: note any inconsistencies, non-physiological signs like Waddell signs, multifocal signs, etc, and observe the patient's affect, cognitive function, and behavior.

risk of ulcer disease, long-term studies have failed to support this.

Acetaminophen

Acetaminophen is one of the most widely used analgesics and is equipotent with aspirin. It can be considered a first line analgesic for a variety of nociceptive pains.[4]

Antidepressants

This class is hypothesized to act via a variety of mechanisms including inhibition of reuptake of noradrenaline (NA) and 5-hydroxytryptamine (5HT) in the brainstem projections to the spinal cord, opioid effect,[4] calcium and sodium channel blockade,[5] and N-methyl-D-aspartate receptor (NMDA) antagonism.[6] Their analgesic effects are independent of their antidepressant effect.

Tricyclic antidepressants (TCAs) have the lowest number needed to treat (NNT) for neuropathic pain. Sedation, anticholinergic, autonomic, and cardiovascular effects may affect tolerability, but imipramine, desipramine, nortriptyline, are well tolerated and have a low number needed to harm (NNH).

The serotonin norepinephrine reuptake inhibitors like venlafaxine, duloxetine, and milnacipram have emerged as alternatives to TCAs. Studies have shown venlafaxine to be as effective as other tricyclics and gabapentin in the treatment of neuropathic pain.[7] In addition to neuropathic pain, they have been shown to be effective in the treatment of fibromyalgia and musculoskeletal and osteoarthritis pain.

All patients initiated on antidepressants should be monitored for the emergence of suicidal thoughts. The common antidepressants and their doses are listed in **Table 1**.

ANTIEPILEPTICS

Antiepileptics have been shown to be effective in the treatment of a variety of neuropathic conditions, including diabetic neuropathy, postherpetic neuralgia, spinal cord injury–related neuropathic pain, and radicular pain. Other musculoskeletal conditions like fibromyalgia have been shown to respond to gabapentin and pregabalin. Valproate, gabapentin, and topiramate are used in the preventive management of migraines and other cephalgias. Carbamazepine and oxcarbazepine are used in trigeminal neuralgia. **Table 2** provides more details of use.

OPIOIDS

Opioids are effective in the management of acute pain. While they have been used for decades in the management of chronic pain, there is limited data on long term use, mostly due to a paucity of studies. The emergence of greater mortality and morbidity related to prescription opiates has mired this issue in further controversy. Additional risks like interactions, additive effects, addiction, development of hyperalgesia, and death are increasingly coming into focus. Opioid analgesics are best used with close monitoring

for improvement in pain and function along with emergence of signs of harm. They are considered to be a good option in well-selected patients with monitoring for improvement in activity and analgesia without aberrant behavior or adverse effects. A full discussion of the use of opioid medications is beyond the scope of this article.

NONPHARMACOLOGIC TREATMENT OPTIONS

Non–biologic based treatments play an important role in achieving optimum outcomes for chronic pain. For decades, many of these modalities were viewed as being outside the mainstream of treatment. Increasing evidence of the effectiveness of these therapies has pushed more patients and providers toward acknowledging their utility, thereby moving them into the mainstream.

Misinformation about chronic pain frequently leads to kinesophobia (fear of movement). Patients with chronic pain often equate hurt with harm and take on an increasingly sedentary lifestyle, leading to splinting of the painful area. This process inadvertently leads to deconditioning, wasting of muscles, and weakening of ligaments and bones, making any attempts at remobilization more challenging. Reduced activity and self-efficacy lead to loss of self-esteem, changes in the patient's role within their family and society and leading to psychological sequelae like depression, anxiety, anger, etc, as discussed elsewhere in this issue.

A review of literature by the American College of Physicians found good evidence to support cognitive behavior therapy (CBT), spinal manipulation, and interdisciplinary rehabilitation for chronic back pain. Other therapies, including acupuncture, yoga, and functional restoration, also seemed to have modest benefit. A key concept of treatment

Table 1
Common antidepressants and their dosages

	Initiating Dosage	Therapeutic Range	Notes
Amitriptyline	10–25 mg at night	50–150 mg/d	1. Strongly anticholinergic and sedating 2. Administer at night 3. Check QTc before initiation
Nortriptyline	25 mg at night	50–150 mg/d	1. Take larger dose at night 2. Check QTc before initiation
Desipramine	100 mg/d	100–300 mg/d	Can monitor levels
Imipramine	50–75 mg/d	150 mg/d	—
Venlafaxine	37.5 mg/d	150–225 mg/d	Monitor for hypertension at higher doses
Duloxetine	30 mg/d	60–120 mg/d	Increased sweating
Milnacipran	12.5 mg/d	100–200 mg/d	Starter pack available

Table 2
Antiepileptic drugs and their dosages

	Initiating Dosage	Therapeutic Range	Notes
Gabapentin	300 mg, 2–3 times a day	1800–3600 mg/d	1. Use larger doses at night to help sleep and reduce the risk of dose-related daytime sedation. Avoid aggressive titration. Aim to reach the therapeutic range over 4–6 wk 2. Safe in liver disease
Pregabalin	50 mg 1–2 times a day	300–600 mg/d	Similar to gabapentin
Valproate	250 mg 1–2 times a day	1000–2000 mg/d	1. There are a few versions available 2. Check hepatic function before initiation and monitor 6 mo 3. Check blood levels for toxicity. Weak correlation between levels and analgesic effects
Topiramate	25–50 mg, 1–2 times/d	100–200 mg/d	1. Monitor for cognitive deterioration, depression, psychosis 2. Use with caution if history of nephrolithiasis (calcium phosphate)
Carbamazepine	100 mg BID	600–1200 mg/d	1. Increased risk of Stevens-Johnson syndrome, toxic epidermal necrolysis 2. Increased risk of aplastic anemia and agranulocytosis
Oxcarbazepine	300 mg BID	1200 mg/d	Risk of hyponatremia

Abbreviation: BID, twice a day.

is to help the patient overcome kinesophobia using all available modalities.

PHYSICAL THERAPY

Reactivation of the body to improve function is important in the successful management of chronic pain. An increase in the pain is expected as patients increase their physical activity. In the absence of an acute disorder, the patient can be reassured and taught psychological techniques like relaxation, biofeedback and guided imagery to push through the pain. As patients increase their strength and endurance, they typically see a reduction in pain. Evidence suggests that using fear-reducing psychological strategies during physical therapy (PT) leads to improved pain and function and fewer pain days for 2 years following the intervention, highlighting the importance of using multiple approaches concurrently.[8] A key aspect is to help patients time and pace their activities. Overstraining in the first few days of treatment can lead to increased pain and a reinforcement of the belief that physical activity is more harmful than helpful.

Either water-based or land-based therapies can be used. In the deconditioned patient with chronic

pain, we often recommend initiation of water therapy first, to take advantage of the buoyancy. Once patients develop some confidence in their physical abilities, land-based therapies can be introduced. Hayden and colleagues's[9] systematic review found the following to be associated with better outcomes:

- Individualized treatment programs
- Supervised individual or group exercise
- Supervised home exercise
- High-dose PT
- Combination of PT with other treatment modalities

OCCUPATIONAL THERAPY

In conjunction with PT, occupational therapy can help the patient improve function by improving sensory discrimination, posture, and ergonomics; optimizing sensory experiences (fluidotherapy for allodynia and hyperalgesia); and improving hand coordination, computer ergonomics, home care tasks, etc.

Being able to return to activities, including driving, playing golf, doing home and yard work, can have the additional psychological benefit of improved self-esteem and efficacy, further feeding the positive reinforcement cycle and accelerating wellness.

NUTRITION

There is an increasing acknowledgment of the role of nutrition in the management of chronic pain. Some of the obvious benefits of healthy eating include weight loss, increased energy levels, improved sleep, and improved management of other diet-related diseases, all of which may contribute to overall emotional and physical well-being.

High doses of omega-3 fatty acids were found to have analgesic properties in patients with neck and low back pain. Laboratory studies have shown that rats on a soy diet were less likely to develop laboratory-induced neuropathic pain.

PSYCHOLOGICAL THERAPIES

Psychosocial factors have consistently been found to be the best predictors of outcomes in pain-related conditions. Maladaptive coping mechanisms, catastrophization, external locus of control etc have been found to be predictors of poor outcome. Various approaches in psychotherapy can help address these. However, no single type of therapy may be sufficient to address all the maladaptive patterns seen in the same patient. It may require a combination of approaches to bring about an optimum outcome. Some of the common therapies and the data supporting them are discussed here.

Cognitive Behavioral Therapy

People's feelings are governed by their thoughts and behaviors rather than by external forces. People can change the way they feel by changing their thoughts and behaviors, and this can have a profound effect on the interpretation of pain. Patients with chronic pain experience helplessness and lack of control, which influence their feelings. Cognitive Behavioral Therapy (CBT) has been shown to be very effective when combined with PT, medications, and occasionally surgery. A systematic review showed an improvement in pain experience, cognitive coping, and appraisal (positive coping measures), and reduced behavioral expression of pain.[10] CBT is also favorable because it can be a manual-based therapy and trained providers are accessible in most parts of the country. In addition, the time-limited nature of it also makes it economically viable.

Other Psychotherapies

A variety of other psychotherapies, including psychodynamic psychotherapy, interpersonal therapies, and family therapies, have been shown to be effective in improving pain and function in selected patients. Guided imagery, relaxation, and distraction therapies can be beneficial and it is easy to train patients in their use. The body of evidence in these forms of psychotherapies is not as robust as in CBT. In addition, these therapies can depend heavily on the skill of the provider and access may be limited.

Biofeedback

Patients train to gain greater awareness of their physiologic states by measurement of brain activity (electroencephalogram), heart rate, muscle tension (electromyogram), palmar sweating, pain, etc, and then learn to self-regulate these physiologic functions. Biofeedback works on the hypothesis that when under stress, the above parameters are increased and self-control is possible. Over time, the patient may not need any additional equipment to practice biofeedback and along with relaxation and guided imagery can make it a part of their daily wellness regimen.

Biofeedback has shown efficacy over the past 4 decades in muscle pain, headaches, low back and neck pain, phantom pain, etc. The advantage of this therapy is patient buy-in because patients are able to see the physiologic responses to their pain and stressors. The lack of availability of well-trained therapists and the reluctance of many insurance payers to cover it are obstacles.

Mindfulness Therapy

There is increasing acceptance of this meditation-based therapy that has its origins in the eastern religions (Hinduism and Buddhism). There is evidence of improved outcomes in patients with fibromyalgia[11] and low back pain.

ADJUNCTIVE THERAPIES
Tai Chi

Tai chi uses adaptive exercises, mind-body interaction, and meditation to help manage chronic pain. There is evidence that it is effective in osteoarthritis, fibromyalgia, and low back pain, although weaker evidence suggests efficacy in headaches and rheumatoid arthritis too.[12]

Yoga

This ancient physical-meditative technique has been gaining increasing popularity in the management of pain. A meta-analysis and systematic review found strong evidence of both short-term and long-term improvement in pain and back-specific disability.[13]

COMBINATION THERAPIES

Sometimes, permutations of a few therapies may not be sufficient to break the cycle of pain and functional impairment and in those cases it is best to treat the patient in a multidisciplinary pain rehabilitation program, as described elsewhere in this book.

SUMMARY/DISCUSSION

The complex disorder of chronic pain lends itself better to a biopsychosocial model of assessment and care. Ignoring the multiple confounding factors is likely to lead to a poor outcome and wasteful use of health care resources. The strongest support in the literature is for a multimodal approach and perhaps with the changing health care landscape, providers will be more motivated to work toward an outcomes-based model.

REFERENCES

1. Boulanger A, Clark JA, Squire P, et al. Chronic pain in Canada: have we improved our management of chronic noncancer pain? Pain Res Manag 2007; 12(1):39–47.
2. Malaty A, Sabharwal J, Lirette LS, et al. How to assess a new patient for a multidisciplinary chronic pain rehabilitation program: a review article. Ochsner J 2014;14(1):96–100.
3. Yaksh TL, Dirig DM, Malmberg AB. Mechanism of action of nonsteroidal anti-inflammatory drugs. Cancer Invest 1998;16:509–27.
4. Eschalier A, Ardid D, Dubray C. Tricyclic and other antidepressants as analgesics. In: Sawnyok J, Cowan A, editors. Novel aspects of pain management: opioids and beyond. New York: Wiley; 1999. p. 303–20.
5. Pancrazio JJ, Kamatchi GL, Roscoe AK, et al. Inhibition of neuronal Na+ channels by antidepressant drugs. J Pharmacol Exp Ther 1998;284(1): 208–14.
6. Eisenach JC, Gebhart GF. Intrathecal amitriptyline acts as an N-methyl-D-aspartate receptor antagonist in the presence of inflammatory hyperalgesia in rats. Anesthesiology 1995;83(5):1046–54.
7. Rowbotham MC, Goli V, Kunz NR, et al. Venlafaxine extended release in the treatment of painful diabetic neuropathy: a double-blind, placebo-controlled study. Pain 2004;110(3):697–706.
8. Von Korff M, Balderson BH, Saunders K. A trial of an activating intervention for chronic back pain in primary care and physical therapy settings. Pain 2005;113(3):323–30.
9. Hayden JA, van Tulder MW, Tomlinson G. Systematic review: strategies for using exercise therapy to improve outcomes in chronic low back pain. Ann Intern Med 2005;142:776–85.
10. Morley S, Eccleston C, Williams A. Systematic review and meta-analysis of randomized controlled trials of cognitive behaviour therapy and behaviour therapy for chronic pain in adults, excluding headache. Pain 1999;80:1–13.
11. Henke M, Chur-Hansen A. The effectiveness of mindfulness-based programs on physical symptoms and psychological distress in patients with fibromyalgia: a systematic review. International Journal of Wellbeing 2014;4(1):28–45.
12. Peng PW. Tai chi and chronic pain. Reg Anesth Pain Med 2012;37(4):372–82.
13. Holger C, Romy L, Heidemarie H, et al. A systematic review and meta-analysis of yoga for low back pain. Clin J Pain 2013;29(5):450–60.

Nerve Blocks for Chronic Pain

Salim M. Hayek, MD, PhD[a],*, Atit Shah, MD[b]

KEYWORDS

- Nerve block • Chronic pain • Diagnosis • Therapy

KEY POINTS

- Nerve blocks can be performed for a variety of conditions, providing diagnostic and therapeutic modalities.
- Whenever considering nerve blocks, risks and benefits must be considered before intervention.

INTRODUCTION

Nerve blocks are often performed as therapeutic or palliative interventions for pain relief. However, they are often performed for diagnostic or prognostic purposes. When considering nerve blocks for chronic pain, clinicians must always consider the indications, risks, benefits, and proper technique, in order to provide maximal benefit for the patients. Nerve blocks encompass a wide variety of interventional procedures. The most common nerve blocks for chronic pain and that may be applicable to the neurosurgical patient population are reviewed in this article. This article is an introduction and brief synopsis of the different available blocks that can be offered to a patient.

DIAGNOSTIC VERSUS THERAPEUTIC NERVE BLOCKS

In general, nerve blocks may be divided into diagnostic and therapeutic interventions. Pain is a subjective unpleasant sensation, the exact pathophysiology of which is uncertain or multifactorial in most clinical situations. In human beings, chronic pain is a complex process that is compounded by psychosocial, financial, and sometimes legal

matters.[1] When the cause of pain is unclear despite appropriate history taking, physical examination, and imaging or electrodiagnostic studies, diagnostic or prognostic nerve blocks may be in order. For instance, pain originating in the zygapophyseal joints or the sacroiliac joint cannot reliably be diagnosed by clinical examination or imaging studies and diagnostic local anesthetic blocks are frequently called on to confirm the diagnosis.[2,3] However, there are significant limitations to nerve blocks in making the leap from pain relief to establishing that pain is mediated by the targeted nerve, because performance of a nerve block takes into consideration many assumptions:

1. The nerve being blocked is responsible for generation, conduction, or maintenance of the painful stimulus
2. The operator performing the procedure is skilled in the performance of the block
3. The needle is placed in the exact and correct anatomic location
4. The patient does not have anatomic variations or aberrant physiologic or pharmacologic responses to the medication used
5. The volume of the medication injected is appropriate for the nerve/space

Disclosures: All authors report and declare no support from any organization for the submitted work; no financial relationships with any organizations that might have an interest in the submitted work in the previous 3 years; no other relationships or activities that could have influenced the submitted work.
[a] Division of Pain Medicine, Department of Anesthesiology, University Hospitals of Cleveland, Case Western Reserve University, 11100 Euclid Avenue, Cleveland, OH 44106, USA; [b] Department of Anesthesiology, Case Western University, 450 East Waterside Drive Unit 1511, Chicago, IL 60601, USA
* Corresponding author.
E-mail address: salim.hayek@uhhospitals.org

neurosurgery.theclinics.com

6. The medication injected will remain in place and anesthetize only the targeted nerve and no other nerves or structures or act systemically

7. The patient is able to understand and interpret the response to the block appropriately

Nonetheless, when properly performed in the appropriate clinical setting, nerve blocks can provide valuable adjunct information that, when taken together with the patient's complete clinical picture, may help in decision making about the cause of pain.

The most commonly performed diagnostic nerve blocks include:

1. Selective nerve blocks. These may be indicated in the presence of radicular symptoms and questionable or multiple levels of abnormalities on imaging studies. Assessing selective nerve root blocks is challenging given that no loss of cutaneous sensation occurs following surgical division of a single nerve root.[1] Multiple studies attest to the high positive predictive value of selective nerve root blocks and their accuracy is superior to that of imaging and electrodiagnostic testing.[4–7] Nonetheless, accuracy of these blocks awaits authentication in controlled blinded trials.

2. Joint injections. Controlled diagnostic blocks have been used successfully to identify the sacroiliac joint and other joints as a source of pain and represent the most reliable way of diagnosing painful joint syndromes. Sacroiliac joint pain accounts for between 15% and 20% of patients presenting with axial low back pain. Even though their validity has yet to be proved, small-volume local anesthetic blocks are still the most used method for diagnosing sacroiliac joint pain.[8]

3. Medial branch blocks. Medial branches of posterior rami supply zygapophyseal (facet) joints at the same level and the level below. Hence, blocking a single facet joint requires blockade of 2 medial branches. Diagnostic medial nerve branch blocks are the gold standard to establish facet-mediated pain. Lumbar zygapophyseal pain accounts for up to 15% of patients with axial low back pain.[9]

4. Differential nerve blocks. These blocks are often performed in the setting of abdominal or pelvic pain of unknown cause. An anatomic (nerve-by-nerve block) or pharmacologic approach may be used. The pharmacologic approach is preferred and involves epidural blockade of all innervation to the target area (typically T4 level) and evaluation of the pain response as the epidural block resolves. It is most useful to differentiate organic peripheral pain that would be amenable to further interventions from central pain.[10]

False-positive responses occur with blocks even with the use of imaging. For instance, a placebo response rate of 38% (false-positives) has been shown for uncontrolled lumbar facet joint blocks and a low positive predictive value of 31%.[11] To curtail the rate of false-positive responses, repeat blocks or comparative local anesthetic blocks have been performed, resulting in refinement of diagnostic accuracy.[12,13]

Diagnostic blocks typically provide a patient with relief limited to the duration of action of the local anesthetic used, although longer-lasting responses are occasionally noted.

THERAPEUTIC NERVE BLOCKS

Therapeutic interventions allow longer-term pain relief. The many common therapeutic nerve interventions include epidural steroid injections, radiofrequency ablations, and sympathetic nerve neurolysis.

Epidural Steroid Injection

Introduction

Epidural steroid injections have been used for chronic spinal pain relief for decades. Depositing steroids in the epidural space helps reduce inflammation around nerve roots contributing to pain. Epidural steroids can be delivered by several approaches, including the interlaminar, transforaminal, and caudal approaches.[14,15]

Epidural steroid injection can be performed as a more conservative approach than surgery, when surgery is not indicated or as a palliative bridge to surgery. Epidural injections can benefit a patient when the pain is secondary to disc herniation, discogenic pain, or spinal stenosis.[15] Benefits involve predominantly short-term pain relief, although occasionally long-term pain relief occurs. A series of 3 injections can be done in a 6-month span; however, this standard relates to limiting steroid toxicity. The main concern with repeated epidural steroid injections centers on the amount of total steroid injected and the possibility of causing adrenal suppression and affecting bone reabsorption.[14–16]

Indications

Indications for epidural steroid injection include radiculopathy secondary to disc herniation, isolated spondylotic spurring of the foramina, or neurogenic claudication associated with spinal stenosis.[15]

Efficacy

Moderate to strong evidence exists for interlaminar and transforaminal epidural steroid injections, at least in the short-term relief of radicular pain.[15]

Multiple studies of transforaminal epidural steroid injections in patients with herniated discs, radiculopathy, and stenosis reported significant benefit in pain scores, walking tolerance, and standing.[17,18]

In 2010, the American Society of Anesthesiologist Task Force on Chronic Pain Management published a practice guideline that stated, "Epidural Steroid injections with or without local anesthetics may be used as part of a multimodal treatment regimen to provide pain relief in selected patients with radicular pain or radiculopathy. Shared decision making regarding epidural steroid injections should include a specific discussion of potential complications, particularly with regard to the transforaminal approach."[19]

Procedure

There are multiple approaches to delivering steroid into the epidural space. The interlaminar epidural steroid injection uses a midline approach and delivers medications centrally with some spread to surrounding nerve roots. It is useful in central canal stenosis and in patients with diffuse disorder. The transforaminal approach is a directed injection, either right or left sided, and delivers medication that surrounds the affected nerve root with spread into the anterior epidural space. The caudal approach uses the opening at the sacral hiatus to deliver medication to the lower lumbar spine area. These procedures are done under fluoroscopic guidance and confirmation is obtained with contrast dye before injection of steroid (**Fig. 1**).[15,16]

Complications

When considering an epidural steroid injection, the risks versus benefits must be assessed. Potential risks of the procedure include, but are not limited to, dural puncture, postdural headache, bleeding, infection, nerve damage, epidural hematoma, epidural abscess, and paralysis. Transforaminal injections of particulate steroids carry a small but significant risk of embolization of large steroid particles into radicular arteries and from there into arterial spinal cord artery or vertebral arteries. Catastrophic events have occurred, in particular with cervical transforaminal injection of particulate steroids. Nonparticulate steroids are now advocated in transforaminal epidural steroid injections in the cervical region. Even though the risks are low, all patients must be well informed and consented before the procedure.[14–16]

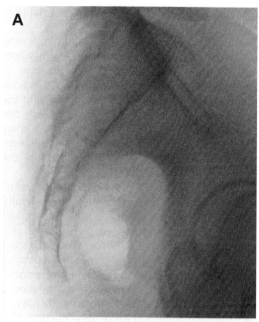

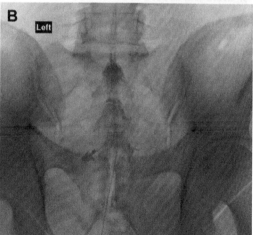

Fig. 1. Caudal epidural; (*A*) lateral and (*B*) anteroposterior (AP) views.

Facet Joint Nerve Blocks

Introduction

Zygapophyseal or facet joints are a source of pain for many patients.[20] A common cause of this joint pain is degeneration and arthritis of the spine and joint.[14,15]

Pain that is caused by facet joints typically presents with axial pain that increases with movement. Pain is worse with bending, extending, and rotational movements. Radiation of pain toward the extremity is an uncommon presentation but pain is often referred to the buttocks or shoulders.[15]

Patients typically have insidious onset of pain over time; however, a subgroup of patients has sudden onset of facet pain that occurs after some sort of trauma or deceleration (whiplash) injury.[16]

Though facet arthropathy is a common finding on imaging, correlation must be made with history and physical examination. When suspicion of facet-related pain is high, a diagnostic medial branch block must be performed to confirm the diagnosis. A unilateral or bilateral approach can be performed, depending on the patient's character of pain.[9] The facet joint is provided with sensory innervation by the medial branch of the posterior primary ramus.[14,16]

Medial branch blocks provide diagnostic value, indicating whether the joint is the pain generator for a patient. Patients are asked to perform movements that normally cause them pain after the procedure and their pain is reassessed. Significant pain relief, 50% or greater, is considered a positive response and a patient can return for a radiofrequency ablation at a later date. Radiofrequency ablation provides a much longer duration of pain relief, averaging about 6 to 9 months in duration.[14,15]

Procedure

A diagnostic medial branch block is conducted with local anesthetic only. Using fluoroscopic guidance, the needles are positioned along the posterior spine at a consistent location where the medial branch is known to travel.[21]

In the cervical region, the needles are advanced toward the middle of the articular pillars. After correct location has been verified, 0.25 mL of local anesthetic is injected. In the thoracic and lumbar regions, after correct location has been verified, 0.5 mL of local anesthetic is injected.[15]

Radiofrequency ablation is performed in a similar manner to medial branch blocks; however, sensory and motor testing is typically performed before the ablation (**Fig. 2**).[15]

Efficacy

Good evidence exists in support of radiofrequency lesioning of the medial branch nerves given that properly performed diagnostic tests have provided significant temporary relief.

Numerous placebo-controlled trials have examined lumbar facet pain and shown that radiofrequency ablation yielded positive results in lumbar pain in selected patients.[22,23]

Complications

Complications include pain at the injection site, injury to spinal nerves, uncomfortable dysesthesia, and sensory loss. Use of fluoroscopic guidance, proper testing before ablation, and performance of the procedure in an awake or minimally sedated patient results in near elimination of major risks.[14,16]

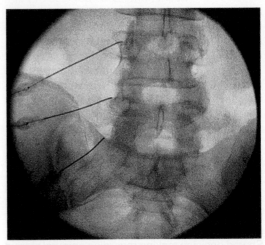

Fig. 2. Medial branch probe positioning; AP view.

Sympathetic Blocks

Introduction

These are multiple neural pathways that are involved in the perception and maintenance of pain. Following neuronal injury, the sympathetic nervous system is involved in pain perception and maintenance of chronic pain.[14,16]

The sympathetic chain extends from the first thoracic level to the second or third lumbar level. Its target area covers the cervical to the sacral region, providing sympathetic stimulation throughout the body.[14,16] Targeting different sympathetic ganglia allows blockade of sympathetic fibers in various regions throughout the body that may be contributing to or maintaining a patient's chronic pain.[14,16]

Efficacy

Limited evidence exists in support of the use of sympathetic blocks in pain relief of extremity pain.[24–27] There is stronger evidence for efficacy in neurolytic celiac plexus blocks in patients with pancreatic cancer pain.[28–30] There are multiple studies investigating the use of neurolysis in patients with cancer. One study comparing celiac plexus neurolysis versus sham showed significant pain relief at follow-up at 6 weeks.[29] A meta-analysis of 21 retrospective studies in patients undergoing celiac plexus neurolysis reported that 89% of patients received excellent pain relief in the follow-up visit at 2 weeks and 90% of patients received pain relief at the 3-month visit. When investigating superior hypogastric plexus blocks, it has been reported that 70% of patients with pelvic pain associated with cancer received significant pain relief in terms of visual analog scores.[31]

Stellate Ganglion Block

Introduction

The cervical sympathetic trunk contains 3 ganglia: the superior, middle, and inferior cervical ganglia. In 80% of people the lowest cervical ganglia is fused with the upper thoracic ganglion to form the cervicothoracic ganglion, also known as the stellate ganglion.[32] The cervicothoracic ganglion is on or just lateral to the longus colli muscle between the base of the seventh cervical transverse process and the neck of the first rib. The cervicothoracic ganglion receives preganglionic fibers from the lateral gray column of the spinal cord. The preganglionic fibers for the head and neck emerge from the upper 5 thoracic spinal nerves, ascending in the sympathetic trunk to synapse in the cervical ganglia. The preganglionic fibers supplying the upper extremity originate from the upper thoracic segments between T2 and T6 and in turn synapse in the cervicothoracic ganglion.

Procedure

The block is generally conducted at the sixth or seventh cervical vertebra using ultrasonography or fluoroscopic guidance. Ultrasonography allows a physician to visualize the soft tissue, artery, vein, and neural bundle. Fluoroscopy allows better visualization of bony structures.[15]

Regardless of the technique, after appropriate positioning of the needle is confirmed, approximately 2 to 5 mL of 0.25% bupivacaine or ropivacaine are injected. Injection is done slowly, in increments, being aware of any signs of local anesthetic toxicity. Signs of appropriate spread include increased temperature in the affected upper extremity, venodilatation in the ipsilateral arm, nasal congestion, anhidrosis, and Horner syndrome.[14,15] For a successful sympathetic block, a temperature increase in the hand to at least 34°C is recommended to achieve meaningful interruption of the postganglionic sympathetic supply.[33] The many indications for the blockade of the stellate ganglion include, but are not limited to, complex regional pain syndrome of the upper extremity, vascular insufficiency of the upper extremity, hyperhydrosis, acute pain of herpes zoster, postherpetic neuralgia, congenital prolonged QT syndrome (left cervicothoracic ganglion blockade), migraines, tension and cluster headaches, cerebral angiospasm, and cerebral thrombosis (**Fig. 3**).

Complications

Because of the close proximity of many critical and important structures in the neck, numerous complications are possible. Minor complications include recurrent laryngeal nerve paralysis or

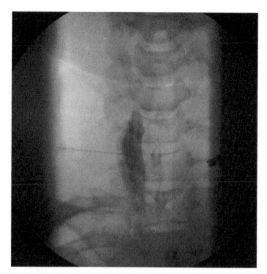

Fig. 3. Stellate ganglion needle positioning; AP view.

phrenic nerve paralysis from local anesthetic spread, and self-resolving somatic block. Pneumothorax may occur, especially on the right side (higher lung apex). Major complications result from intraspinal spread (subdural or epidural injection) typically resulting in ventilatory inadequacy; or from intravascular injection, usually the vertebral artery, with loss of consciousness, convulsions, ventilatory inadequacy, and hypotension. Use of image guidance may curtail many of these complications.

Celiac Plexus

Introduction

The celiac plexus is another sympathetic plexus that is generally found at the level of T12 and L1, just lateral to the aorta. The celiac plexus is formed by a combination of the greater, lesser, and least splanchnic nerves with parasympathetic contribution from the vagus nerve. This important plexus is responsible for conducting afferent visceral pain signals typically covering the abdomen with distal bowel and pelvic structures excluded.[14,16]

Celiac plexus blocks can provide diagnostic value to a physician by identifying pain that is conducted by sympathetic fibers. If a patient receives short-lived significant benefit, the patient may be a candidate for neurolytic celiac plexus block, which has long-lasting benefit in 70% to 90% of patients with visceral pain from upper intra-abdominal malignancies.[14,16]

Neurolytic block is generally performed using alcohol or phenol. Ethyl alcohol is less viscous than phenol and allows easier injection through small-diameter needles. Ethyl alcohol has a high concentration that can be appreciated by patients as pain on injection, and therefore injection of local anesthetic precedes ethanol injection. After injection, alcohol can also cause an inflammatory reaction that can persist and cause pain for a short time after the procedure.[14,16]

Phenol is typically prepared by combining carbolic acid, oxybenzene, hydroxybenzene, phenyl hydroxide, phenylic acid, and phenic acid. Phenol, unlike alcohol, is very viscous and difficult to inject. On injection, patients generally experience little pain.[25]

Procedure

The procedure is conducted under fluoroscopic guidance with the patient in the prone position. Once the needle is in the correct location, confirmation with contrast is obtained. Spread to the anterolateral surface of the aorta is desired.[15]

Diagnostic celiac plexus block is performed before neurolysis. When performing diagnosis, a total volume of 20 to 30 mL of 0.25% bupivacaine is injected. An identical volume is injected when performing neurolysis with frequent aspiration (**Fig. 4**).[15]

Complications

The most common side effects known after celiac plexus block include orthostatic hypotension and diarrhea. Complications include local anesthetic toxicity, kidney injury, pneumothorax, and aortic injury. With neurolysis, complications are similar and also include increased blood alcohol concentration, cardiovascular collapse, and paraplegia.[1–3] Paraplegia may occur secondary to damage or occlusion of the artery of Adamkiewicz and occurs at a rate of 1 in 683 blocks, predominantly with ethanol.[34] However, there has been 1 case report of paraplegia following a neurolytic celiac plexus block with phenol.[35]

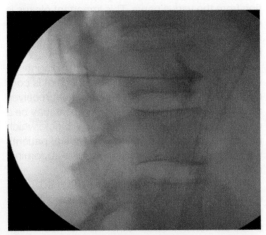

Fig. 4. Celiac plexus needle positioning; lateral view.

Lumbar Sympathetic Block

Introduction

The lumbar sympathetic plexus is involved in pain that is sympathetically maintained in the lower extremities. The lumbar sympathetic chain lies at the level of the second to fourth lumbar vertebral bodies. The most common indication for a lumbar sympathetic block include complex regional pain syndrome of the lower extremity with sympathetically maintained pain. Patients may benefit most when sympathetic plexus block is combined with a treatment plan involving physical therapy; however, evidence is scarce, with only 1 study in children showing short-term relief.[14,16,27]

Procedure

Similar to celiac plexus block, the patient starts in the prone position and the procedure is conducted under fluoroscopic guidance. The needle is typically placed over the inferior portion of the second or third lumbar vertebrae. Once the needle is verified in correct position, 15 to 20 mL of 0.25% bupivacaine or ropivacaine are injected incrementally. Proper spread yields a lower extremity sympathetic block that results in venodilatation and a temperature increase to within 3°C of the patient's core temperature.[15,36]

When a patient perceives only short-term benefit from local anesthetic injections, neurolysis can be performed. For neurolysis, phenol or alcohol can be used. Needles are positioned at the level of L2, L3, and L4, which represent the most common location of the lumbar sympathetic chain. After proper positioning has been confirmed, 2 to 3 mL of phenol or alcohol are injected at each site.[15]

Radiofrequency ablation is another option to short-lived pain control with local anesthetic injection. With this approach, radiofrequency probes are inserted over the anterolateral surfaces of the second, third, and fourth lumbar vertebrae.[15,37]

Complications

Complications include local anesthetic toxicity, kidney injury, intrathecal injection, and partial neurolysis of adjacent nerves, including predominantly the genitofemoral nerve.[14–16]

Superior Hypogastric Block

Introduction

The superior hypogastric plexus is responsible for sympathetically maintained pain in the pelvic region, which includes the uterus, vagina, rectum, prostate, and bladder. The plexus is located at the level of the fourth and fifth lumbar vertebrae and first sacral vertebrae.[14,16] Limited evidence exists in support of its use in visceral pelvic pain.

Procedure

Superior hypogastric blocks are performed in a similar manner to lumbar sympathetic blocks with needle placement at the level of the fifth lumbar vertebrae. After correct needle location is confirmed, 8 to 10 mL of 0.25% bupivacaine local anesthetic are injected. The procedure is repeated bilaterally and, for those patients who do not receive significant duration of pain relief, neurolysis can be performed.[15]

Complications

Complications include nerve injury, local anesthetic toxicity, puncture of surrounding organs, bleeding, and partial neurolysis of adjacent nerves.[14–16]

Intercostal Nerve Block

Introduction

Underneath each thoracic rib (T1–T12) runs an intercostal nerve that provides sensory input from the thoracic and abdominal dermatomal regions. These nerves are branches of the anterior primary rami that lie underneath the respective rib in the subcostal groove. The intercostal artery and nerve run alongside the nerve. The location of these 3 structures from superior to inferior typically includes vein, artery, and nerve. Along the course of the intercostal nerve there are multiple branches, such as the posterior, lateral cutaneous, and anterior branches.[14,16]

These nerves can be blocked with local anesthetic or frozen and deactivated with cryoablation. Indications include surgical thoracic pain, rib pain from fracture, neuropathic pain from herpes zoster, and cancer pain attributable to rib metastases.[14,16]

Procedure

Intercostal nerve blocks can be performed using either ultrasonography or fluoroscopic guidance. The block can be performed anywhere along the course of the nerve; however, it is recommended to block the nerves proximal to the branching of the posterior cutaneous nerve to obtain posterior coverage.[15]

Using fluoroscopy, the patient is placed in the prone position. A needle is advanced to the subcostal groove. Careful attention must be paid to the lung anatomy in order to avoid the risk of pneumothorax. Contrast is injected to verify correct placement and 2 to 4 mL of local anesthetic can be injected for diagnostic purposes. The procedure can be repeated at multiple levels; however, be aware of local anesthetic toxicity because both artery and vein are in close proximity.[14,15]

After a positive diagnostic intercostal block, cryoablation can be performed. Cryoablation uses an active probe tip that is cooled to −20°C. Cryoablation damages the vasa nervorum, causing edema and nerve injury. Patients can obtain weeks to months of pain relief, depending on the speed of nerve regeneration. Cryoablation minimizes the risk of neuroma formation and deafferentation pain (**Fig. 5**).[14,15]

Efficacy

Studies of intercostal nerve block for pain relief have been reported with positive results. One retrospective study of pain control in patients with cancer reported that 80% of patients received optimal pain control, whereas 56% of patients reported a reduction in their analgesic use. Thirty-two percent of the patients did not have recurrence of pain until the end of their lives.[38]

Complications

Complications include local anesthetic toxicity, infection, pneumothorax, nerve damage, hematoma, and spinal anesthesia.[14–16]

Occipital Nerve Block

Introduction

As the greater occipital nerve or lesser occipital nerve becomes irritated, the patient may experience headaches. Occipital nerve headaches present with paroxysmal pain that can be stabbing in nature. The pain occurs along the distribution of the greater and lesser occipital nerves.[14,16]

Possible causes for occipital nerve headaches include trauma to the nerves, spondylosis, cervical disc disease, myofascial pain, and tumors in the occipital scalp.[14,16]

When approaching a patient with head pain for the first time, a systematic and complete history and physical should be completed. At first, conservative modalities can be attempted, which

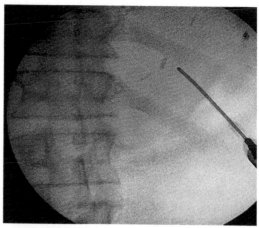

Fig. 5. Intercostal nerve cryoablation needle positioning; AP view.

include massages, physical therapy, heat, ice, nonsteroidal antiinflammatory drugs, muscle relaxants, anticonvulsants, and antidepressants. Patients with significant pain without relief from conservative approaches can be offered occipital nerve blockade if the cause is thought to arise from the occipital nerve.[14,16]

Procedure

The greater occipital nerve arises from the dorsal ramus of the second cervical nerve and passes between the inferior capitis oblique and semispinalis capitis muscles.[14]

The occipital nerve block is performed with the patient in the sitting position. The occipital artery runs lateral to the occipital nerve and is found approximately at one-third the distance between the occipital protuberance and the mastoid process along the nuchal ridge. Palpation of the artery is performed and a needle is inserted just medial to the artery and advanced until bony contact is made along the nuchal ridge. After negative aspiration, approximately 3 to 5 mL of local anesthetic are injected. The lesser occipital nerve can be blocked as well; however, the insertion point is more lateral.[14]

Efficacy

An uncontrolled study of 180 patients with cervicogenic headaches reported that 94% of patients experienced complete relief of their headaches lasting from 10 to 77 days.[39]

Complications

Complications include bleeding, infection, nerve damage, and allergy.[14]

SUMMARY

Nerve blocks can be performed for a variety of conditions, providing diagnostic and therapeutic modalities. Whenever considering nerve blocks, risks and benefits must be considered before intervention. This article discusses a variety of nerve blocks that can be offered to patients when appropriate.

REFERENCES

1. Hogan QH, Abram SE. Neural blockade for diagnosis and prognosis. A review. Anesthesiology 1997;86:216–41.
2. Schwarzer AC, Aprill CN, Derby R, et al. Clinical features of patients with pain stemming from the lumbar zygapophysial joints. Is the lumbar facet syndrome a clinical entity? Spine 1994;19:1132–7.
3. Maigne JY, Aivaliklis A, Pfefer F. Results of sacroiliac joint double block and value of sacroiliac pain provocation tests in 54 patients with low back pain. Spine 1996;21:1889–92.
4. Schutz H, Lougheed WM, Wortzman G, et al. Intervertebral nerve-root in the investigation of chronic lumbar disc disease. Can J Surg 1973;16:217–21.
5. Dooley JF, McBroom RJ, Taguchi T, et al. Nerve root infiltration in the diagnosis of radicular pain. Spine 1988;13:79–83.
6. Stanley D, McLaren MI, Euinton HA, et al. A prospective study of nerve root infiltration in the diagnosis of sciatica. A comparison with radiculography, computed tomography, and operative findings. Spine 1990;15:540–3.
7. Haueisen DC, Smith BS, Myers SR, et al. The diagnostic accuracy of spinal nerve injection studies. Their role in the evaluation of recurrent sciatica. Clin Orthop Relat Res 1985;(198):179–83.
8. Cohen SP. Sacroiliac joint pain: a comprehensive review of anatomy, diagnosis, and treatment. Anesth Analg 2005;101(5):1440–53.
9. Cohen SP, Srinivasa RN. Pathogenesis, diagnosis, and treatment of lumbar zygapophysial (facet) joint pain. Anesthesiology 2007;106(3):591–614.
10. Garcia J, Veizi E, Hayek S. Differential diagnostic nerve blocks. In: Deer T, editor. Interventional and neuromodulatory techniques for pain management. Philadelphia: Elsevier/Saunders; 2012.
11. Schwarzer AC, Aprill CN, Derby R, et al. The false-positive rate of uncontrolled diagnostic blocks of the lumbar zygapophysial joints. Pain 1994;58:195–200.
12. Barnsley L, Lord S, Bogduk N. Comparative local anaesthetic blocks in the diagnosis of cervical zygapophysial joint pain. Pain 1993;55:99–106.
13. Barnsley L, Lord S, Wallis B, et al. False-positive rates of cervical zygapophysial joint blocks. Clin J Pain 1993;9:124–30.
14. Benzon HT. Essentials of pain medicine. Philadelphia: Elsevier/Saunders; 2011.
15. Rathmell JP. Atlas of image-guided intervention in regional anesthesia and pain medicine. Philadelphia: Wolters Kluwer/Lippincott Williams & Wilkins Health; 2012.
16. Benzon HT, Raj PP. Raj's practical management of pain. Philadelphia: Mosby-Elsevier; 2008.
17. Ghahreman A, Ferch R, Bogduk N. The efficacy of transforaminal injection of steroids for the treatment of lumbar radicular pain. Pain Med 2010;11(8):1149–68.
18. Riew KD, Yin Y, Gilula L, et al. The effect of nerve-root injections on the need for operative treatment of lumbar radicular pain. A prospective, randomized, controlled, double-blind study. J Bone Joint Surg Am 2000;82-A(11):1589–93.
19. Rosenquist RW, Benzon HT, Connis RT. Practice guidelines for chronic pain management: an updated report by the American Society of Anesthesiologists

Task Force on chronic pain management and the American Society of Regional Anesthesia and Pain Medicine. Anesthesiology 2010;112:810–33.

20. Kuslich SD. The tissue origin of low back pain and sciatica: a report of pain response to tissue stimulation during operations on the lumbar spine using local anesthesia. Orthop Clin North Am 1991;22(2): 181–7.

21. Lau P, Mercer S, Govind J, et al. The surgical anatomy of lumbar medial branch neurotomy. Pain Med 2004;5(3):289–98.

22. Stovner LJ, Kolstad F, Helde G. Radiofrequency denervation of facet joints C2–C6 in cervicogenic headache. a randomized, double-blind, sham-controlled study. Cephalalgia 2004;24:821–30.

23. Van WR, Geurts JW, Wynne HJ. Radiofrequency denervation of lumbar facet joints in the treatment of chronic low back pain. a randomized, double-blind, sham lesion-controlled trial. Clin J Pain 2005; 21:335–44.

24. Day M. Sympathetic blocks: the evidence. Pain Pract 2008;8:98–109.

25. Forouzanfar T, Van Kleef M, Weber WE. Radiofrequency lesions of the stellate ganglion in chronic pain syndromes: retrospective analysis of clinical efficacy in 86 patients. Clin J Pain 2000;16:164–8.

26. Price DD, Long S, Wilsey B. Analysis of peak magnitude and duration of analgesia produced by local anesthetic injected into sympathetic ganglia of complex regional pain syndrome patients. Clin J Pain 1998;14:216–8.

27. Meier PM, Zurakowski D, Berde CB, et al. Lumbar sympathetic blockade in children with complex regional pain syndromes: a double blind placebo-controlled crossover trial. Anesthesiology 2009; 111(2):372–80.

28. Lillemoe KD, Cameron JL, Kaufman HS, et al. Chemical splanchnicectomy in patients with unresectable pancreatic cancer. A prospective randomized trial. Ann Surg 1993;217(5):447–55.

29. Wong GY, Schroeder DR, Carns PE. Effect of neurolytic celiac plexus block on pain relief, quality of life, and survival in patients with unresectable pancreatic cancer: a randomized controlled trial. JAMA 2004; 291:1092–9.

30. Eisenberg E, Carr DB, Chalmers TC. Neurolytic celiac plexus block for treatment of cancer pain: a meta-analysis. Anesth Analg 1995;80:290–5.

31. Plancarte R, Amescua C, Patt RB, et al. Superior hypogastric plexus block for pelvic cancer pain. Anesthesiology 1990;73:236–9.

32. Marples IL, Atkinson RE. Stellate ganglion block. Pain Rev 2001;8:3–11.

33. Malmqvist EL, Bengtsson M, Sorensen J. Efficacy of stellate ganglion block: a clinical study with bupivacaine. Reg Anesth 1992;17:340–7.

34. Davies DD. Incidence of major complications of neurolytic coeliac plexus block. J R Soc Med 1993; 86(5):264–6.

35. Galizia EJ, Lahiri SK. Paraplegia following coeliac plexus block with phenol. Case report. Br J Anaesth 1974;46(7):539–40.

36. Tran KM, Frank SM, Raja SN, et al. Lumbar sympathetic block for sympathetically maintained pain: changes in cutaneous temperatures and pain perception. Anesth Analg 2000;90(6):1396–401.

37. Rocco A. Anatomy of the lumbar sympathetic chain for radiofrequency lesioning. Reg Anesth Pain Med 1995;17(1):28.

38. Wong FC, Lee TW, Yuen KK, et al. Intercostal nerve blockade for cancer pain: effectiveness and selection of patients. Hong Kong Med J 2007;13(4): 266–70.

39. Anthony M. Cervicogenic headache. Prevalence and response to local steroid therapy. Clin Exp Rheumatol 2000;18(19):59–64.

Transcranial Magnetic Stimulation for Chronic Pain

Nicole A. Young, PhD[a,1], Mayur Sharma, MD[b,1],
Milind Deogaonkar, MD[b,*]

KEYWORDS

- Transcranial magnetic stimulation • Neuromodulation • Chronic pain • Neuropathic pain
- Fibromyalgia • Migraine

KEY POINTS

- Current data suggest that transcranial magnetic stimulation (TMS) has the potential to be an effective and complimentary treatment of patients with chronic neuropathic pain syndromes.
- The success of TMS for pain relief depends on the parameters of the stimulation delivered, the location of the neural target, and the duration of the treatment.
- TMS can be used to excite or inhibit underlying neural tissue that depends on long-term potentiation and long-term depression respectively.
- Multiple sessions of repetitive TMS (rTMS) and increased number of pulses per session have cumulative analgesic effects with long-lasting pain control in patients with chronic pain syndromes.
- Long-term randomized controlled studies investigating the optimal rTMS parameters, cortical targets, long-term efficacy of rTMS, interindividual variability, effect of oral analgesics, and predictors of analgesic efficacy are warranted to establish the efficacy of rTMS in patients with various chronic pain syndromes.

INTRODUCTION

Chronic pain is a common condition worldwide; affecting approximately one-third of the adult population in the United States.[1,2] This complex clinical conundrum poses significant management challenges to physicians. In epidemiologic studies, the prevalence of chronic pain is approximately 48% and that of chronic neuropathic pain varies from 6% to 8%.[3,4] Given its high prevalence in the general population, economists estimate that the annual cost of chronic pain ranges from $560 billion to $635 billion a year in the United States alone.[5] The International Association for the Study of Pain defined neuropathic pain as "pain initiated or caused by a primary lesion or dysfunction in the nervous system."[6,7] Neuropathic pain can be further classified as peripheral or central (depending on the site of the disorder) and acute or chronic (lasting >3 months).[6,7] Based on imaging studies, there is accruing evidence that chronic pain results from alteration in neural networks and central pain mechanisms including perception, sensitization, and pain modulation pathways.[8,9] Therefore, modulation of these neural networks may provide clinical benefits in patients with chronic pain syndromes.

[a] Department of Neuroscience, Center of Neuromodulation, Wexner Medical Center, The Ohio State University, 480 Medical Center Drive, Columbus, OH 43210, USA; [b] Department of Neurosurgery, Center of Neuromodulation, Wexner Medical Center, The Ohio State University, 480 Medical Center Drive, Columbus, OH 43210, USA
[1] Contributed equally.
* Corresponding author.
E-mail address: milind.deogaonkar@osumc.edu

neurosurgery.theclinics.com

In 1991, Tsubokawa and colleagues[10] showed the efficacy of motor cortex stimulation in patients with deafferentation pain. Since then, numerous investigators have explored this domain to alleviate symptoms in patients with chronic neuropathic pain.[11–13] The introduction of noninvasive brain stimulation reduced the morbidity associated with invasive stimulation techniques and fostered interest in this modality for chronic pain syndromes. The noninvasive modalities of neuromodulation include repetitive transcranial magnetic stimulation (rTMS), transcranial direct current stimulation, cranial electrotherapy stimulation, and reduced impedance noninvasive cortical electrostimulation.[14] Of these, rTMS is the most frequently used and studied modality in patients with chronic pain, with variable outcomes.[9,14–19] A recent systematic review on the utility of transcranial magnetic stimulation (TMS) in patients with fibromyalgia syndrome concluded that high-frequency rTMS at the left primary motor cortex (M1) significantly reduces the pain associated with fibromyalgia syndrome and has a lasting impact beyond the duration of stimulation.[20] Contrary to this, a recent Cochrane Systematic Review concluded that single doses of rTMS may provide short-term beneficial effects in patients with chronic pain; however, multiple doses of rTMS for chronic pain did not show consistent benefits across different studies.[14,18] To date, 30 studies have evaluated the efficacy of rTMS in 528 patients with chronic pain syndromes (fibromyalgia, complex regional pain syndrome, phantom limb pain, thalamic pain, poststroke pain, pain related to injury of spinal cord/brachial plexus).[14] This article focuses on the efficacy of rTMS in patients with different pain syndromes and the physiology and technique of rTMS with a review of the pertinent literature.

MECHANISM OF ACTION AND PARAMETERS OF rTMS RELEVANT TO CHRONIC PAIN MANAGEMENT

The technique of TMS was introduced in the 1950s, but it was not until the introduction of noninvasive magnetic stimulation by Barker and colleagues[21] in 1985 that the scope of this therapy was widened. Since then TMS has been evaluated for refractory depression, chronic pain, neuropathic pain, schizophrenia, and obsessive compulsive disorders, with varied success.[15,16,22–24] TMS involves generation of action potentials with either activation or inhibition of various cortical and subcortical neural networks by generating a magnetic field that penetrates the skull of the patient. High-frequency rTMS of the M1 has been shown to induce rapid changes and modulation of the sensorimotor networks in

healthy individuals.[25] It differs from conventional electrical stimulation in the way currents are induced in the underlying neural tissue. Simple electrical stimulation requires that current flow from an anode to a cathode placed on the scalp activates/inhibits neural tissue below; however, the impedance associated with the scalp and cranium limits the reach of electrical current to the most superficial layers of cortex (without increasing the electrical current to levels that are painful for patients). TMS uses electromagnetic induction to generate an electrical current. A high-current pulse is discharged from a stimulator to a wire coil to produce a magnetic field. When the wire coil is placed tangentially to the scalp, the magnetic field passes unobstructed through the scalp and cranium to excite or inhibit the neural tissue below. Compared with electrical stimulation, magnetic stimulation allows the study of focal neural tissue activation in which the signal is not impeded by other tissues and is minimally invasive to the patient.

As with other types of stimulation, the effect of TMS depends strongly on positioning of the source (ie, position of the coil), the orientation of the underlying cell structure, duration of stimulation, and the stimulation parameters used to activate the underlying neural tissue.[26] The currents induced by TMS flow parallel to the plane of the wire coil.[27,28] It has been suggested that there is preferential activation of cells that are horizontally positioned within the cortex when the coil placed tangentially to the scalp (**Figs. 1** and **2**), such that cortical interneurons are preferentially stimulated and cortical pyramidal neurons are activated transsynaptically because of their vertical orientation within the cortex[29–31]; however, this may be a generalization because it is difficult to accurately estimate the area of activation because of variation in the cortical geometry, currents generated, cerebral plasticity, membrane potentials, and ion channel activity.[32]

The ability of TMS to modify the synaptic characteristics of neural networks depends on stimulation parameters. The frequency at which the stimulation is delivered largely determines whether the stimulation produces an excitatory or inhibitory effect on the underlying neural tissue. In general, high-frequency stimulation increases the cortical excitability, whereas low-frequency stimulation has inhibitory control on the neural circuits.[33] High-frequency rTMS (>5 Hz) produces an excitatory effect on neural tissue by inducing a form of long-term potentiation (LTP)[34] that increases efficacy at the synapse that can last beyond the duration of a treatment session. High-frequency rTMS delivered to the left M1 has been shown to be effective in the treatment of widespread chronic

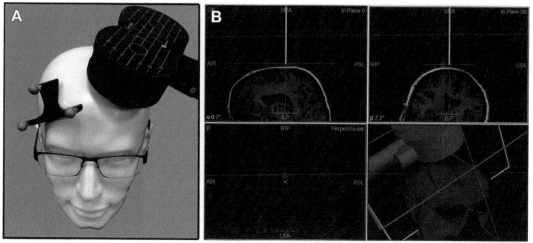

Fig. 1. (*A*) The positioning of a wire coil (MagVenture) when delivering TMS to motor cortex. The head tracker is adhered to the forehead on the opposite side to where stimulation is to be delivered. The 3 reflecting spheres are used in conjunction with an infrared camera to visualize the target location. (*B*) We use software from Localite to identify stimulation targets. Data from the orientation of the reflective spheres and camera are merged with a T1 magnetic resonance imaging of a patient. When the coil is positioned over the patient's cranium, the software displays the position of the coils in the sagittal, coronal, and horizontal planes, as well as providing a three-dimensional representation of the patient's cranium reconstructed from the MRI with the coil position registered in real time.

pain in patients with fibromyalgia, while simultaneously increasing short intracortical inhibition and intracortical facilitation in the motor cortex.[35] Patients with neuropathic pain who had received high-frequency TMS to motor cortex also had reduced intracortical inhibition that correlated with pain relief in the corresponding hand.[36] The ability of high-frequency TMS to increase synaptic efficacy is likely to depend on modulation of both the GABAergic and glutamatergic systems,[37–39]

which have been shown to be important in the modulation of function in motor cortex.[40,41] Low-frequency rTMS (≤ 1 Hz) produces an inhibitory effect on neural tissue via a long-term depression (LTD)–like mechanism.[42] However, the excitatory and inhibitory effects of high-frequency and low-frequency rTMS respectively depend on the target and the state of the polarization of the neural tissues being stimulated.[43] Patients with fibromyalgia who received low-frequency rTMS to the right

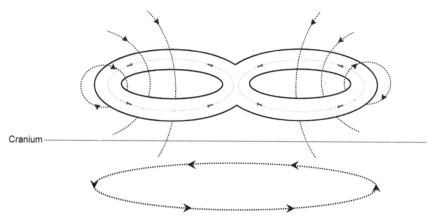

Fig. 2. Simplified diagram of the electrical and magnetic fields generated during TMS. The 2 circular figures represent a butterfly coil configuration for this example (*solid black lines*). Red dashed lines indicate the direction of the flow of current through the wire coils during TMS. Blue dashed lines indicate the direction of the magnetic field generated by the wire coil during stimulation. The black dashed line represents the direction of the currents generated in neural tissue as a result of TMS. The size of the field, penetrating depth through tissue, and level of activation depend on stimulation parameters and coil configuration.

dorsal prefrontal cortex reported improvements in both pain and mood.[44] Low-frequency magnetic stimulation can also be used successfully in the periphery for neuropathic pain management when stimulation is delivered at the site of nerve entrapment.[45] Both high-frequency and low-frequency TMS are effective for pain management and the effectiveness depends on target selection, which suggests that the neural networks involved in pain perception are both widespread and complex.

Theta burst stimulation (TBS) is a form of TMS that also modulates neural function in a way that reflects LTP-like and LTD-like mechanisms that last longer than those induced by rTMS.[46] TBS uses high-frequency bursts (3 pulses at 50 Hz) that are repeated at intervals of 200 milliseconds. Intermittent TBS (iTBS) increases the amplitude of neuron responses[46] and increases cortical excitability in human motor cortex,[47] whereas a continuous TBS (cTBS) pattern suppresses evoked responses.[48] Although the pattern of delivery was thought to determine its excitatory or inhibitory effect on neural tissue, recent work has shown that the effects of iTBS and cTBS may not be as clear.[49] Likewise, the success of TBS for pain management has been mixed. cTBS delivered to the M1 had been reported to reduce laser-evoked pain perception[50]; however, other studies have not shown either cTBS or iTBS to be effective when applied to M1 alone in patients with neuropathic pain.[49]

Successful pain management with magnetic stimulation may rely on a combination of stimulation types and targets that are tailored to the disease and specific symptoms. For instance, a recent study showed that the analgesic effects of high-frequency TMS are enhanced when iTBS is first delivered to M1, a paradigm known as priming.[49] Although this is an interesting perspective on stimulation-based therapies, more studies are needed to evaluate this approach.

Activation of cortical structures in turn transmits action potentials to various limbic and other pain modulation pathways such as cingulate gyrus, orbitofrontal cortex, insula, hippocampus, caudate nucleus, and periaqueductal areas in either an orthodromic or antidromic direction.[9,19,51] rTMS has been shown to induce the release of dopamine in the ipsilateral caudate nucleus, which might have implications in the clinical role of this therapy.[19] rTMS of the M1 and dorsolateral prefrontal cortex has been shown to have antinociceptive and antidepressants effects, respectively.[15,16] Release of endogenous opioids in the anterior cingulate cortex and periaqueductal gray matter has been implicated in the nociceptive effects of rTMS of M1.[52,53]

SAFETY PROFILE OF TMS

The excellent safety profile of TMS is the major advantage of this noninvasive treatment modality and led to the expansion of this therapy for a variety of indications. The most serious of the reported complications is the occurrence of seizures, and most of these complications occurred either because of nonadherence to recommended stimulation parameters or in patients who were on medications (tricyclic antidepressants, antipsychotics, theophylline, cocaine, alcohol, amphetamines, MDMA [3,4-methylenedioxy-N-methylamphetamine]) that are known to lower seizure threshold.[54] The risk of epilepsy following TMS is <1% in healthy individuals which increases to 1.4% in patients with history of epilepsy.[9,54] In addition, TMS in patients with intracranial implants can result in heating or magnetization of these implants and impaired functioning. Therefore TMS is relatively contraindicated in patients with DBS (Deep brain stimulation) electrodes, cochlear implants, or aneurysm clips, whereas it is safer in patients with titanium implants or implants containing ferromagnetic alloys.[9] Other reported adverse effects include histotoxicity, hearing disorders, persistent local pain, transient headache or discomfort at the TMS coil application, impaired cognition, psychiatric symptoms, and biological alterations.[9,20,54] In our study, the safety profile of TMS was assessed by noting the occurrence of any of the adverse effects mentioned earlier during the treatment sessions that may or may not have resulted in discontinuation of therapy in either of the groups.

TMS FOR CHRONIC PAIN

High-frequency rTMS of the M1 has been shown to induce rapid changes and modulation of the sensorimotor networks in healthy individuals.[25] High-frequency rTMS has also been shown to have a direct effect on sensory thresholds for both cold and hot temperature sensations and thus may be effective in alleviating symptoms in patients with chronic pain.[55] Low-frequency rTMS (1 Hz) over the M1 has been shown to induce early recovery from capsaicin-induced acute pain mediated by C fibers in healthy volunteers compared with sham stimulation and control cohorts.[56] This low-frequency stimulation over M1 was also associated with decreased regional cerebral blood flow (rCBF) in the right medial prefrontal cortex (Brodmann area [BA] 9) and a significant increase in rCBF in the right caudal anterior cingulate cortex (BA 24) and the left premotor area (BA 6).[56] However, the same study group reported facilitation of A-delta fiber–mediated acute pain by low-frequency rTMS over the motor cortex in 13 normal subjects using thulium:yttrium-aluminum-garnet laser stimulation.[57] High-frequency rTMS (10 Hz) of the M1 has similarly not been able to control A-delta fiber–mediated experimental electrically induced acute pain with an increase in the pain scores.[58] In contrast with this, continuous TBS of the M1 has been shown to significantly reduce the perception of laser-induced acute pain in both hands.[50] High-frequency rTMS of the medial (medial frontal cortex) and lateral (motor cortex) pain-regulating pathways has been shown to have variable effects on sensory perception and pain threshold levels.[59] High-frequency stimulation of lateral pain pathways resulted in increase in both sensory perception and pain threshold levels, whereas stimulation of medial pain pathways resulted in decrease in pain threshold levels with an increase in sensory perception levels.[59] There are conflicting reports of TMS of the medial frontal cortex on pain perception, with some of the studies reporting suppression and others facilitating perception of pain following stimulation.[60,61] There are similarly discordant findings regarding the efficacy of TMS of the sensorimotor cortex on the perception of experimentally induced pain.[59,60,62] Low-frequency (1 Hz) rTMS of the right dorsolateral prefrontal cortex (DLPFC) has been shown to increase pain tolerance and threshold to cold pressure test in 180 right-handed healthy volunteers.[63] High-frequency (10 Hz) rTMS over the left prefrontal cortex has been reported to increase thermal pain threshold in 20 healthy adults.[64] Therefore DLPFC can be explored as a potential cortical target to alleviate chronic pain. The results of these studies based on experimentally induced acute pain need to be interpreted cautiously because of the heterogeneity in the rTMS protocol, the cortical target stimulated, and the difference in the pathophysiology of acute and chronic pain mechanisms.

rTMS of M1 for Chronic Pain

In one of the initial studies on the utility of motor cortex stimulation using electrodes in patients with chronic pain, 8 of the 12 patients (67%) benefitted from this therapy after 1 year of stimulation.[10] In 1995, Migita and colleagues[65] reported the utility of rTMS (0.2 Hz using circular coils) applied to the contralateral M1 in 2 patients with central pain. One patient with central pain secondary to left putaminal hemorrhage reported significant pain relief following rTMS of contralateral M1, which was comparable with electrical cortical stimulation. However, another patient with cerebral palsy who underwent left thalamotomy twice at ages 9 and 13 years did not report attenuation of pain following rTMS of motor cortex.[65] Lefaucher and colleagues[66] in 2001 reported significant pain relief in 18 patients with chronic neurogenic pain (thalamic or brainstem stroke, n = 12; brachial plexus lesion, n = 6) following 10-Hz rTMS over the motor cortex compared with 0.5-Hz or sham stimulation. Later, the same group reported transient pain relief for about a week in 14 patients with thalamic stroke (n = 7) and trigeminal nerve lesion pain (n = 7) following a 20-minute session of 10-Hz rTMS over the motor cortex.[67] In 2003, Canavero and colleagues[68] reported that 50% of patients responded to motor cortex stimulation using rTMS (0.2 Hz, figure-of-eight and double-cone coils) in the long term in their series of 9 patients with central pain (poststroke pain n = 5, and spinal cord lesion pain n = 4). Another study using 20-Hz rTMS of the primary cortex in 12 patients with chronic pain (spinal cord lesion n = 2, osteomyelitis n = 1, complex regional pain syndrome n = 2, phantom limb pain n = 1, peripheral nerve lesion n = 6) did not reveal a significant difference between active (mean visual analog scale [VAS] reduction, −4.0% ± 15.6%) and sham stimulation (mean VAS reduction, −2.3% ± 8.8%) in terms of pain relief.[69] Numerous studies have reported the efficacy of rTMS (10 Hz) of the M1 in relieving chronic pain related to thalamic/brainstem stroke, trigeminal nerve, brachial plexus, nerve trunk, and spinal cord lesions compared with sham stimulation.[17,36,70–73] One of the studies reported that rTMS is more effective when applied to an area adjacent to the cortical representation of the painful zone compared with stimulation of the motor cortex corresponding with the painful area (facial pain improved instead of hand pain when the hand motor cortical area was stimulated).[71] Pleger and colleagues[74] reported transient pain relief in 70% of patients (7 of 10 patients) with complex regional pain syndrome following rTMS (10 Hz) of the motor cortex, with maximum benefits being observed 15 minutes after stimulation. Similar results were reported by Picarelli and colleagues[75] in 23 patients with refractory complex regional pain syndrome affecting the upper limbs, and rTMS was recommended as an add-on therapy in such patients. In contrast with this, Irlbacher and colleagues[76] reported no significant difference in pain relief following sham stimulation or rTMS (1 Hz or 5 Hz) in 27 patients with central (n = 13) and phantom limb pain (n = 14). High-frequency (20 Hz) rTMS of the motor cortex has been shown to have long-lasting effects (2 weeks) on pain control in patients with poststroke or trigeminal nerve lesion pain.[77] Low-frequency rTMS (1 Hz) has been shown to have a proalgesic effect, whereas

Table 1
Studies showing the efficacy of rTMS in patients with chronic pain syndromes

Study	Origin of Pain (and # Patients)	Target	Stimulation Parameters	Pain Outcome
Migita et al,[65] 1995	Cerebral palsy and thalamotomy (n = 1) and putamen hemorrhage (n = 1)	M1	0.2 Hz, 80% of stimulator output	Successful pain relief in 1 patient
Lefaucheur et al,[66] 2001	Neuropathic pain (n = 18)	M1	0.5 Hz or 10 Hz, 80% RMT	20% reduction in pain symptoms at 10 Hz
Lefaucheur et al,[67] 2001	Thalamic stroke (n = 7) and trigeminal neuropathy (n = 7)	M1	10 Hz, 80% RMT	30% reduction in pain symptoms for up to 8 d
Reid et al,[81] 2001	Teeth removal (n = 1)	Left prefrontal cortex	20 Hz, 100% RMT	42% decrease in pain lasting for 1 mo
Canavero et al,[68] 2003	Stroke (n = 5) and lesion (n = 4)	M1	0.2 Hz, 100% of stimulator output	50% of patients were responsive to treatment
Rollnik et al,[69] 2002	Varying chronic pain syndromes (n = 12)	M1	20 Hz, 80% RMT	Analgesic effects in only some patients
Topper et al,[82] 2003	Root avulsion (n = 2)	Posterior parietal cortex	1 Hz or 10 Hz, 110% RMT	Transient pain relief only
Lefaucheur et al,[17] 2004	Stroke (n = 24) and trigeminal nerve, brachial plexus, and spinal cord lesion (n = 36)	M1	10 Hz, 80% RMT	Pain level reduction in 65% of patients, better results with facial pain
Lefaucheur et al,[17] 2004	Brachial plexus lesion (n = 1)	M1	10 Hz, 80% RMT	Pain controlled with monthly sessions of rTMS for 16 mo
Pleger et al,[74] 2004	Complex regional pain syndrome (n = 10)	M1	10 Hz, 110% RMT	Pain decreased in 70% of patients, but effect was transient
Kheder et al,[77] 2005	Neuropathic pain (n = 48)	M1 hand area	20 Hz, 80% RMT	Pain relief that lasted 2 wk
Fregni et al,[83] 2005	Chronic pancreatitis (n = 5)	Secondary somatosensory cortex	1 Hz or 20 Hz, 90% RMT	36% improvement in pain with 1-Hz, improvement with left-side stimulation only
Andre-Obadia et al,[78] 2006	Stroke (n = 10) and lesion (n = 4)	M1	1 Hz or 20 Hz, 90% RMT	Repetitive 20 Hz most effective for analgesia

Study	Condition (n)	Target site	Parameters	Outcome
Lefaucheur et al,[71] 2006	Chronic neuropathic pain of face and hand, stroke (n = 9) and lesion (n = 27)	M1	10 Hz, 90% RMT	Best efficacy with stimulation to the hand and face area of M1
Hirayama et al,[84] 2006	Deafferentation pain	M1, S1, premotor, SMA	5 Hz, 90% RMT	Pain relief in 50% of patients stimulated in M1 only, relief lasted 3 h
Sampson et al,[97] 2006	Fibromyalgia (n = 4)	DLPFC	1 Hz, 110% RMT	Good analgesic effect that lasts >15 wk
Passard et al,[100] 2007	Fibromyalgia (n = 30)	M1	10 Hz, 80% RMT	Long-lasting decrease in chronic widespread pain
Lefaucheur et al,[73] 2008	Neuropathic pain (n = 48)	M1	1 Hz or 10 Hz, 90% RMT	Improvement in thermal sensory perception to the painful region that correlated with pain relief
Brockardt et al,[85] 2009	Chronic neuropathic pain (n = 4)	Prefrontal cortex	10 Hz, 100% RMT	Decrease of 19% in daily pain
Carretero et al,[96] 2009	Fibromyalgia (n = 28)	DLPFC	1 Hz, 110% RMT	No difference
Lefaucheur et al,[72] 2010	Chronic neuropathic pain in 1 upper limb (n =32)	M1, hand area	10 Hz, 90% RMT	Reduction of laser-induced pain scores in patients with pain
Picarelli et al,[75] 2010	Complex regional pain syndrome type 1 (n = 23)	M1	10 Hz, 100% RMT	Reduction in pain intensity
Mhalla et al,[35] 2011	Fibromyalgia (n = 40)	M1	10 Hz, 80% RMT	Long-term, reduced pain intensity
Short et al,[98] 2011	Fibromyalgia (n = 20)	Prefrontal cortex	10 Hz, 120% RMT	29% reduction in pain symptoms
Lee et al,[44] 2012	Fibromyalgia (n = 15)	DLPFC (1-Hz group), and M1 (10-Hz group)	1 Hz, 110% RMT or 10 Hz, 80% RMT	Low-frequency group (DLPFC) had greater improvement in pain and antidepressant effects relative to high-frequency group (M1)
Hosomi et al,[79] 2013	Neuropathic pain (n = 70)	M1	5 Hz, 90% RMT	Transient, modest pain relief
Tzabazis et al,[99] 2013	Fibromyalgia (n = 16)	Dorsal anterior cingulate cortex	1 Hz or 10 Hz, 110% RMT	43% reduction in pain score at 10 Hz, no effect at 1 Hz

Abbreviations: RMT, resting motor threshold; S1, postcentral gyrus or primary somatosensory cortex; SMA, supplementary motor area.

high-frequency rTMS (20 Hz) predicted the efficacy of subsequent motor cortex stimulation in a double-blind study.[78] A randomized double-blind, sham-controlled, crossover study (7 centers, n = 70 patients) concluded that daily multisession (10 sessions) high-frequency (5 Hz) rTMS of M1 provides short-term and modest pain relief in patients with neuropathic pain.[79] Therefore, low-frequency (1 Hz or 5 Hz) rTMS of M1 is unlikely to induce significant beneficial effects in terms of pain control compared with high-frequency (10 Hz or 20 Hz) stimulation (**Table 1**).[76,80]

rTMS of Other Cortical Areas for Chronic Pain

In 2001, Reid and Pridmore[81] reported 42% pain relief following high-frequency rTMS of left dorsolateral prefrontal cortex in a patient with pain associated with teeth extraction, and this pain relief lasted for 4 weeks. rTMS (1 Hz and 10 Hz) of the posterior parietal cortex similarly led to a reduction in pain intensity in patients with arm pain associated with cervical nerve root avulsion, which lasted for up to 10 minutes.[82] However, this study did not recommend the use of rTMS in the treatment of phantom pain. Fregni and colleagues[83] reported the efficacy of rTMS of right and left secondary sensory cortex (S2) in 5 patients with pain associated with chronic pancreatitis. In this study, low-frequency (1 Hz) rTMS of the right S2 region was associated with 62% reduction in pain, whereas high-frequency (20 Hz) rTMS of left S2 worsened the pain associated with chronic pancreatitis.[83] Hirayama and colleagues[84] performed 5-Hz rTMS of M1, postcentral gyrus (S1), premotor area, and supplementary motor area in 20 patients with refractory deafferentation pain (thalamic/brainstem stroke, trigeminal nerve, brachial plexus, or spinal cord lesion pain). Fifty percent of patients (10 of 20 patients) who received rTMS of M1 reported significant and beneficial pain relief that lasted for 3 hours; however, none of the other stimulated cortical regions was effective in controlling pain.[84] In contrast, high-frequency (10 Hz) rTMS of the prefrontal cortex in patients with chronic neuropathic pain has been shown to decrease daily pain on an average and pain at its worst by 19% compared with sham stimulation.[85] A single 20-minute session of 10-Hz rTMS over the left DLPFC was associated with significant (40%) reduction in postoperative patient-controlled morphine use following gastric bypass surgery (see **Table 1**).[86,87]

TMS FOR FIBROMYALGIA

Fibromyalgia syndrome (FMS) is the second most common rheumatologic disorder, affecting approximately 4 to 10 million people in the United States.[9,20,88–91] According to the American college of Rheumatology (ACR) in 1990 the diagnosis of FMS requires the presence of chronic diffuse pain and painful response to 11 of 18 tender points.[92] Other symptoms include excessive fatigue, nonrestorative sleep, mood and cognitive disturbances, and diminished physical reserves.[20,92,93] FMS is more common in women (75%–90%) compared with men.[20,93] Various pharmacologic and nonpharmacologic interventions have been shown to have a clinical benefit in patients with this syndrome.[94] This complex syndrome requires a multidisciplinary approach with emphasis on patients' education, use of pharmacotherapeutic agents (tricyclic antidepressants), cardiovascular exercise, and cognitive-behavior therapy in varying combinations.[94,95] rTMS of the M1 and dorsolateral prefrontal cortex has been shown to be efficacious in reducing pain associated with fibromyalgia in various studies.[35,44,96–100]

Sampson and colleagues[97] reported the efficacy of low-frequency (1-Hz) rTMS of the right DLPFC in 4 patients with depression and fibromyalgia. Average pain reduced from a pretreatment level of 8.2 (Likert scale) to 1.5 after rTMS and 2 patients reported complete resolution of pain in this study.[97] Another study reported significant reduction in pain intensity with long-term (day 5 to week 25) maintenance of analgesic effects and improvement in items related to quality of life following 10-Hz rTMS of left primary cortex in patients with fibromyalgia.[35] Likewise, Short and colleagues[98] reported 29% reduction in pain symptoms following 10-Hz rTMS of prefrontal cortex in 20 patients with fibromyalgia. In contrast with these studies, Carretero and colleagues[96] reported no significant difference between 1-Hz rTMS of the dorsolateral prefrontal cortex and sham stimulation in patients with fibromyalgia. Lee and colleagues[44] evaluated the efficacy of low-frequency (1 Hz) rTMS of DLPFC, high-frequency (10 Hz) rTMS of left primary cortex, and sham stimulation in patients with fibromyalgia and reported that the low-frequency group (DLPFC) had greater improvement in pain and antidepressant effects compared with the high-frequency group (left M1). In addition to M1 and DLPFC, dorsal anterior cingulate cortex has been evaluated as a potential target for rTMS with beneficial effects at 10 Hz compared with 1 Hz in patients with fibromyalgia (see **Table 1**).[99]

TMS FOR MIGRAINE

Migraine is a debilitating condition with prevalence of 11.7% in the general population.[101] This condition is more prevalent in women (17.1%) compared with men (5.6%).[101] Migrainous attacks may or may not be associated or preceded by transient neurologic symptoms and are classified as with or without aura, respectively. Based on animal studies, altered cortical excitability has been implicated in the pathophysiology of migraine.[102–104] There are conflicting reports of hyperexcitability or hypoexcitability of the visual cortex during interictal periods.[103,105–107] Studies have reported different responses to visual motor cortex stimulation at different stimulation intensities in patients with migraine.[108] Cortical spreading depression and trigeminovascular activation are the likely mechanisms responsible for migranous auras and attacks respectively, but the exact pathogenesis of migraine remains to be elucidated.[109] TMS has been investigated to study the physiology of the visual cortex and to evaluate the efficacy of cortical stimulation in patients with migraine.[107,110–112] Phosphene threshold (PT) is used to gauge the excitability of visual cortex in various studies.[112] In a recent meta-analysis of studies evaluating the efficacy of rTMS in patients with migraine, a significant difference was reported in the PT in patients with migraine with aura and healthy controls, whereas no statistically significant difference was noted between patients with migraine without aura and the control group.[111] Using a figure-of-eight coil for rTMS, no significant difference in PT was noted between patients with migraine with or without aura and healthy controls.[111] However, with a circular coil for rTMS, a lower threshold for phosphene generation was noted in patients with migraine with or without aura compared with healthy control groups.[111] Significant clinical and methodological heterogeneity was noted across different clinical studies in this meta-analysis. In a randomized, double-blind, sham-controlled trial, single-pulse TMS has been shown to be efficacious in reducing pain at 2 hours in patients with migraine attacks with aura compared with sham stimulation.[113] In addition, the pain relief was sustained at 24 hours and 48 hours after stimulation.[113] High-frequency rTMS over the left dorsolateral prefrontal cortex has been shown to be efficacious as preventive treatment in patients with chronic migraine compared with placebo.[114] In another study, low-frequency rTMS of the vertex was not effective in migraine prophylaxis compared with placebo stimulation.[115] Neuromodulation using rTMS is a useful modality in understanding the pathophysiology and offering pain relief to patients with acute migranous attacks with aura. The utility of this modality as a prophylactic treatment of migraine needs further investigation. Further large prospective randomized controlled trials are required to establish the efficacy of rTMS in patients with migraine.

SUMMARY

rTMS has been shown to have significant analgesic effects and can be used as a complementary treatment modality in patients with chronic refractory pain syndromes such as poststroke pain (thalamic/brainstem), trigeminal neuropathy pain, nerve root/brachial plexus avulsion pain, spinal cord injury pain, fibromyalgia, or migraine. The efficacy of rTMS according to the diagnosis of different pain syndromes has not yet been elucidated. In terms of cortical targets, high-frequency stimulation of M1 has been shown to have significant analgesic effects in patients with various pain syndromes compared with sham stimulation. rTMS of DLPFC has significant analgesic effects in patients with fibromyalgia. Advances in neuroimaging and navigation techniques have made it possible to target these cortical structures precisely and to explore other targets such as anterior cingulate cortex and other cortical areas for rTMS. Low-frequency rTMS has been shown to have less favorable outcomes in terms of pain control compared with high-frequency stimulation. rTMS can also be used to select patients with chronic refractory pain syndromes who can benefit from surgically implanted motor cortex stimulation.[16]

The major limitation of rTMS is the short duration of analgesia achieved with transcranial stimulation and therefore the efficacy of this modality is not established in patients with chronic pain syndromes. Nevertheless, rTMS has been shown to be effective in achieving significant analgesia in patients with postoperative pain or acute pain syndromes. Multiple sessions of rTMS and increased number of pulses per session have cumulative analgesic effects with long-lasting pain control in patients with chronic pain syndromes.[77,100,116] However, long-term randomized controlled studies investigating the optimal rTMS parameters, cortical targets, long-term efficacy of rTMS, interindividual variability, effect of analgesics, and predictors of analgesic efficacy are warranted to establish the efficacy of rTMS in patients with various chronic pain syndromes.

REFERENCES

1. Johannes CB, Le TK, Zhou X, et al. The prevalence of chronic pain in United States adults: results of an Internet-based survey. J Pain 2010;11(11):1230–9.

2. Wong WS, Fielding R. Prevalence and characteristics of chronic pain in the general population of Hong Kong. J Pain 2011;12(2):236–45.

3. Torrance N, Smith BH, Bennett MI, et al. The epidemiology of chronic pain of predominantly neuropathic origin. Results from a general population survey. J Pain 2006;7(4):281–9.

4. Smith BH, Torrance N. Epidemiology of neuropathic pain and its impact on quality of life. Curr Pain Headache Rep 2012;16(3):191–8.

5. Gaskin DJ, Richard P. The economic costs of pain in the United States. J Pain 2012;13(8):715–24.

6. Dworkin RH. An overview of neuropathic pain: syndromes, symptoms, signs, and several mechanisms. Clin J Pain 2002;18(6):343–9.

7. Merskey H, Bogduk N. Classification of chronic pain. Descriptions of chronic pain syndromes and definitions of pain terms. 2nd edition. Seattle (WA): IASP Press; 1994.

8. Williams DA, Gracely RH. Biology and therapy of fibromyalgia. Functional magnetic resonance imaging findings in fibromyalgia. Arthritis Res Ther 2006;8(6):224.

9. Perocheau D, Laroche F, Perrot S. Relieving pain in rheumatology patients: Repetitive transcranial magnetic stimulation (rTMS), a developing approach. Joint Bone Spine 2014;81:22–6.

10. Tsubokawa T, Katayama Y, Yamamoto T, et al. Chronic motor cortex stimulation for the treatment of central pain. Acta Neurochir Suppl (Wien) 1991;52:137–9.

11. Cioni B, Meglio M. Motor cortex stimulation for chronic non-malignant pain: current state and future prospects. Acta Neurochir Suppl 2007; 97(Pt 2):45–9.

12. Bolognini N, Olgiati E, Maravita A, et al. Motor and parietal cortex stimulation for phantom limb pain and sensations. Pain 2013;154(8):1274–80.

13. Nguyen JP, Nizard J, Keravel Y, et al. Invasive brain stimulation for the treatment of neuropathic pain. Nature reviews. Neurology 2011;7(12):699–709.

14. O'Connell NE, Wand BM, Marston L, et al. Non-invasive brain stimulation techniques for chronic pain. Cochrane Database Syst Rev 2014;(4): CD008208.

15. Lefaucheur JP. The use of repetitive transcranial magnetic stimulation (rTMS) in chronic neuropathic pain. Neurophysiol Clin 2006;36(3):117–24.

16. Lefaucheur JP, Antal A, Ahdab R, et al. The use of repetitive transcranial magnetic stimulation (rTMS) and transcranial direct current stimulation (tDCS) to relieve pain. Brain Stimul 2008;1(4):337–44.

17. Lefaucheur JP, Drouot X, Menard-Lefaucheur I, et al. Neurogenic pain relief by repetitive transcranial magnetic cortical stimulation depends on the origin and the site of pain. J Neurol Neurosurg Psychiatr 2004;75(4):612–6.

18. O'Connell NE, Wand BM, Marston L, et al. Non-invasive brain stimulation techniques for chronic pain. A report of a Cochrane systematic review and meta-analysis. Eur J Phys Rehabil Med 2011; 47(2):309–26.

19. Strafella AP, Paus T, Barrett J, et al. Repetitive transcranial magnetic stimulation of the human prefrontal cortex induces dopamine release in the caudate nucleus. J Neurosci 2001;21(15): RC157.

20. Marlow NM, Bonilha HS, Short EB. Efficacy of transcranial direct current stimulation and repetitive transcranial magnetic stimulation for treating fibromyalgia syndrome: a systematic review. Pain Pract 2013;13(2):131–45.

21. Barker AT, Jalinous R, Freeston IL. Non-invasive magnetic stimulation of human motor cortex. Lancet 1985;1(8437):1106–7.

22. George MS, Nahas Z, Kozel FA, et al. Improvement of depression following transcranial magnetic stimulation. Curr Psychiatry Rep 1999;1(2):114–24.

23. Martin JL, Barbanoj MJ, Perez V, et al. Transcranial magnetic stimulation for the treatment of obsessive-compulsive disorder. Cochrane Database Syst Rev 2003;(3):CD003387.

24. Zaman R, Thind D, Kocmur M. Transcranial magnetic stimulation in schizophrenia. Neuro Endocrinol Lett 2008;29(Suppl 1):147–60.

25. Yoo WK, You SH, Ko MH, et al. High frequency rTMS modulation of the sensorimotor networks: behavioral changes and fMRI correlates. Neuroimage 2008;39(4):1886–95.

26. Maccabee PJ, Amassian VE, Eberle LP, et al. Magnetic coil stimulation of straight and bent amphibian and mammalian peripheral nerve in vitro: locus of excitation. J Physiol 1993;460: 201–19.

27. Roth BJ, Saypol JM, Hallett M, et al. A theoretical calculation of the electric field induced in the cortex during magnetic stimulation. Electroencephalogr Clin Neurophysiol 1991;81(1):47–56.

28. Saypol JM, Roth BJ, Cohen LG, et al. A theoretical comparison of electric and magnetic stimulation of the brain. Ann Biomed Eng 1991;19(3):317–28.

29. Day BL, Thompson PD, Dick JP, et al. Different sites of action of electrical and magnetic stimulation of the human brain. Neurosci Lett 1987;75(1): 101–6.

30. Amassian VE, Quirk GJ, Stewart M. A comparison of corticospinal activation by magnetic coil and electrical stimulation of monkey motor cortex. Electroencephalogr Clin Neurophysiol 1990;77(5): 390–401.

31. Amassian VE, Stewart M, Quirk GJ, et al. Physiological basis of motor effects of a transient stimulus to cerebral cortex. Neurosurgery 1987;20(1): 74–93.

32. Pell GS, Roth Y, Zangen A. Modulation of cortical excitability induced by repetitive transcranial magnetic stimulation: influence of timing and geometrical parameters and underlying mechanisms. Prog Neurobiol 2011;93(1):59–98.

33. Fitzgerald PB, Fountain S, Daskalakis ZJ. A comprehensive review of the effects of rTMS on motor cortical excitability and inhibition. Clin Neurophysiol 2006;117(12):2584–96.

34. Esser SK, Huber R, Massimini M, et al. A direct demonstration of cortical LTP in humans: a combined TMS/EEG study. Brain Res Bull 2006;69(1): 86–94.

35. Mhalla A, Baudic S, Ciampi de Andrade D, et al. Long-term maintenance of the analgesic effects of transcranial magnetic stimulation in fibromyalgia. Pain 2011;152(7):1478–85.

36. Lefaucheur JP, Drouot X, Menard-Lefaucheur I, et al. Motor cortex rTMS restores defective intracortical inhibition in chronic neuropathic pain. Neurology 2006;67(9):1568–74.

37. Kapogiannis D, Wassermann EM. Transcranial magnetic stimulation in clinical pharmacology. Cent Nerv Syst Agents Med Chem 2008;8(4): 234–40.

38. Reis J, Swayne OB, Vandermeeren Y, et al. Contribution of transcranial magnetic stimulation to the understanding of cortical mechanisms involved in motor control. J Physiol 2008;586(2):325–51.

39. Ziemann U, Rothwell JC, Ridding MC. Interaction between intracortical inhibition and facilitation in human motor cortex. J Physiol 1996;496(Pt 3): 873–81.

40. Young NA, Vuong J, Flynn C, et al. Optimal parameters for microstimulation derived forelimb movement thresholds and motor maps in rats and mice. J Neurosci Methods 2011;196(1):60–9.

41. Young NA, Vuong J, Teskey GC. Development of motor maps in rats and their modulation by experience. J Neurophysiol 2012;108(5):1309–17.

42. Chen R, Classen J, Gerloff C, et al. Depression of motor cortex excitability by low-frequency transcranial magnetic stimulation. Neurology 1997;48(5): 1398–403.

43. Siebner HR, Lang N, Rizzo V, et al. Preconditioning of low-frequency repetitive transcranial magnetic stimulation with transcranial direct current stimulation: evidence for homeostatic plasticity in the human motor cortex. J Neurosci 2004;24(13): 3379–85.

44. Lee SJ, Kim DY, Chun MH, et al. The effect of repetitive transcranial magnetic stimulation on fibromyalgia: a randomized sham-controlled trial with 1-mo follow-up. Am J Phys Med Rehabil 2012;91(12): 1077–85.

45. Leung A, Fallah A, Shukla S. Transcutaneous magnetic stimulation (tMS) in alleviating post-traumatic peripheral neuropathic pain states: a case series. Pain Med 2014. [Epub ahead of print].

46. Huang YZ, Edwards MJ, Rounis E, et al. Theta burst stimulation of the human motor cortex. Neuron 2005;45(2):201–6.

47. Di Lazzaro V, Pilato F, Dileone M, et al. The physiological basis of the effects of intermittent theta burst stimulation of the human motor cortex. J Physiol 2008;586(16):3871–9.

48. Di Lazzaro V, Pilato F, Saturno E, et al. Theta-burst repetitive transcranial magnetic stimulation suppresses specific excitatory circuits in the human motor cortex. J Physiol 2005;565(Pt 3):945–50.

49. Lefaucheur JP, Ayache SS, Sorel M, et al. Analgesic effects of repetitive transcranial magnetic stimulation of the motor cortex in neuropathic pain: influence of theta burst stimulation priming. Eur J Pain 2012;16(10):1403–13.

50. Poreisz C, Csifcsak G, Antal A, et al. Theta burst stimulation of the motor cortex reduces laser-evoked pain perception. Neuroreport 2008;19(2):193–6.

51. Paus T, Castro-Alamancos MA, Petrides M. Cortico-cortical connectivity of the human mid-dorsolateral frontal cortex and its modulation by repetitive transcranial magnetic stimulation. Eur J Neurosci 2001;14(8):1405–11.

52. de Andrade DC, Mhalla A, Adam F, et al. Neuropharmacological basis of rTMS-induced analgesia: the role of endogenous opioids. Pain 2011;152(2): 320–6.

53. Maarrawi J, Peyron R, Mertens P, et al. Motor cortex stimulation for pain control induces changes in the endogenous opioid system. Neurology 2007;69(9): 827–34.

54. Lefaucheur JP, Andre-Obadia N, Poulet E, et al. French guidelines on the use of repetitive transcranial magnetic stimulation (rTMS): safety and therapeutic indications. Neurophysiol Clin 2011;41(5–6): 221–95 [in French].

55. Johnson S, Summers J, Pridmore S. Changes to somatosensory detection and pain thresholds following high frequency repetitive TMS of the motor cortex in individuals suffering from chronic pain. Pain 2006;123(1–2):187–92.

56. Tamura Y, Okabe S, Ohnishi T, et al. Effects of 1-Hz repetitive transcranial magnetic stimulation on acute pain induced by capsaicin. Pain 2004; 107(1–2):107–15.

57. Tamura Y, Hoshiyama M, Inui K, et al. Facilitation of A[delta]-fiber-mediated acute pain by repetitive transcranial magnetic stimulation. Neurology 2004;62(12):2176–81.

58. Mylius V, Reis J, Knaack A, et al. High-frequency rTMS of the motor cortex does not influence the nociceptive flexion reflex but increases the unpleasantness of electrically induced pain. Neurosci Lett 2007;415(1):49–54.

59. Yoo WK, Kim YH, Doh WS, et al. Dissociable modulating effect of repetitive transcranial magnetic stimulation on sensory and pain perception. Neuroreport 2006;17(2):141–4.

60. Kanda M, Mima T, Oga T, et al. Transcranial magnetic stimulation (TMS) of the sensorimotor cortex and medial frontal cortex modifies human pain perception. Clin Neurophysiol 2003;114(5):860–6.

61. Mylius V, Reis J, Kunz M, et al. Modulation of electrically induced pain by paired pulse transcranial magnetic stimulation of the medial frontal cortex. Clin Neurophysiol 2006;117(8):1814–20.

62. Poreisz C, Antal A, Boros K, et al. Attenuation of N2 amplitude of laser-evoked potentials by theta burst stimulation of primary somatosensory cortex. Exp Brain Res 2008;185(4):611–21.

63. Graff-Guerrero A, Gonzalez-Olvera J, Fresan A, et al. Repetitive transcranial magnetic stimulation of dorsolateral prefrontal cortex increases tolerance to human experimental pain. Brain Res Cogn Brain Res 2005;25(1):153–60.

64. Borckardt JJ, Smith AR, Reeves ST, et al. Fifteen minutes of left prefrontal repetitive transcranial magnetic stimulation acutely increases thermal pain thresholds in healthy adults. Pain Res Manag 2007;12(4):287–90.

65. Migita K, Uozumi T, Arita K, et al. Transcranial magnetic coil stimulation of motor cortex in patients with central pain. Neurosurgery 1995;36(5):1037–9 [discussion: 1039–40].

66. Lefaucheur JP, Drouot X, Keravel Y, et al. Pain relief induced by repetitive transcranial magnetic stimulation of precentral cortex. Neuroreport 2001; 12(13):2963–5.

67. Lefaucheur JP, Drouot X, Nguyen JP. Interventional neurophysiology for pain control: duration of pain relief following repetitive transcranial magnetic stimulation of the motor cortex. Neurophysiol Clin 2001;31(4):247–52.

68. Canavero S, Bonicalzi V, Dotta M, et al. Low-rate repetitive TMS allays central pain. Neurol Res 2003; 25(2):151–2.

69. Rollnik JD, Wustefeld S, Dauper J, et al. Repetitive transcranial magnetic stimulation for the treatment of chronic pain - a pilot study. Eur Neurol 2002; 48(1):6–10.

70. Lefaucheur JP, Drouot X, Menard-Lefaucheur I, et al. Neuropathic pain controlled for more than a year by monthly sessions of repetitive transcranial magnetic stimulation of the motor cortex. Neurophysiol Clin 2004;34(2):91–5.

71. Lefaucheur JP, Hatem S, Nineb A, et al. Somatotopic organization of the analgesic effects of motor cortex rTMS in neuropathic pain. Neurology 2006; 67(11):1998–2004.

72. Lefaucheur JP, Jarry G, Drouot X, et al. Motor cortex rTMS reduces acute pain provoked by laser stimulation in patients with chronic neuropathic pain. Clin Neurophysiol 2010;121(6):895–901.

73. Lefaucheur JP, Drouot X, Menard-Lefaucheur I, et al. Motor cortex rTMS in chronic neuropathic pain: pain relief is associated with thermal sensory perception improvement. J Neurol Neurosurg Psychiatr 2008;79(9):1044–9.

74. Pleger B, Janssen F, Schwenkreis P, et al. Repetitive transcranial magnetic stimulation of the motor cortex attenuates pain perception in complex regional pain syndrome type I. Neurosci Lett 2004;356(2):87–90.

75. Picarelli H, Teixeira MJ, de Andrade DC, et al. Repetitive transcranial magnetic stimulation is efficacious as an add-on to pharmacological therapy in complex regional pain syndrome (CRPS) type I. J Pain 2010;11(11):1203–10.

76. Irlbacher K, Kuhnert J, Roricht S, et al. Central and peripheral deafferent pain: therapy with repetitive transcranial magnetic stimulation. Nervenarzt 2006;77(10):1196, 1198–203. [in German].

77. Khedr EM, Kotb H, Kamel NF, et al. Longlasting antalgic effects of daily sessions of repetitive transcranial magnetic stimulation in central and peripheral neuropathic pain. J Neurol Neurosurg Psychiatr 2005;76(6):833–8.

78. Andre-Obadia N, Peyron R, Mertens P, et al. Transcranial magnetic stimulation for pain control. Double-blind study of different frequencies against placebo, and correlation with motor cortex stimulation efficacy. Clin Neurophysiol 2006;117(7): 1536–44.

79. Hosomi K, Shimokawa T, Ikoma K, et al. Daily repetitive transcranial magnetic stimulation of primary motor cortex for neuropathic pain: a randomized, multicenter, double-blind, crossover, sham-controlled trial. Pain 2013;154(7):1065–72.

80. Saitoh Y, Hirayama A, Kishima H, et al. Reduction of intractable deafferentation pain due to spinal cord or peripheral lesion by high-frequency repetitive transcranial magnetic stimulation of the primary motor cortex. J Neurosurg 2007;107(3): 555–9.

81. Reid P, Pridmore S. Improvement in chronic pain with transcranial magnetic stimulation. Aust N Z J Psychiatry 2001;35(2):252.

82. Topper R, Foltys H, Meister IG, et al. Repetitive transcranial magnetic stimulation of the parietal cortex transiently ameliorates phantom limb pain-like syndrome. Clin Neurophysiol 2003;114(8): 1521–30.

83. Fregni F, DaSilva D, Potvin K, et al. Treatment of chronic visceral pain with brain stimulation. Ann Neurol 2005;58(6):971–2.

84. Hirayama A, Saitoh Y, Kishima H, et al. Reduction of intractable deafferentation pain by navigation-guided repetitive transcranial magnetic stimulation

of the primary motor cortex. Pain 2006;122(1–2): 22–7.

85. Borckardt JJ, Smith AR, Reeves ST, et al. A pilot study investigating the effects of fast left prefrontal rTMS on chronic neuropathic pain. Pain Med 2009; 10(5):840–9.

86. Borckardt JJ, Weinstein M, Reeves ST, et al. Postoperative left prefrontal repetitive transcranial magnetic stimulation reduces patient-controlled analgesia use. Anesthesiology 2006;105(3):557–62.

87. Borckardt JJ, Reeves ST, Weinstein M, et al. Significant analgesic effects of one session of postoperative left prefrontal cortex repetitive transcranial magnetic stimulation: a replication study. Brain Stimul 2008;1(2):122–7.

88. Crofford LJ, Clauw DJ. Fibromyalgia: where are we a decade after the American College of Rheumatology classification criteria were developed? Arthritis Rheum 2002;46(5):1136–8.

89. Bannwarth B, Blotman F, Roue-Le Lay K, et al. Fibromyalgia syndrome in the general population of France: a prevalence study. Joint Bone Spine 2009;76(2):184–7.

90. Branco JC, Bannwarth B, Failde I, et al. Prevalence of fibromyalgia: a survey in five European countries. Semin Arthritis Rheum 2010;39(6):448–53.

91. Schochat T, Raspe H. Elements of fibromyalgia in an open population. Rheumatology (Oxford) 2003; 42(7):829–35.

92. Wolfe F, Smythe HA, Yunus MB, et al. The American College of Rheumatology 1990 criteria for the classification of fibromyalgia. Report of the Multicenter Criteria Committee. Arthritis Rheum 1990; 33(2):160–72.

93. Wolfe F, Hawley DJ, Goldenberg DL, et al. The assessment of functional impairment in fibromyalgia (FM): Rasch analyses of 5 functional scales and the development of the FM Health Assessment Questionnaire. J Rheumatol 2000;27(8):1989–99.

94. Goldenberg DL, Burckhardt C, Crofford L. Management of fibromyalgia syndrome. JAMA 2004; 292(19):2388–95.

95. Hauser W, Thieme K, Turk DC. Guidelines on the management of fibromyalgia syndrome - a systematic review. Eur J Pain 2010;14(1):5–10.

96. Carretero B, Martin MJ, Juan A, et al. Low-frequency transcranial magnetic stimulation in patients with fibromyalgia and major depression. Pain Med 2009;10(4):748–53.

97. Sampson SM, Rome JD, Rummans TA. Slow-frequency rTMS reduces fibromyalgia pain. Pain Med 2006;7(2):115–8.

98. Short EB, Borckardt JJ, Anderson BS, et al. Ten sessions of adjunctive left prefrontal rTMS significantly reduces fibromyalgia pain: a randomized, controlled pilot study. Pain 2011;152(11): 2477–84.

99. Tzabazis A, Aparici CM, Rowbotham MC, et al. Shaped magnetic field pulses by multi-coil repetitive transcranial magnetic stimulation (rTMS) differentially modulate anterior cingulate cortex responses and pain in volunteers and fibromyalgia patients. Mol Pain 2013;9(1):33.

100. Passard A, Attal N, Benadhira R, et al. Effects of unilateral repetitive transcranial magnetic stimulation of the motor cortex on chronic widespread pain in fibromyalgia. Brain 2007;130(Pt 10): 2661–70.

101. Lipton RB, Bigal ME, Diamond M, et al. Migraine prevalence, disease burden, and the need for preventive therapy. Neurology 2007;68(5):343–9.

102. Welch KM, Barkley GL, Tepley N, et al. Central neurogenic mechanisms of migraine. Neurology 1993;43(6 Suppl 3):S21–5.

103. Cosentino G, Fierro B, Vigneri S, et al. Cyclical changes of cortical excitability and metaplasticity in migraine: evidence from a repetitive transcranial magnetic stimulation study. Pain 2014; 155(6):1070–8.

104. van den Maagdenberg AM, Pizzorusso T, Kaja S, et al. High cortical spreading depression susceptibility and migraine-associated symptoms in Ca(v) 2.1 S218L mice. Ann Neurol 2010;67(1):85–98.

105. Shepherd AJ. Increased visual after-effects following pattern adaptation in migraine: a lack of intracortical excitation? Brain 2001;124(Pt 11): 2310–8.

106. Cosentino G, Brighina F, Talamanca S, et al. Reduced threshold for inhibitory homeostatic responses in migraine motor cortex? A tDCS/TMS study. Headache 2014;54(4):663–74.

107. Schoenen J, Ambrosini A, Sandor PS, et al. Evoked potentials and transcranial magnetic stimulation in migraine: published data and viewpoint on their pathophysiologic significance. Clin Neurophysiol 2003;114(6):955–72.

108. Brighina F, Cosentino G, Vigneri S, et al. Abnormal facilitatory mechanisms in motor cortex of migraine with aura. Eur J Pain 2011;15(9):928–35.

109. Brighina F, Cosentino G, Fierro B. Brain stimulation in migraine. Handb Clin Neurol 2013;116: 585–98.

110. Fumal A, Bohotin V, Vandenheede M, et al. Transcranial magnetic stimulation in migraine: a review of facts and controversies. Acta Neurol Belg 2003;103(3):144–54.

111. Brigo F, Storti M, Nardone R, et al. Transcranial magnetic stimulation of visual cortex in migraine patients: a systematic review with meta-analysis. J Headache Pain 2012;13(5):339–49.

112. Merabet LB, Theoret H, Pascual-Leone A. Transcranial magnetic stimulation as an investigative tool in the study of visual function. Optom Vis Sci 2003;80(5):356–68.

113. Lipton RB, Dodick DW, Silberstein SD, et al. Single-pulse transcranial magnetic stimulation for acute treatment of migraine with aura: a randomised, double-blind, parallel-group, sham-controlled trial. Lancet Neurol 2010;9(4):373–80.

114. Brighina F, Piazza A, Vitello G, et al. rTMS of the prefrontal cortex in the treatment of chronic migraine: a pilot study. J Neurol Sci 2004;227(1):67–71.

115. Teepker M, Hotzel J, Timmesfeld N, et al. Low-frequency rTMS of the vertex in the prophylactic treatment of migraine. Cephalalgia 2010;30(2):137–44.

116. Defrin R, Grunhaus L, Zamir D, et al. The effect of a series of repetitive transcranial magnetic stimulations of the motor cortex on central pain after spinal cord injury. Arch Phys Med Rehabil 2007;88(12): 1574–80.

Technological Innovations in Implants Used for Pain Therapies

Andrew Shaw, MD, Mayur Sharma, MBBS,
Milind Deogaonkar, MD, Ali Rezai, MD*

KEYWORDS

- Peripheral field stimulation • Neuromodulation • Innovation • Technology • Spinal cord stimulation

KEY POINTS

- Spinal cord stimulation was first attempted in 1967 to relieve the pain of a patient dying with cancer. Since that time electrodes, implanted pulse generators, patient programmers, and techniques have drastically improved with the progress of technology.
- Implanters have a wide armamentarium of devices to implant electrodes in any part of the body. Traditional Tuohy needles have been adapted for not only spinal cord stimulation but also peripheral/field stimulation. The Epimed Coudé, Abbocath catheters, and ON-Q tunnelers have found new applications in neuromodulation and provide safe and effective alternatives to traditional approaches.
- There are a variety of electrodes available from percutaneous cylindrical electrodes to paddle leads. Through innovation there are now percutaneous paddle leads, paddle leads with five-column arrays, and 16-contact cylindrical electrodes that provide implanters and programmers greater ability to provide adequate pain coverage.
- Lead anchoring is essential to avoid lead migration with resultant loss of efficacy and need for revision surgery. There are compression and screw restraint devices that have significantly reduced rates of lead migration compared with suture anchoring alone.
- Implanted pulse generators have acquired new abilities with adaptive stimulation, MRI compatibility, rechargeability, and update capable devices. Adaptive stimulation changes stimulation automatically based on the patient's position. MRI compatibility allows for full-body MRIs, so patients requiring serial imaging can benefit from this therapy. Most recently, an IPG has been developed whose software can be updated remotely allowing for the most up-to-date algorithms to be applied to a battery that can last up to 10 years.
- Innovation is a result of dissatisfaction with the current paradigm and driven by curiosity to explore new avenues to relieve the suffering of patients.

INTRODUCTION

Pain management has experienced tremendous growth in implantable therapies secondary to the innovations of bioengineers, implanters, and industry. From the first trial of spinal cord stimulation (SCS) in 1967 using an externalized electrode and generator for intractable cancer pain to the introduction of positional stimulation using three-axis accelerometers, the treatment of chronic pain continues to evolve with the constant introduction

Conflict of Interest: We declare no conflict of interest.
Department of Neurological Surgery, Wexner Medical Center, Center for Neuromodulation, Ohio State University, 410 West 10th Avenue, Columbus, OH 43210, USA
* Corresponding author.
E-mail address: Ali.Rezai@osumc.edu

of new innovations and technologies.[1,2] Every aspect of neuromodulation is amenable to innovation from implanting devices to anchors, electrodes, programming, and even patient programmers. Patients with previously refractory neuropathic pain syndromes have new and effective pain management strategies that are a direct result of innovations in implantable devices.

SCS and peripheral nerve field stimulation have been used for the treatment of numerous refractory chronic pain conditions including occipital neuralgia, trigeminal neuralgia, failed back surgery syndrome, chronic inguinal neuralgia, postherpetic neuralgia, and refractory angina.[3–14] Patients with severe refractory pain are often managed with a variety of treatment modalities that include narcotics, anticonvulsants, antidepressants, nerve blocks, and destructive procedures with limited or short-term benefit.[3–8,10–12] SCS and field stimulation have consistently been shown to reduce pain significantly in appropriately selected patients.[3–8,10–14] The mechanism of pain relief from neurostimulation has not been completely elucidated, but is based on the gate control theory of pain initially published by Melzack and Wall[15] with the blockade of distal nociceptive information and C fiber inhibition.[9,10] Later, the "neuromatrix theory of pain" was proposed by Melzack in 1989, which described the "neurosignature" patterns of nerve impulses by a widely distributed neural network in response to noxious stimuli.[16,17] Since the initial description of SCS in 1967, implanters, scientists, and innovators continue to change the face of neuromodulation with advances in implantable pain management technologies.

IMPLANTING DEVICES

Percutaneous implantation techniques for subcutaneous and SCS cylindrical electrodes involves the use of slightly curved 14- to 15-gauge Tuohy needles.[3–8,10–12,14,18]

From a historical perspective, field stimulators were placed in an open fashion with direct visualization of nerves and associated significant complications and poor efficacy.[19,20] Subcutaneous implantation started with tunneling using a curved hemostat.[10] The initial SCS experience also involved an open approach with a thoracic laminectomy and placement of electrodes under direct visualization.[1]

Tuohy needles are hollow hypodermic needles with a stylet and are of appropriate gauge to allow implantation of electrodes in a variety of locations (**Fig. 1**C). Several percutaneous techniques have been developed for the implantation of peripheral nerve/field stimulators including the use of curved

Tuohy needles, intravenous catheters (Abbocath; Abbott Ireland), and the Epimed Coudé (Epimed, NY).[21,22] For percutaneous spinal cord stimulator implantation, Tuohy needles remain one of the primary instruments chosen for implantation of electrodes.

The Epimed Coudé has been chosen by some implanters because it is malleable and allows for improved steering and test stimulation before lead implantation.[22] It has a 14-gauge circular profile that facilitates the passage of multipolar electrodes without the risk of lead shearing. There is an associated 5-mm stimulating tip with an end connector at the proximal part of the needle that allows connection to standard regional-anesthesia nerve stimulators. This is especially useful in field or peripheral nerve stimulation when using test stimulation to determine the optimal site for electrode implantation.

Abbocath IV catheters (Abbott Ireland) have also been used for implantation of subcutaneous electrodes for peripheral nerve and field stimulation. Abbocaths come in two sizes and several different gauges. For neuromodulation a 14-gauge cannula is chosen because it is of sufficient size to accommodate an electrode. There are two different lengths (50- and 150-mm cannula) to choose from depending on the desired application. Here a sharp needle is used to make the preliminary trajectory through the subcutaneous tissues and a softer catheter is left behind for the implantation of the electrodes.

The ON-Q (Braun Melsungen AG, Pfieffewiesen, Germany) Pain Relief System and ON-Q Tunneling System have been used to deliver local anesthesia to surgical sites and have been shown to provide improved postoperative pain relief from orthopedic to cardiothoracic surgery.[23,24] Recently, ON-Q Tunneling System has been used for the implantation of peripheral nerve and field stimulators. This system involves the use of a blunt needle with a soft flexible silastic peel-away sheath that is left in place following tunneling. Multiple sheaths can be implanted with a single needle in the event multiple electrodes are planned. Furthermore, the stylet of the ON-Q is malleable and can be made to conform to specific body angles (see **Fig. 1** A and B). There are a variety of lengths of ON-Q systems available (3.25, 5, 8, and 12 inches), which can be tailored according to the region of interest. The 17-gauge cannula is preferred for peripheral field stimulators.

St. Jude Medical introduced the Epiducer (St. Jude Medical, Plano, TX) in 2009 as an innovative product to deliver an array of SCS leads including paddle leads, cylindrical leads, or combination of leads without the need for an open laminectomy or laminotomy (**Fig. 2**). This device has been shown to be safe in a multicenter trial involving 34 patients with no adverse events related to this

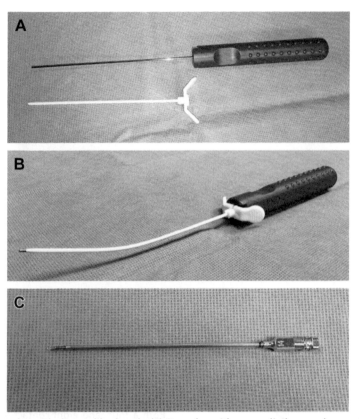

Fig. 1. (*A*) ON-Q tunneler with disposable sheath. (*B*) Tunneler with an applied curve demonstrating the malleability of the tunneler. (*C*) Traditional Tuohy needle used for implanting peripheral nerve and field stimulators.

lead delivery system.[25] This system still requires a Tuohy needle to access the epidural space. Once the epidural space is accessed a guidewire is inserted and the Tuohy needle is removed. The Epiducer involves an inner dilator, an outer sheath, and a flexible radiopaque tip that is designed to avoid penetrating the dura. The inner dilator is then passed over the guidewire and through the ligamentum flavum. The outer sheath does not contact the dura. Once this occurs, the inner stylet and guidewire can be removed leaving a sheath to insert an array of electrodes including the S series percutaneous paddle lead (St. Jude Medical).

The goal of surgery is to implant electrodes safely and efficiently at appropriate locations so as to achieve desired outcomes. All described tools have been used effectively with good outcomes. Ultimately, implanters must decide what tools they are comfortable with and the appropriateness of the application.

ELECTRODES

The S series Percutaneous Paddle Lead by St. Jude Medical is the first paddle lead to be introduced into the epidural space in a percutaneous manner (**Fig. 3**). Both paddle and cylindrical electrodes are used regularly by implanters with each having their own benefits. Paddle leads are flat two-dimensional insulated electrodes that provide stimulation in a unidirectional manner with lower rates of lead migration; improved coverage and outcomes; and lower amplitude, which could prolong battery life.[26,27] Cylindrical electrodes provide stimulation circumferentially and can be implanted in a percutaneous manner. This affords the advantage of lower postoperative pain and need for open neurosurgical implantation.

The S Series Percutaneous paddle lead requires the use of the Epiducer (described previously) for implantation. This paddle lead comes with a stylet and thus can be steered to the desired location. It has a single bank of contacts and is available in two different models (four and eight contacts). The paddle lead can also be implanted surgically if required. The lead has been shown to be safe and effective with low migration rates in 81 patients. This same study showed that it can be implanted percutaneously under local anesthesia, which allows for intraoperative test stimulation to ensure adequate pain coverage.[28]

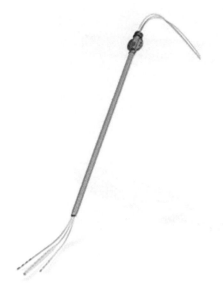

Epiducer with Leads.

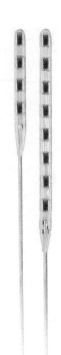

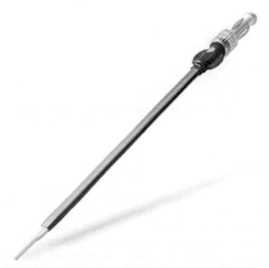

Fig. 2. Epiducer with an electrode array and as a single unit. (*Reprinted* with permission of St. Jude Medical, © 2014. All rights reserved.)

The first percutaneous 16-contact lead was introduced in 2011 by Boston Scientific (Natick, MA) named the Infinion (**Fig. 4**). This is a cylindrical lead that can be implanted percutaneously and individually, paired, or as a part of an electrode array. Boston Scientific developed the Precision Spectra implanted pulse generators (IPG), which can accommodate 32 contacts affording greater variability in electrode arrays and programming compared with the standard 16-contact IPGs.

The Penta paddle lead (St. Jude Medical) is the only paddle lead with a five-column array with four rows that provides 20 contacts of coverage

Fig. 3. The S series Percutaneous Paddle lead can be used with the Epiducer to introduce a paddle lead into the epidural space in a percutaneous manner. Both a four- and eight-contact lead is demonstrated here. (*Reprinted* with permission of St. Jude Medical, © 2014. All rights reserved.)

(**Fig. 5**). The profile of this lead provides wide lateral coverage of 9 mm and precise field control because it has more options for programming. This is especially beneficial because the actual midline of the spinal cord is 1 to 2 mm to the right or left of the midline.[29] The wide profile ensures the ability for programming to steer current to the actual position of the spinal cord.

ANCHORS

Clik Anchor (Boston Scientific; **Fig. 6**A) and Swift-Lock Anchor (St. Jude Medical; see **Fig. 6**B)

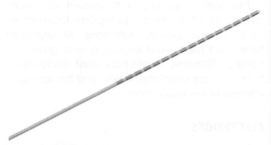

Fig. 4. The Infinion lead is the first 16-contact percutaneous lead introduced by Boston Scientific in 2011. (*Courtesy of* Boston Scientific, Natick, MA.)

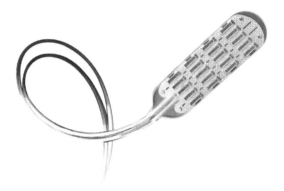

Fig. 5. The Penta paddle lead shown here as the only paddle lead with a five-column array with four rows that provides 20 contacts of coverage in a single lead. (*Reprinted* with permission of St. Jude Medical, © 2014. All rights reserved.)

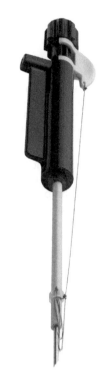

Fig. 7. FiXate Tissue band was developed as a semiautomatic suturing device that can be used for lead and catheter anchoring. (*Courtesy of* Boston Scientific, Natick, MA.)

provide a mechanism for securing the anchor to the lead and then the anchor to the fascia. These anchors are radiopaque making them visible under fluoroscopy. In addition they have a low profile, and the Clik Anchor has a polyether urethane sleeve internally that protects the lead from ever being touched by the plastic when securing the lead with a set screw restraint and torque hex wrench. There is a hole on each side allowing for two sutures to be used to secure the lead to underlying fascia. These anchors afford the advantage of easy reversibility allowing the anchor to move up and down the lead if needed.

FiXate Tissue band (Boston Scientific) is a semiautomatic suturing device that can be used for lead or catheter anchoring (**Fig. 7**). It was designed to be an efficient, simple, and secure method of securing lead anchors to the underlying fascia.

Titan anchor (Medtronic Inc, Minneapolis, MN) is a cylindrical low-profile anchor that has been used for securing cylindrical percutaneous spinal cord

stimulator leads (**Fig. 8**). It requires the placement of three nonabsorbable sutures. The first suture is used to crimp the anchor on the lead. The other two are then used to secure the anchor to the underlying fascia. There are undulations on the body of the anchor that prevent the sutures from moving after implantation. Kim and colleagues[30] showed similar rates of lead migration for percutaneous and paddle leads when using these anchors.

Injex anchor (Medtronic) is an injectable anchor that comes as a bi-wing or bumpy model and is intended to compress along the lead instead of

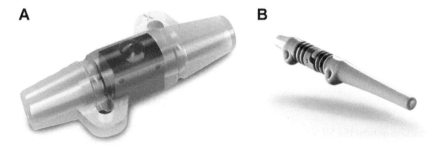

Fig. 6. (*A*) Clik Anchor by Boston Scientific and (*B*) Swift-Lock Anchor by St. Jude Medical are mechanical locking anchors that are radiopaque and low profile for patient comfort. There are also two anchoring points to secure them to the underlying fascia. (*Courtesy of* Boston Scientific, Natick, MA; and *Reprinted* with permission of St. Jude Medical, © 2014. All rights reserved.)

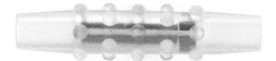

Fig. 8. Titan anchor is a cylindrical low-profile anchor that secures leads by circumferential compression. This has largely been replaced by the Injex anchor system. (*Reprinted* with the permission of Medtronic, Inc. Copyright © 2009.)

requiring a set screw restraint system (**Fig. 9**). It is low profile, flexible, and soft unlike its counterparts and made up of silicone/barium sulfate. The bi-wing has two wings for securing sutures. The bumpy anchor can be anchored directly to the fascia. To remove the anchor the Injex must be cut with an anchor removal tool that contains a blunt tip and protected blade. This anchoring system has replaced Titan anchors because Medtronic testing data showed a 58% greater retention strength with Injex anchor compared with Titan anchor. St. Jude Medical created the Cinch anchor, which is also a flexible, radiopaque silicone anchor that is similar to the bumpy Injex anchor in that it can be sutured across the anchor to the fascia.

Anchoring devices have undergone several rounds of evolution. Initially sutures were used alone to secure the lead to the fascia and maintain strain relief loops. Now there are a variety of anchors to choose from depending on implanter preference and preferred product. Each comes with its own advantages and shortcomings including profile, securing method (compression vs screw restraint), and ease of use. Anchoring and strain relief loops are essential in providing a secure lead and to avoid lead migration with resultant loss of efficacy and need for revision surgery.

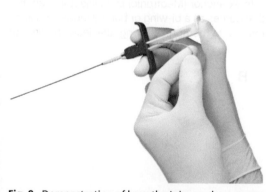

Fig. 9. Demonstration of how the Injex anchor secures a cylindrical electrode by passing the lead through the anchor and "injecting" it onto the fascia. This must then be anchored with nonabsorbable suture. (*Reprinted* with the *permission* of Medtronic, Inc. Copyright © 2012.)

IPGs

IPGs have improved significantly over the years. North and colleagues[18] in the 1990s showed that multichannel devices have improved clinical results when compared with single-channel devices. Then in 2007 using a patient-interactive computer system, standard programming and interleaved stimulation were compared in a double-blind randomized study.[31] They showed that paresthesia and pain coverage with interleaved stimulation was superior to standard programming in part because of frequency doubling.[31] As programming continues to improve so do the IPGs. They are now smaller, rechargeable, adaptable, compatible with magnetic resonance imaging (MRI), and have greater programming capabilities and battery life.

ADAPTIVE STIMULATION

Up to 71% of patients report discomfort when changing positions that results in changing stimulation parameters or adjusting position. To adapt to these changes patients must use their programmers to change stimulation settings.

Holsheimer and colleagues[32] reported on the normal position of the spinal cord in the spinal canal in 26 healthy volunteers in the prone and supine positions. They noted that there is a greater than two-fold variation in the dorsal cerebrospinal fluid layers with significant variation in the medio-lateral position of the spinal cord between prone and supine positioning. Further studies have shown that energy requirements do change based on positioning with supine requiring the lowest amplitudes.[33]

Medtronic developed the Restore Sensor Neurostimulator, which provides Adaptive stimulation (**Fig. 10**). The IPG can detect patient position based on three-axis accelerometers similar to those seen in smart phones. This IPG also records patient activity that allows programmers and implanters to evaluate and optimize stimulation parameters. Different programs can then be provided based on patient positioning and therapeutic benefit. This is typically done after 6 weeks to allow surgical changes to resolve. Once programmed the IPG changes stimulation based on patient positioning.

BURST STIMULATION

Innovation is not limited to hardware alone. In fact, St. Jude with the Prodigy TM Chronic Pain System with Burst Technology is conducting the Success Using Neuromodulation with Burst study. This is a randomized crossover study aimed at looking at safety and efficacy of

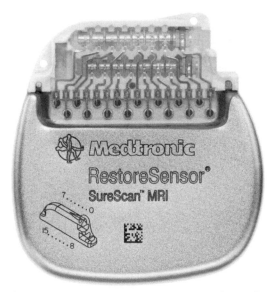

Fig. 10. Restore Sensor Surescan MRI combines the advantage of adaptive stimulation based on patient positioning with MRI compatibility when used with Medtronic Vectris leads. The IPG can hold 16 contacts and boasts MRI compatibility. (*Reprinted* with the permission of Medtronic, Inc. Copyright © 2013.)

burst stimulation compared with tonic stimulation in spinal cord stimulators. Tonic stimulation works by interrupting pain signals and replacing it with paresthesias. Some patients lose efficacy over time, and the tingling sensation may fluctuate with position. The Prodigy system then offers the combination of both tonic and burst stimulation. Burst stimulation was developed to not only improve pain but also reduce paresthesias that may be bothersome to some patients. Burst stimulation adds another layer of options for programmers to further tailor therapy and improve patient quality of life, especially those who have lost efficacy over time. The Prodigy system also boasts the advantage of being smaller in size and has the longest-lasting battery life for a rechargeable SCS in its class.

MRI COMPATIBILITY

Most companies have conditions in which their SCS system can undergo an MRI of the brain with a head coil alone. Please refer to the specifics of the implanted equipment and manufacturers' recommendations.

Medtronic developed the Restore Sensor Sure Scan MRI, which is compatible with a full-body MRI when used with Vectris leads (see **Fig. 10;** **Fig. 11**). This is the first full-body MRI-compatible SCS system that avoids the need for explantation to obtain an MRI. This technology may

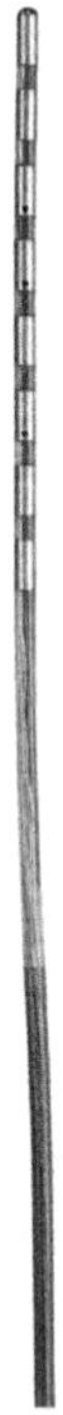

Fig. 11. The Vectris lead is a standard eight-contact cylindrical electrode that when combined with a Surescan MRI IPG can undergo MRI safely. (*Reprinted* with the permission of Medtronic, Inc. Copyright © 2013.)

allow SCS therapies to be used in patients requiring serial MRI scans that were previously not eligible for these procedures. In addition it combines MRI compatibility with adaptive stimulation to maximize ease of use. MRI guidelines have been developed that should be referenced before undergoing any MRI and at a hospital where radiology clinicians are familiar with the technology.

Other Advances in IPGs

Boston Scientific developed the Precision Spectra System, which has the option of using 32 contacts and four lead inputs (**Fig. 12**). It also uses their proprietary software, Bionic Navigator Programming, with Illumina 3D, which boasts control in three-dimensional space. It has the advantage of using Fluorosync interface (**Fig. 13**) where leads can be placed on a map as they appear on fluoroscopic images to allow for customized programming via their algorithm. Furthermore, Lead Sync technology allows for the programming software to adjust for lead offset by synchronizing parallel contacts and detecting relative lead position.

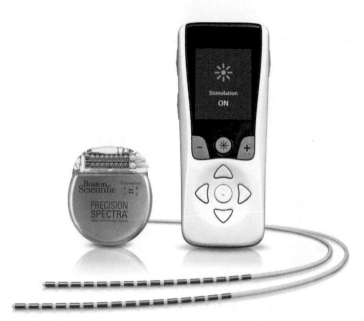

Fig. 12. The Precision Spectra System has the option of using 32 contacts with four-lead inputs on its IPG. This system can be used with Bionic Navigator Programming with Illumina 3D, which boasts control in three-dimensional space. (*Courtesy of* Boston Scientific, Natick, MA.)

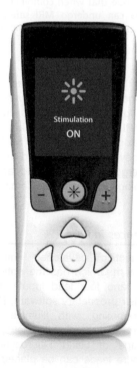

Fig. 13. The Fluorosync interface allows for virtual lead placement on a fluoroscopic map to allow programmers to sync the actual lead locations as determined by fluoroscopy with software to allow for customized programming via their algorithm. (*Courtesy of* Boston Scientific, Natick, MA.)

An upgradeable IPG has been developed by St. Jude Medical in their Protégé Spinal Cord Stimulator (**Fig. 14**). This product recently received Food and Drug Administration approval and is the first of its kind to allow software updates as technology advances. With its 10-year battery life, the ability to upgrade the software can allow patients to benefit from the newest and most innovative programming algorithms.

PATIENT PROGRAMMER

Patient programmers have greater capabilities with more options that can be controlled directly by the patient beyond simple amplitude and on/off state. The programmers have also become smaller, lighter, and wireless (see **Fig. 12**).

ELECTRICAL NERVE BLOCK

Neuros Medical TM (Willoughby, OH) has developed the patented platform of electrical nerve blockade. Residual limb pain (stump pain) is less common than phantom limb pain and affects up to 25% of amputees following surgery. The few options available include field stimulation, SCS, and the use of transcutaneous electrical nerve stimulation units. Neuros Medical developed the Altius System High Frequency Nerve Block therapy for the management of postamputation pain. Currently, this system is not available commercially and is still in the development

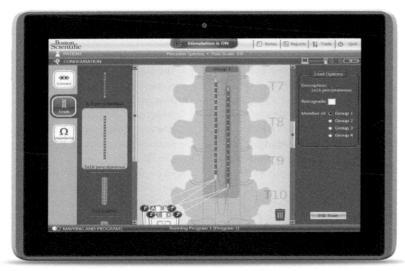

Fig. 14. Protégé Spinal Cord Stimulator is the first IPG that can have a software upgrade. With a life of around 10 years this will prove beneficial to patients and programmers allowing them to apply the latest techniques to further tailor therapy. (*Reprinted* with permission of St. Jude Medical, © 2014. All rights reserved.)

stages. This technology requires surgery where the nerve that had been cut during the amputation or suspected to have a neuroma is identified with ultrasound. The nerve is then dissected and the stimulator placed in direct contact with that nerve. High-frequency stimulation (10,000 Hz) is then applied for short periods of time to effectively block nerve signal transmission for 12 to 18 hours. A multicenter clinical trial is being developed to evaluate the safety and efficacy of this therapy.

SUMMARY

There's a way to do it better—find it.
　　　　　　　　　　　— Thomas Edison

We keep moving forward, opening new doors, and doing new things, because we're curious and curiosity keeps leading us down new paths.
　　　　　　　　　　　— Walt Disney

Innovation requires determination, dedication, and dissatisfaction with the current situation. Implantable pain management devices need innovative implanters to drive the field into the future. Technology will only continue to improve if clinicians are not satisfied with what they have now. Wires, contacts, and batteries are currently very effective in alleviating the suffering of patients. But can it be done better, faster, safer, and less invasive? Innovation continues to change neuromodulation and will continue to do so as the understanding of technology and the nervous system continues to grow.

ACKNOWLEDGMENTS

A special thanks to Medtronic Inc (Santa Clara, California, Epimed Johnstown, NY), St. Jude Medical(Plano, TX, USA), and Boston Scientific (Boston Scientific, Natick, MA, USA) for providing images of their various innovations. Protégé, S-Series, Swift-Lock, Epiducer, and St. Jude Medical are trademarks of St. Jude Medical, Inc., or its related companies.

REFERENCES

1. Shealy CN, Mortimer JT, Reswick JB. Electrical inhibition of pain by stimulation of the dorsal columns: preliminary clinical report. Anesth Analg 1967; 46(4):489–91.
2. Schultz DM, Webster L, Kosek P, et al. Sensor-driven position-adaptive spinal cord stimulation for chronic pain. Pain Physician 2012;15(1):1–12.
3. Burns B, Watkins L, Goadsby PJ. Treatment of medically intractable cluster headache by occipital nerve stimulation: long-term follow-up of eight patients. Lancet 2007;369(9567):1099–106.
4. Dunteman E. Peripheral nerve stimulation for unremitting ophthalmic postherpetic neuralgia. Neuromodulation 2002;5(1):32–7.
5. Johnstone CS, Sundaraj R. Occipital nerve stimulation for the treatment of occipital neuralgia-eight case studies. Neuromodulation 2006;9(1):41–7.
6. Monti E. Peripheral nerve stimulation: a percutaneous minimally invasive approach. Neuromodulation 2004;7(3):193–6.
7. Oh MY, Ortega J, Bellotte JB, et al. Peripheral nerve stimulation for the treatment of occipital neuralgia

and transformed migraine using a c1-2-3 subcutaneous paddle style electrode: a technical report. Neuromodulation 2004;7(2):103–12.

8. Paicius RM, Bernstein CA, Lempert-Cohen C. Peripheral nerve field stimulation in chronic abdominal pain. Pain Physician 2006;9(3):261–6.

9. Slavin KV, Colpan ME, Munawar N, et al. Trigeminal and occipital peripheral nerve stimulation for craniofacial pain: a single-institution experience and review of the literature. Neurosurg Focus 2006;21(6):E5.

10. Slavin KV, Wess C. Trigeminal branch stimulation for intractable neuropathic pain: technical note. Neuromodulation 2005;8(1):7–13.

11. Stinson LW Jr, Roderer GT, Cross NE, et al. Peripheral subcutaneous electrostimulation for control of intractable post-operative inguinal pain: a case report series. Neuromodulation 2001;4(3):99–104.

12. Weiner RL, Reed KL. Peripheral neurostimulation for control of intractable occipital neuralgia. Neuromodulation 1999;2(3):217–21.

13. Murray S, Carson KG, Ewings PD, et al. Spinal cord stimulation significantly decreases the need for acute hospital admission for chest pain in patients with refractory angina pectoris. Heart 1999;82(1):89–92.

14. North RB, Kidd DH, Zahurak M, et al. Spinal cord stimulation for chronic, intractable pain: experience over two decades. Neurosurgery 1993;32(3):384–94 [discussion: 394–5].

15. Melzack R, Wall PD. Pain mechanisms: a new theory. Science 1965;150(3699):971–9.

16. Melzack R. Pain and the neuromatrix in the brain. J Dent Educ 2001;65(12):1378–82.

17. Iannetti GD, Mouraux A. From the neuromatrix to the pain matrix (and back). Exp Brain Res 2010;205(1):1–12.

18. North RB, Ewend MG, Lawton MT, et al. Spinal cord stimulation for chronic, intractable pain: superiority of "multi-channel" devices. Pain 1991;44(2):119–30.

19. Kirsch WM, Lewis JA, Simon RH. Experiences with electrical stimulation devices for the control of chronic pain. Med Instrum 1975;9(5):217–20.

20. Nielson KD, Watts C, Clark WK. Peripheral nerve injury from implantation of chronic stimulating electrodes for pain control. Surg Neurol 1976;5(1):51–3.

21. Goroszeniuk T, Pang D, Al-Kaisy A, et al. Subcutaneous target stimulation-peripheral subcutaneous field stimulation in the treatment of refractory angina: preliminary case reports. Pain Pract 2012;12(1):71–9.

22. Goroszeniuk T, Pang D, Shetty A, et al. Percutaneous peripheral neuromodulation lead insertion using a novel stimulating Coude needle. Neuromodulation 2013. [Epub ahead of print].

23. Dowling R, Thielmeier K, Ghaly A, et al. Improved pain control after cardiac surgery: results of a randomized, double-blind, clinical trial. J Thorac Cardiovasc Surg 2003;126(5):1271–8.

24. Morgan SJ, Jeray KJ, Saliman LH, et al. Continuous infusion of local anesthetic at iliac crest bone-graft sites for postoperative pain relief. A randomized, double-blind study. J Bone Joint Surg Am 2006;88(12):2606–12.

25. Loge D, De Coster O, Washburn S. Technological innovation in spinal cord stimulation: use of a newly developed delivery device for introduction of spinal cord stimulation leads. Neuromodulation 2012;15(4):392–401.

26. North RB, Kidd DH, Olin JC, et al. Spinal cord stimulation electrode design: prospective, randomized, controlled trial comparing percutaneous and laminectomy electrodes-part I: technical outcomes. Neurosurgery 2002;51(2):381–9 [discussion: 389–90].

27. North RB, Kidd DH, Petrucci L, et al. Spinal cord stimulation electrode design: a prospective, randomized, controlled trial comparing percutaneous with laminectomy electrodes: part II-clinical outcomes. Neurosurgery 2005;57(5):990–6 [discussion: 990–6].

28. Kinfe TM, Schu S, Quack FJ, et al. Percutaneous implanted paddle lead for spinal cord stimulation: technical considerations and long-term follow-up. Neuromodulation 2012;15(4):402–7.

29. Struijk JJ, Holsheimer J. Transverse tripolar spinal cord stimulation: theoretical performance of a dual channel system. Med Biol Eng Comput 1996;34(4):273–9.

30. Kim DD, Vakharyia R, Kroll HR, et al. Rates of lead migration and stimulation loss in spinal cord stimulation: a retrospective comparison of laminotomy versus percutaneous implantation. Pain Physician 2011;14(6):513–24.

31. North RB, Kidd DH, Olin J, et al. Spinal cord stimulation with interleaved pulses: a randomized, controlled trial. Neuromodulation 2007;10(4):349–57.

32. Holsheimer J, den Boer JA, Struijk JJ, et al. MR assessment of the normal position of the spinal cord in the spinal canal. AJNR Am J Neuroradiol 1994;15(5):951–9.

33. Abejon D, Feler CA. Is impedance a parameter to be taken into account in spinal cord stimulation? Pain Physician 2007;10(4):533–40.

Index

Note: Page numbers of article titles are in **boldface** type.

Neurosurg Clin N Am 25 (2014) 843–847
http://dx.doi.org/10.1016/S1042-3680(14)00092-8
1042-3680/14/$ – see front matter © 2014 Elsevier Inc. All rights reserved.

United States Postal Service

Statement of Ownership, Management, and Circulation
(All Periodicals Publications Except Requestor Publications)

1. Publication Title: Neurosurgery Clinics of North America

2. Publication Number: 0 1 3 - 1 2 4

3. Filing Date: 9/14/14

4. Issue Frequency: Jan, Apr, Jul, Oct

5. Number of Issues Published Annually: 4

6. Annual Subscription Price: $380.00

7. Complete Mailing Address of Known Office of Publication (*Not printer*) (*Street, city, county, state, and ZIP+4®*)

Elsevier Inc.
360 Park Avenue South
New York, NY 10010-1710

Contact Person: Stephen R. Bushing

Telephone (*Include area code*): 215-239-3688

8. Complete Mailing Address of Headquarters or General Business Office of Publisher (*Not printer*)

Elsevier Inc., 360 Park Avenue South, New York, NY 10010-1710

9. Full Names and Complete Mailing Addresses of Publisher, Editor, and Managing Editor (*Do not leave blank*)

Publisher (*Name and complete mailing address*)

Linda Belfus, Elsevier Inc., 1600 John F. Kennedy Blvd., Suite 1800, Philadelphia, PA 19103-2899

Editor (*Name and complete mailing address*)

Jennifer Flynn-Briggs, Elsevier Inc., 1600 John F. Kennedy Blvd., Suite 1800, Philadelphia, PA 19103-2899

Managing Editor (*Name and complete mailing address*)

Adrianne Brigido, Elsevier Inc., 1600 John F. Kennedy Blvd., Suite 1800, Philadelphia, PA 19103-2899

10. Owner (*Do not leave blank. If the publication is owned by a corporation, give the name and address of the corporation immediately followed by the names and addresses of all stockholders owning or holding 1 percent or more of the total amount of stock. If not owned by a corporation, give the names and addresses of the individual owners. If owned by a partnership or other unincorporated firm, give its name and address as well as those of each individual owner. If the publication is published by a nonprofit organization, give its name and address.*)

Full Name	Complete Mailing Address
Wholly owned subsidiary of	1600 John F. Kennedy Blvd. Ste. 1800
Reed/Elsevier, US holdings	Philadelphia, PA 19103-2899

11. Known Bondholders, Mortgagees, and Other Security Holders Owning or Holding 1 Percent or More of Total Amount of Bonds, Mortgages, or Other Securities. If none, check box ☐ None

Full Name	Complete Mailing Address
N/A	

12. Tax Status (*For completion by nonprofit organizations authorized to mail at nonprofit rates*) (*Check one*)
The purpose, function, and nonprofit status of this organization and the exempt status for federal income tax purposes:
☐ Has Not Changed During Preceding 12 Months
☐ Has Changed During Preceding 12 Months (*Publisher must submit explanation of change with this statement*)

PS Form 3526, August 2012 (Page 1 of 3 (Instructions Page 3)) PSN 7530-01-000-9931 PRIVACY NOTICE: See our Privacy policy in www.usps.com

---

13. Publication Title: Neurosurgery Clinics of North America

14. Issue Date for Circulation Data Below: July 2014

15. Extent and Nature of Circulation

		Average No. Copies Each Issue During Preceding 12 Months	No. Copies of Single Issue Published Nearest to Filing Date
a. Total Number of Copies (*Net press run*)		602	614
b. Paid Circulation (By Mail and Outside the Mail)	(1) Mailed Outside-County Paid Subscriptions Stated on PS Form 3541. (*Include paid distribution above nominal rate, advertiser's proof copies, and exchange copies*)	199	167
	(2) Mailed In-County Paid Subscriptions Stated on PS Form 3541 (*Include paid distribution above nominal rate, advertiser's proof copies, and exchange copies*)		
	(3) Paid Distribution Outside the Mails Including Sales Through Dealers and Carriers, Street Vendors, Counter Sales, and Other Paid Distribution Outside USPS®	108	128
	(4) Paid Distribution by Other Classes Mailed Through the USPS (e.g. First-Class Mail®)		
c. Total Paid Distribution (*Sum of 15b (1), (2), (3), and (4)*)		307	295
d. Free or Nominal Rate Distribution (By Mail and Outside the Mail)	(1) Free or Nominal Rate Outside-County Copies Included on PS Form 3541	88	144
	(2) Free or Nominal Rate In-County Copies Included on PS Form 3541		
	(3) Free or Nominal Rate Copies Mailed at Other Classes Through the USPS (e.g. First-Class Mail)		
	(4) Free or Nominal Rate Distribution Outside the Mail (Carriers or other means)		
e. Total Free or Nominal Rate Distribution (*Sum of 15d (1), (2), (3) and (4)*)		88	144
f. Total Distribution (*Sum of 15c and 15e*)		395	439
g. Copies not Distributed (*See instructions to publishers #4 (page #3)*)		207	175
h. Total (*Sum of 15f and g*)		602	614
i. Percent Paid (*15c divided by 15f times 100*)		77.72%	67.20%

16. Total circulation includes electronic copies. Report circulation on PS Form 3526-X worksheet.

17. Publication of Statement of Ownership
If the publication is a general publication, publication of this statement is required. Will be printed in the October 2014 issue of this publication.

18. Signature and Title of Editor, Publisher, Business Manager, or Owner

[signature] Stephen R. Bushing – Inventory Distribution Coordinator

Date: September 14, 2014

I certify that all information furnished on this form is true and complete. I understand that anyone who furnishes false or misleading information on this form or who omits material or information requested on the form may be subject to criminal sanctions (including fines and imprisonment) and/or civil sanctions (including civil penalties).

PS Form 3526, August 2012 (Page 2 of 3)

Moving?

Make sure your subscription moves with you!

To notify us of your new address, find your **Clinics Account Number** (located on your mailing label above your name), and contact customer service at:

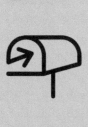

Email: journalscustomerservice-usa@elsevier.com

800-654-2452 (subscribers in the U.S. & Canada)
314-447-8871 (subscribers outside of the U.S. & Canada)

Fax number: 314-447-8029

Elsevier Health Sciences Division
Subscription Customer Service
3251 Riverport Lane
Maryland Heights, MO 63043

ELSEVIER

Moving?

Make sure your subscription moves with you!

To notify us of your new address, find your Clinics Account Number (located on your mailing label above your name), and contact customer service at:

Email: journalscustomerservice-usa@elsevier.com

800-654-2452 (subscribers in the U.S. & Canada)
314-447-8871 (subscribers outside of the U.S. & Canada)

Fax number: 314-447-8029

Elsevier Health Sciences Division
Subscription Customer Service
3251 Riverport Lane
Maryland Heights, MO 63043

To ensure uninterrupted delivery of your subscription, please notify us at least 4 weeks in advance of move.

Printed and bound by CPI Group (UK) Ltd, Croydon, CR0 4YY

03/10/2024

01040375-0002